The AmFAR AIDS Handbook

The Complete Guide to Understanding HIV and AIDS

■ *Darrell E. Ward, M.S.* ■

Introduction by
Mathilde Krim, Ph.D.

W · W · Norton & Company
New York · London

This book is intended only as a source of general information and reference; it is not a substitute for professional medical advice for individuals with HIV infection. Readers who wish to use the information presented here should always consult with their physician or healthcare provider.

Copyright © 1999 by American Foundation for AIDS Research and Darrell E. Ward

For information about permission to reproduce selections from this book, write to Permissions, W. W. Norton & Company, Inc., 500 Fifth Avenue, New York, NY 10110.

The text of this book is composed in Minion
with the display set in Trade Gothic Bold
Composition by ComCom
Manufacturing by the Haddon Craftsmen
Book design by Sabrina Bowers
Illustrations by David Schumick

LIBRARY OF CONGRESS CATALOGING-IN-PUBLICATION DATA
Ward, Darrell E., 1947–
    The AmFAR AIDS handbook : the complete guide to understanding HIV and AIDS / Darrell E. Ward ; introduction by Mathilde Krim.
        p. cm.
    Includes bibliographical references and index.
    ISBN 0-393-31636-X (pbk.)
    1. AIDS (Disease)—Popular works.   I. Title.
RC607.A26W368   1998   98-6985
616.97′92—dc21   CIP

W. W. Norton & Company, Inc.,
500 Fifth Avenue, New York, N.Y. 10110
http://www.wwnorton.com

W. W. Norton & Company Ltd.,
10 Coptic Street, London WC1A 1PU

1 2 3 4 5 6 7 8 9 0

To the researchers and physicians working to end the HIV pandemic

and

*To the people in AIDS clinical trials,
without whom advances in treatment and
vaccine development cannot be made*

CONTENTS

WHAT YOU NEED TO KNOW ABOUT HIV/AIDS

THE MEDICAL SCIENCE OF HIV/AIDS

LIST OF ILLUSTRATIONS

FOREWORD AND ACKNOWLEDGMENTS

HIV disease is one of the most complex diseases for physicians to treat, and one of the most bewildering for laypeople to understand. *The AmFAR AIDS Handbook: The Complete Guide to Understanding HIV and AIDS* is intended to help eliminate that bewilderment. It is written primarily for people with HIV, and their families and loved ones, but it should also be helpful to anyone who would like a comprehensive understanding of the disease. This could include public-health workers, social workers, counselors and others who provide ancillary services to people with HIV, and reporters who write about issues relating to HIV/AIDS. It also provides an overview of the disease to nurses and primary-care physicians.

In addition to helping people make sense of the complexities of HIV infection, its diagnosis, treatment, and prevention, *The AmFAR AIDS Handbook* can help people with HIV talk with their doctor, make informed decisions about their medical care and daily life, and better evaluate new HIV/AIDS-related medical discoveries and issues debated in the media.

The goal of *The AmFAR AIDS Handbook* is to make the science of HIV disease comprehensible. As such, it packs more scientific detail in its pages than most books on the subject for general readers, but less detail than that found in scientific or medical texts. In fact, it is hoped that the book will make the scientific literature accessible to many of those who would like to use it but who are discouraged or intimidated by the jargon and seemingly impenetrably difficult concepts.

The book contains three sections. The first presents topics of medical—clinical—interest. These chapters cover the testing and diagnosis of HIV infection, HIV transmission, the course of untreated disease, the opportunistic infections and cancers that can occur, anti-HIV treatment, how new drugs are developed and the clinical trial process, as well as prevention of HIV transmission. The section closes with chapters describing the challenges of vaccine development, how HIV disease affects women and children, and lifestyle issues to help the HIV-positive person maintain a high quality of life during different phases of his or her HIV disease.

The second section explores the scientific evidence acquired through basic research, the sum of which underlies the facts and recommendations covered in the first section. These chapters describe the cell and its components and the relationship between DNA, RNA, and protein, familiarity of which will help readers understand such things as HIV replication and how anti-HIV therapies work. There is an overview of the immune system and how it works, and another of viruses in general. This chapter is followed by one devoted specifically to HIV, its structure, diversity, and origin. That is followed by a brief chapter on human genes and how HIV interacts with them. Last, there is a discussion of the evidence that implicates HIV as the cause of AIDS.

The third section is a comprehensive glossary of terms used in the text. The glossary is followed by two appendices. Appendix 1 provides information on using the scientific literature, and on books, hotlines, and Internet sources for additional information on HIV/AIDS; Appendix 2 reproduces the 1993 classification system for HIV/AIDS, which lists the clinical criteria used by the Centers for Disease Control and Prevention (CDC) and public-health departments to identify and report cases of AIDS.

A book like this, of course, cannot be written alone. Many outstanding people gave their time to reviewing entire chapters or parts of chapters. It was my privilege to work with them, and I truly appreciate their contributions. These people include the following:

- Jonathan Allan, Southwest Foundation for Biomedical Research

- Arthur Ammann, American Foundation for AIDS Research

- Warren Andiman, Yale University School of Medicine

- Marcel A. Baluda, University of California, Los Angeles

- Ronald Bayer, Columbia University

- Tom Coates, University of California, San Francisco

- Matthew Coles, American Civil Liberties Union Foundation

- Ellen Cooper, National Institutes of Health

- Paul Corser, American Foundation for AIDS Research

- James Curran, Emory School of Public Health

- Anke Ehrhardt, Columbia College of Physicians and Surgeons

- Allen Gifford, San Diego Veterans Administration Medical Center

- Michael Giordano, Cornell University Medical College

- David Gold, AIDS Vaccine Advocacy Coalition

- Erica Gollub, Department of Public Health, Philadelphia

- Joan Kreiss, University of Washington

- Merry Krempasky, Columbus (Ohio) City Health Department

- Jay Levy, University of California, San Francisco Cancer Research Institute

- Kenneth Mayer, Brown University

- Valerie Ng, University of California, San Francisco

- Joel Palefsky, University of California, San Francisco

- Michael Para, Ohio State University

- Jeremy Paul, Cadus Pharmaceutical Corporation

- William Powderly, Washington University School of Medicine

- David Purchase, North American Syringe Exchange Network

- Charles Rabkin, National Cancer Institute

- Lee Ratner, Washington University School of Medicine

- Robert Schooley, University of Colorado Health Sciences Center

- Frederick Siegal, Institute of Oncology, Long Island Jewish Medical Center

- David Volsky, St. Luke's-Roosevelt Hospital Center

- Bruce Walker, Harvard Medical School

- Harrison Weed, Ohio State University

- Lowell S. Young, University of California, San Francisco, and Kuzell Institute for Arthritis and Infectious Diseases, California Pacific Medical Center

My thanks, too, to Earle Holland, associate executive director of University Communications and my supervisor at Ohio State University, for the encouragement and help he provided in many, many ways during this project. I also want to thank Dave Schumick, who is an extraordinary illustrator and a pleasure to work with; the staff of the CDC's National Center for HIV, STD, and TB Prevention; and the reference and circulation staff of Ohio State's Prior Health Sciences Library.

Special thanks to Ardith Chang, Ph.D., who lined up reviewers for each chapter and contributed helpful comments to the manuscript, all with unfailing cheerfulness. Special thanks also to Jeffrey Laurence, M.D., Ph.D., director of the Cornell University AIDS Research Laboratory and senior scientific consultant to AmFAR, who read the entire manuscript and provided many thoughtful comments.

But this book would not be what it is—and perhaps wouldn't exist at all—without the interest and dedication of Mathilde Krim, Ph.D., AmFAR's co-founder and chairman of the board. What is it like working with Mathilde Krim? Matthew Coles, director of the ACLU Foundation AIDS/HIV Project, summed it up well when I mentioned during our first conversation that I was working closely with Mathilde Krim on the project. "You're fortunate," he said, "she's a wonderful person." It couldn't be said better. I have indeed been fortunate. Dr. Krim and I spent many hours working shoulder-to-shoulder reviewing manuscript pages, and discussing changes and updates by phone and fax. The book is inexpressibly richer for her direction, insights, comments, and contributions.

Last, a special thank you to my wife, Barbara, and my children, Alicia and Matthew, for their forbearance during my many months of reading, interviewing, writing, and revising. Now, for that vacation I promised you. . . .

CDC ■ Centers for Disease Control and Prevention

CIN ■ cervical intraepithelial neoplasia

CMV ■ cytomegalovirus

CNS ■ central nervous system (i.e., brain and spinal cord)

CPR ■ cardiopulmonary respiration

CTL ■ cytotoxic T lymphocyte

CT scan ■ computed tomography scan

d4T ■ stavudine

ddC ■ zalcitabine

ddI ■ didanosine

DHHS ■ Department of Health and Human Services

DNA ■ deoxyribonucleic acid

DPAHC ■ durable power of attorney for health care

dsDNA ■ double-stranded DNA

dsRNA ■ double-stranded RNA

EBV ■ Epstein-Barr virus

EIA ■ enzyme immunoassay (same as an ELISA)

ELISA ■ enzyme-linked immunosorbent assay

FDA ■ Food and Drug Administration

FDC ■ follicular dendritic cell

FIV ■ feline immunodeficiency virus

G ■ guanine

GI ■ gastrointestinal

gp ■ glycoprotein (always used with a number that represents the mass of the molecule in thousands of units known as daltons; e.g., gp120 is a glycoprotein with a mass of 120,000 daltons)

HAART ■ highly active antiretroviral therapy

HHV-8 ■ human herpesvirus type 8

HIV ■ human immunodeficiency virus*

HPV ■ human papillomavirus

HSV ■ herpes simplex virus

HTLV ■ human T-cell lymphotropic virus

IDSA ■ Infectious Disease Society of America

IDU ■ injection drug user or injection drug use

IFA ■ indirect immunofluorescence assay

IFN ■ interferon

Ig ■ immunoglobulin

IL ■ interleukin

IND ■ investigational new drug

INH ■ isoniazid

IV ■ intravenous

kb ■ kilobases (1,000 bases)

kbp ■ kilobase pairs (1,000 pairs of bases)

KS ■ Kaposi's sarcoma

KSHV ■ KS-associated herpesvirus

LAV ■ lymphadenopathy-associated virus

LIP ■ lymphoid interstitial pneumonitis

LTR ■ long terminal repeat

MA ■ matrix protein, p17

MAC ■ *Mycobacterium avium* complex

MHC ■ major histocompatibility complex

mg ■ milligram (one-thousandth of a gram)

ml ■ milliter (one-thousandth of a liter)

mm³ ■ cubic millimeter (a millimeter equals about 1/25th of an inch)

When the abbreviation "HIV" is used in the text, it refers to HIV type 1 (HIV-1); when reference is made to HIV type 2, the text will refer to that virus as HIV-2.

Chapter 1

DIAGNOSIS OF HIV INFECTION AND INITIAL PHYSICIAN CARE

When a person learns that he or she tested positive for the human immunodeficiency virus (HIV), the world is turned on end. But today, a person infected with HIV has more cause for hope than ever before. "It's important for people diagnosed with HIV not to beat up on themselves," said Michael Para, M.D., an AIDS specialist at Ohio State University Hospitals. "With the help of their physician, they stand a good chance of striking back at the virus and of buying themselves time and a better quality of life. But they have to want to do it; they have to believe that something can be done."

And something truly can be done for people with HIV infection. By finding an experienced physician, working with that physician, taking care of themselves through rest, exercise, and a nutritious diet, most HIV-positive people remain relatively healthy for an average of ten years or more after the infection is diagnosed. And this incubation period is growing longer with the help of new treatments and preventive therapies. People with HIV infection and AIDS remain well longer than was possible just a few years ago. They are enjoying their families and friends, continuing in their careers, and leading fulfilling lives in spite of HIV.

This success is due to research that has delivered a growing understanding of HIV itself and how it causes disease. This new understanding continues to lead to the development of new drugs that target specific stages of the virus's life cycle. Research on HIV led, for example, to the development of several classes of anti-HIV drugs, including protease inhibitors. The use of protease inhibitors in combination with previously approved anti-HIV drugs has given rise to the theory that it might be possible to cure HIV infection in at least some people: It might become possible to eliminate the virus from people who are asymptomatic and who still have a strong and intact immune system and a relatively small number of HIV particles in their body. Newer drugs now under development may bring further improvements in treatment.

Whether current therapy will truly cure the disease in some people remains to be determined, but scientists have recently learned that early diagnosis and early multidrug treatment enable many people with HIV infection to survive significantly longer. It is therefore essential that all people who might have been exposed to HIV have themselves tested so that if infected they can seek early treatment. In addition, people who know they are infected are less likely to transmit the infection to others.

Tests for HIV have also evolved dramatically. Individuals can even collect their own blood sample and be tested with complete anonymity using kits designed for home use. Physicians can better determine when to begin or change anti-HIV treatments in patients using tests that measure the amount of HIV in the bloodstream (see Chapter 2).

■ DIAGNOSIS OF HIV INFECTION

HIV infection is usually diagnosed using a screening test that detects the presence of antibodies to HIV in blood serum (see Chapter 2). HIV testing is available in a variety of settings, including neighborhood clinics, health-department clinics, physician's offices, and hospitals. Home blood-collection kits involve placing a sample of blood on an absorbent material and mailing the sample to a laboratory for analysis. The results are given over the telephone using an identification number that comes with each kit, thereby providing the user complete anonymity. The test result of a person who is HIV positive is given over the telephone by a trained counselor.

■ Proper Use of the HIV Antibody Test

Every person should know his or her HIV status. This is particularly important for people who know they have been in situations that might have exposed them to the virus, either through sex, used hypodermic needles, or even, before 1986, by blood transfusion or treatment with clotting factors.

A sample of blood for testing can be taken by a physician; appropriate samples of blood can also be self-collected after purchasing a home-collection kit, over the counter, in pharmacies. Testing can also be obtained free of charge from all health departments. *The use of home-collection kits or of a health-department's services makes it possible to be tested anonymously, that is, without having to give one's name and address. The results will not appear in the person's medical records, to which insurance companies and perhaps others could obtain access.* (Also see "Reporting Laws.")

A positive result, which is based on a screening *and* a confirmatory test, is definitely a reliable result. However, a negative result does not mean with any certainty that a person is free of HIV. He or she must wait several weeks (during which any sexual or needle-sharing risk behavior must be strictly avoided) and return for a second test. This must be done because a recently acquired infection may be present but not yet detectable by the tests typically used to screen people for HIV (see Chapter 2). For these reasons, while a positive result is not reversible, a negative result is, and the test must be repeated within a few weeks.

Persons who engage in risk behaviors following the confirmation of their negative status should be tested periodically, again, twice each time at several weeks' interval. ■

■ Pretest and Post-test Counseling

Every person who makes the decision to be tested for HIV should receive counseling as part of an HIV test. Pretest counseling is given before the test is done, post-test counseling after the results are disclosed. In some situations, however, little or no counseling may be provided. A person who is tested may simply be told that he or she is HIV positive, with little else said about the meaning or implications of the finding, and the person may not know what to do next. Anyone in this position should read about post-test counseling below, followed by "What to Do after Receiving a Positive HIV Test Result."

Pretest Counseling

Pretest counseling is important because it provides information about HIV disease, about its transmission and prevention, and about the prevention of all sexually transmitted diseases. It is also an opportunity for the counselor to assess how a person is likely to respond to a positive or negative test result, and it makes it more likely that the person being tested will return to learn the test's result. When pretest counseling is completed, and the counseled person wants to proceed with the test, a sample of blood, saliva, or urine (depending on the type of test used) is collected and sent to a laboratory for analysis (see Chapter 2). The person being tested is then asked to return within a few days, a week, or sometimes longer, to learn the result.

Post-test Counseling

Post-test counseling is extremely important. The counselor typically comes to the point without delay: "Your test result is back. You are HIV positive." Or: "Your test result is negative." Post-test counseling immediately follows.

Post-test Counseling for Negative Test Result

Post-test counseling for a negative test result involves talking with the person about the importance of safer sex and of avoiding other risky behaviors, and reminding the person that people at high risk should not donate blood. The counselor may also explain the window period for HIV infection and recommend that the person return for retesting in the near future.

Post-test Counseling for an HIV-Positive Test Result

Post-test counseling is critical for the person who is HIV positive. It can determine whether a person will seek follow-up care or whether they will deny their diagnosis and delay seeking care. (Instead, they may seek escape through alcohol or drug abuse; see "The Psychological Stress of a

Positive HIV Test Result.") Unfortunately, individuals who deny their positive HIV status are also denying themselves the benefits of early anti-HIV therapies, preventive treatment of opportunistic infections, and early emotional and psychological support, all of which will improve their quality of life and chances of prolonged survival. They may also transmit the infection to others.

For these reasons, it is important for post-test counseling to emphasize that much can be done to help the person with HIV infection. It should also accomplish the following:

- Help the person work through his or her feelings about the positive test result and maintain rapport with the counselor.

- Provide the names of physicians with experience in treating people infected with HIV.

- Discuss whom should be told about the person's HIV-positive status (see "Disclosing One's HIV Status").

- Provide written information on personal care, HIV disease, and preventing transmission of the virus to others (see Chapter 9).

- Refer the person to a health-department social worker, case manager, or local AIDS service organization to help in locating needed resources, social and emotional support, and other help.

■ What to Do after Receiving a Positive HIV Test Result

When the results of an HIV test come back positive, what then? Post-test counseling, if done well, will help answer that question. But when little or no counseling is provided, what should a person do? Under these circumstances, there are several things the person who is newly diagnosed with HIV infection should realize:

- Being HIV positive does not mean one has AIDS. AIDS is one of several stages of HIV disease (see Chapter 4). HIV disease begins when a person becomes infected with the virus. On average, ten or more years pass from the time of a person's infection until signs of clinical AIDS appear. With proper care, this long "incubation period" can be prolonged.

- Some people have signs of AIDS when they first learn of their HIV-positive status, but advances in medical research and care are now allowing many people with AIDS to lead comfortable and productive lives.

- Anyone who is HIV positive can transmit his or her infection to others through unsafe sex or needle sharing, or any activity that results in the exchange of body fluids (including the sharing of shaving razors, ear or body piercing, blood-brother rituals)—even though the person may feel healthy and show no outward sign of HIV disease (see Chapter 3). People who are HIV positive must practice safer sex or abstain from sexual activity; injection drug users should never share needles (see Chapter 9).

- HIV-positive individuals should not donate blood and should not be listed as organ donors on their driver's license.

There are three steps that a person with HIV should take to ensure that he or she receives the best care possible: identifying where to go for help and dependable advice, seeking care from a physician experienced in the treatment of HIV disease, and determining whom to tell about one's positive HIV status.

Where to Find Help

There are three invaluable sources of help for the person with HIV infection who does not know where to turn:

- The National AIDS Hotline, operated by the Centers for Disease Control and Prevention (CDC), is an important source of a variety of HIV information. The toll-free number is 1-800-342-2437.

- Your state's HIV/AIDS hotline; obtain the number from the National AIDS Hotline. Calls to the state HIV/AIDS hotline are toll free.

- The nearest AIDS service organization or AIDS task force; obtain the name and phone number through the state HIV/AIDS hotline. Local AIDS service organizations have information on local support groups; financial, legal, and social services; and state HIV drug assistance programs. They can also provide the names of local physicians experienced in treating people with HIV disease.

Obtain Care from an Experienced Physician

The treatment of HIV infection is becoming increasingly complex. Successful treatment depends on a thorough understanding of how HIV causes disease and on how to use the growing number of potent drugs available. Used incorrectly, these drugs not only will be less effective, but also can reduce the effectiveness of other drugs that may be needed in the future. For these reasons, the single most important step in living with HIV is to seek medical care from a physician who has experience with HIV disease. Research reported at the Third Annual Conference on Retroviruses and Opportunistic Infections in 1996 found that people with AIDS whose primary-care physician had no previous experience with HIV disease died more than a year sooner than did patients whose primary-care physician had cared for at least five other HIV-positive patients. Individuals who were treated by these more experienced physicians tended to have the status of their immune system monitored more regularly through CD4 lymphocyte counts (see below), received timely and appropriate prophylaxis for *Pneumocystis carinii* pneumonia (PCP), and received antiretroviral drugs more frequently. Physicians in the study who were experienced with HIV disease also tended to consult more often with specialists.

A good physician is a person's partner in medical care. He or she will be familiar with the latest studies in anti-HIV therapy. Individuals being treated for HIV disease almost always have options. A good physician will describe the treatment options, explain their advantages and disadvantages, make recommendations based on his or her experience and the patient's circumstances, and answer a patient's questions.

The final say as to which treatment option is used, however, belongs to the patient. This is important. The patient must make the decision as to what treatment is pursued because HIV treatments are often complex and adherence may be difficult. For success, the patient must be committed to his or her therapy.

The patient should never be afraid to ask his or her doctor questions. So that nothing is forgotten, the patient should write down questions and concerns as they arise at home and take the list to the next checkup. Also the patient should write down any side effects or other problems that he or she experiences with medication(s), even things that the patient perhaps believes "come with the territory" and that he or she should simply tolerate. These may include such things as difficulty in taking a medication, the need for better pain control, trouble sleeping, or feelings of anxiety or depression. The physician can often help solve these problems. The patient can ask questions of nurses, too. An experienced nurse can often be easier to talk to and provide information in a less hurried manner than a physician. If the doctor doesn't mind the presence of a tape recorder, it can be helpful to record what the doctor says so his or her recommendations can be listened to again at home.

The Initial Physical Exam

The first visit to a physician following the HIV test involves a thorough physical examination that includes a number of laboratory tests. It should also include a discussion of how HIV is transmitted (see Chapter 3), and how to prevent transmission (see Chapter 9). The initial exam should include the following:

- A detailed medical and drug-use history (a sexual history is also important, but some physicians postpone it until a bond of trust is developed with the patient).

- Weight of the person. This baseline measure is important in HIV-positive patients because unexplained weight loss is an indication of infection or wasting (cachexia), a common occurrence in HIV disease (see Chapters 4 and 13).

- Oral exam. Examination of the mouth should be done during every physical exam. The earliest signs of HIV disease, disease progression, and onset of AIDS often occur in the mouth. Conditions that can be present include the following:

    Candidiasis, a yeast infection. See Chapter 7.

    Kaposi's sarcoma, a type of cancer. See Chapter 8.

    Hairy leukoplakia, a viral infection. See Chapter 7.

    Herpes simplex virus. See Chapter 7.

    Oral warts, a viral infection.

    HIV-associated gingivitis and HIV-associated periodontitis, both of which are bacterial infections.

- Eye exam. This includes a detailed history of visual disturbances and careful examination of the retina, the light-sensitive tissue that lines the inside of the eye. The physician looks in particular for signs of cytomegalovirus (CMV) infection of the eye, or CMV retinitis. It is one of the most common opportunistic infections associated with HIV, and it must be treated promptly to prevent or slow vision loss. It is more common during advanced disease (see Chapter 7).

- Genital-urinary exam for the presence of sexually transmitted diseases, which enhance the transmission of HIV (see Chapter 3).

LABORATORY TESTS. A number of laboratory tests are usually ordered during the initial examination of a person who is HIV positive. The tests are done on a blood sample to help determine the health of the person's immune system, the level of activity of HIV in the person, the presence of certain infections, and the risk that certain opportunistic infections might occur. These tests include the following:

- CD4 lymphocyte counts. CD4 lymphocytes, also known as helper T lymphocytes, are essential for initiating and coordinating immune responses. A decline in the number of CD4 lymphocytes occurs during the course of HIV disease (see Chapter 4), and as their numbers drop, the risk of certain opportunistic infections increases (although some individuals can have very low CD4 cell numbers and show few other signs of serious illness). For this reason, CD4 cell counts, which are usually given as the number of CD4 cells per cubic millimeter of blood (cells per mm^3), are often used as a measure of the health of an HIV-infected person's immune system. CD4 cell counts are also used to determine when preventive treatments for PCP and certain other opportunistic infections should begin. Percentages of CD4 lymphocytes (i.e., CD4 lymphocytes as a percentage of total lymphocytes) are used by some physicians to monitor the progression of HIV disease. For the association between helper T-cell numbers and ratios and HIV disease, see Chapter 4 and Appendix 2; for a brief description of how CD4 tests are done, see the box in Chapter 16, "Why They Call It 'CD4': Telling Immune Cells Apart."

- Viral-load testing. Viral load is a measure of the amount of free HIV particles present in a person's blood. Viral load is the best predictor of HIV disease progression, and it is used to determine whether antiretroviral therapy is working or should be changed (see Chapter 5).

Changes in viral load occur relatively quickly compared to changes in CD4 lymphocyte counts. For this reason, a physician might order viral-load testing within two to four weeks after the patient begins antiretroviral therapy, and as often as every three or four months thereafter.

■ Tuberculin skin test. This test, which is also known as the PPD test, is done to diagnose the presence of tuberculosis (TB). Those who test positive harbor the TB bacterium, *Mycobacterium tuberculosis*. Those with a positive test result but who do not have active disease (i.e., the disease is not transmissible to others) should begin prophylactic treatment; those with active TB should be isolated and receive treatment (see Chapter 7).

■ Syphilis test. Syphilis is often present as a coinfection with HIV, and the two are linked epidemiologically. Treatment is begun in those who have the disease.

■ Some physicians also order tests to determine whether the person has been exposed to CMV, toxoplasmosis, or hepatitis. If tests show that a latent infection is present, the physician can be prepared to begin prophylaxis or treatment if needed.

Evaluation of HIV Disease in Women

The evaluation of HIV disease in women should also include the following (see also Chapter 11):

■ A Pap test, because women who are HIV positive have an increased risk of cervical cancer.

■ Rectal-vaginal exams for candidiasis and other infections.

■ Pregnancy counseling. This should include the latest information on preventing transmission of HIV from mother to infant during pregnancy and childbirth. HIV-positive pregnant women should be warned against breast-feeding (see Chapter 12).

The Follow-up Visit

Evaluation of a person who is HIV positive is determined by three measures: viral load, CD4 lymphocyte counts, and the physical findings of the initial examination. These indicators, together with the individual's medical history, provide an overall assessment of the person's health status.

This overall evaluation is conducted during a follow-up medical visit that occurs after laboratory test results have been received. The overall medical and laboratory findings might reveal that the patient is generally in good health (i.e., that treatment need only be discussed for the time being); that anti-HIV therapy is indicated, either alone or concomitant with preventive treatment for opportunistic infections; or that some other intervention is needed.

If the subject was not discussed during the initial examination, the follow-up visit should also include a session with, or referral to, a social worker or case manager (a person who coordinates the various kinds of assistance and resources that can be needed by someone with HIV disease). The physician's office might also direct the person with HIV disease to needed assistance programs. The state HIV/AIDS hotline and the local AIDS service organization can also provide this information.

Disclosing One's HIV Status

One of the first questions that comes to mind after receiving a diagnosis of HIV infection is who should be told about it? One's seropositive status is highly personal information. Deciding whom to tell is often not easy.

Reporting Laws

AIDS is a reportable illness in all 50 states. That is, doctors must report every case of AIDS they diagnose to the state health department, along with the patient's name and address. This information is kept confidential; by law, it cannot be made available to insurance companies, employers, or any others. This policy of confidentiality has been widely respected and rarely breached. And while state health departments report case statistics to the CDC, names, addresses, and other personal identifiers of people infected with HIV are not sent to the CDC. State health departments and the CDC use the statistical information to monitor changes in the AIDS epidemic.

As of late 1996, more than half of the 50 states had laws or regulations requiring similar confidential reporting by name of all persons with HIV infection, not just AIDS cases.

Partner and Spousal Notification

The federal government also requires all states to have a partner and spousal notification system in place. If a person tests HIV positive, that person's spouse, sexual partner(s), and needle-sharing partner(s) should be notified that they have been exposed to HIV, that they might have become infected, and that they should be tested. Partner notification is usually discussed during post-test counseling with all people who are HIV positive. Notification itself can be carried out by the HIV-positive individual, the physician, the social worker, or personnel of the state health department. If a person has been tested at a health-department clinic, the counselor will ask who will inform those to be notified. The counselor may also suggest how disclosure can be made. If the HIV-positive individual declines to contact his or her partner(s), the counselor will ask for their names, contact the appropriate parties, and inform them that they may have been exposed to HIV, might have become infected, and should be tested. If one is tested through the services of a private physician, either the patient or the physician can perform the notification; if neither wishes to, the health department is responsible for contacting the partner(s).

This notification process is similar to that followed for other sexually transmitted infections (e.g., syphilis and gonorrhea) and has effectively limited their spread. It is important to note that while anyone who is HIV positive deserves the best available medical care, he or she also has a personal responsibility to protect the health of current and previous partners and to cooperate with medical and public-health personnel in helping to control the HIV epidemic. An important aspect of this cooperation is helping them carry out the partner notification procedure.

Determining Whom Else to Tell

Disclosing one's HIV status carries significant risks. They can include rejection by one's partner, spouse, family, friends, neighbors, or employer. It can result in loss of child custody, and discrimination in housing, insurance, and employment.

But disclosing one's HIV status to the right people is also often the first step toward a healthy acceptance of the reality of one's HIV-positive status. In addition, it is the first step in developing a firm emotional support system that is important for maintaining psychological well-being in the face of HIV disease. The people who are a part of such a support system are a needed outlet for one's feelings, fears, and anxieties. If the support system includes others who are HIV positive, the latter can affirm that they share the same feelings and fears. They can be a source of encouragement and of ideas on how better to cope with HIV-associated problems, and how to maintain control of one's life. Studies have shown that people who have a strong support system tend to experience a higher quality of life and to do better in the course of their disease.

Meeting other HIV-positive people can be done with the help of one's physician or social worker, or by joining an HIV support group. There also exist buddy programs that team a recently diagnosed person with an HIV-positive person who is more experienced in dealing with the issues that come from learning one's HIV-positive status.

People to turn to for support other than (or in addition to) family and friends include the following:

- Social workers

- Professional counselors and therapists

- Volunteers serving as buddies in programs run by AIDS service organizations

- HIV support groups

Help to locate these sources of support can be obtained through local AIDS service organizations or by calling the state HIV/AIDS hotline (obtain this phone number from the National AIDS Hotline, listed above and in Appendix 1).

■ The Psychological Stress of a Positive HIV Test Result

SOME PEOPLE REACT to a diagnosis of HIV infection with such despair that they deny the diagnosis and turn to drugs or alcohol to cope with it. Pretest and post-test counseling sessions are intended to reduce this risk. David G., 26 years old, is an example of someone who received neither pretest nor post-test counseling as part of his HIV antibody test—although by law both should have been provided. His reaction upon learning he was HIV positive illustrates why counseling is an important part of HIV testing.

In June 1992, David was driving home from a vacation when he developed nausea, diarrhea, and stomach pain. He attributed it to a recurring stomach problem. He lost weight and developed a fever that spiked at 104°F. His lover convinced him to be tested for HIV.

He went to a health-department clinic for an anonymous test. A staff member drew a blood sample; he returned two weeks later for the results. A woman asked him to follow her to a room. "We were standing in the hallway and as she opened the door, she said 'You're HIV positive.' I went into shock. She had just told me that my life had ended, and she said it while we were still standing in the hallway." If she told him anything else, he didn't hear it.

David went home—and into denial. He began cleaning the house. "I tried to blow it off as if it weren't true." He worked extra hours as a home-health worker. "I was saying: 'I'm healthy; I'm not sick. Watch me work.' " Marijuana and tranquilizers helped him relax. He didn't see a doctor.

"I wanted to escape from myself. I started drinking; I always kept a bottle handy. I took weekend trips to different towns, where I was a stranger, where I could pretend to be someone else, someone without HIV." He lost weight and grew weaker. One day he looked at himself in a mirror. He was jarred by the skeletal prominence of his collarbone, ribs, and hips. "Look what I've done to myself," he said aloud.

David sought good medical care, and with support from family and friends, he gained weight and began feeling better. He came to be at peace with his illness, though he'd lost his sight to cytomegalovirus infection. But in reflection, he said, "I'm sure my drinking, drug use, and denial robbed years from my life." ■

■ *Chapter 2*

TESTING FOR HIV

Tests for HIV include the enzyme-linked immunosorbent assay (ELISA) for the initial detection of HIV infection, confirmatory tests that verify the positive result of an ELISA, and genome tests that detect the presence of HIV's genetic material in blood.

Note that *there is no blood test for the diagnosis of AIDS.* The ELISA test with, if appropriate, a confirmatory test constitutes what is called "the blood test for HIV." It is sometimes loosely—and wrongly—referred to as "the AIDS test." This is incorrect because the blood test determines only whether a sample of blood serum contains antibodies to HIV. The presence of such antibody indicates that the person who has been tested is infected by HIV, is capable of infecting others, and is likely to develop HIV disease. AIDS, on the other hand, is the advanced stage of HIV disease, and its diagnosis requires, in addition to the presence of HIV, a significant loss of CD4 lymphocytes or the appearance of certain illnesses or cancers—the "AIDS-defining diseases"—that are characteristic of a seriously damaged immune system (see Appendix 2).

■ THE PUBLIC-HEALTH NEED FOR HIV TESTING

The decision to be tested for HIV is always a wrenching one, particularly for those who have reasons to believe that they have or might have been exposed to the virus. In addition to being apprehensive about receiving a positive test result, they may fear stigmatization should the result become known.

Many people—even those who were at high risk of HIV infection—did not feel compelled to take advantage of testing when it first became possible in 1985. At that time, no drug was known to be capable of fighting HIV infection, and the severe stigma attached to AIDS (which often resulted in loss of support from family and friends, loss of employment and health insurance, and loss of housing) contributed powerfully to the belief that being tested amounted to assuming grave hazards while not providing any medical benefit. Furthermore, because adoption of low-risk behavior was recommended to everyone anyway, knowing one's HIV status was considered superfluous. This thinking prevailed for several years, particularly in the gay community. It was, in fact, condoned and even advocated by many AIDS-related organizations.

However, attitudes towards HIV testing are now dramatically different as a result of both social and medical advances. Stigmatization has abated because the public is better educated about HIV/AIDS and has lost much of its early fear of and prejudices against people with HIV disease. The law now protects people with HIV/AIDS from discrimination through the Americans with Disability Act of 1990 and numerous local ordinances. A societal sense of fairness and compassion has spawned a broad variety of supportive services including legal-defense services. Most importantly, since 1987, effective anti-HIV drugs have become available. And, more recently, combination therapies that include a protease inhibitor are greatly improving and prolonging the lives of most people at all stages of HIV disease.

Under these new circumstances, knowing one's HIV status—whether positive or negative—has acquired overriding importance: For the many whose test result turns out to be negative, it can be a powerful incentive to remain HIV negative by consistently practicing low-risk sexual or drug-injection behavior; for any person whose test result is positive, it can be the foundation of self-protective and socially responsible behavior (i.e., personal behavior that is consistently protective of others) as well as the foundation of a well-informed daily lifestyle and of an effective overall health-care program (see Chapter 13).

There are many ways to obtain HIV testing: It can be requested from one's personal physician; it can be obtained free of charge from a health-department "anonymous testing site"; or it can even be initiated through the privacy of one's home, using kits (available over the counter in pharmacies) that allow the self-collection of a small blood or saliva sample for anonymous testing (see below). In all these settings, appropriate pretest and post-test counseling should also be provided.

Learning one's HIV status and being counseled are rapidly acquiring lifesaving importance, not only for the individuals tested, but also for their partners and offspring. Because HIV testing and counseling also promote low-risk behaviors, they slow the further spread of the HIV epidemic and so benefit society as a whole.

A more widespread use of voluntary HIV testing is now strongly recommended by all private AIDS-related organizations as well as public-health agencies.

■ THE SCREENING TEST FOR HIV AND HOW IT WORKS

Screening tests are used for detecting certain medical conditions in populations of people or in large collections of samples. Such tests must be inexpensive and easy to perform. Screening tests for HIV use a technique called "ELISA." ELISA-type tests are usually designed to detect antibodies produced in response to infection with viral, bacterial, or other microbial pathogens. Blood banks use HIV ELISA tests for screening all samples of donated blood, and the military uses them to screen the blood of recruits. Through the services of specially certified laboratories, similar ELISA tests are also available to health-department clinics, physicians' offices, hospitals, and others as a first step in identifying individuals infected with HIV (see Chapter 1).

Because most HIV ELISA tests reveal only the presence of antibodies, they do not directly detect HIV. But because antibodies are produced only in response to infection—not to mere exposure—a positive result on an ELISA test for HIV is a strong indication of HIV infection. It also requires verification with a confirmatory test. A person who is tested and found not to have antibodies to HIV is said to be seronegative for HIV (the prefix "sero" indicates "serum"). A person who tests positive is said to be seropositive for HIV.

A drawback to antibody tests, however, is that a person can be infected with a pathogen such as HIV for several weeks before antibodies are produced in sufficient quantities to be detectable.[1] This period, during which infection may be present but before antibodies are detectable, is known as the "window period."

Screening tests must ideally be able to detect all cases of infection. Therefore, they are designed to produce an extremely low number of false-negative results. Consequently, they yield a relatively high number of false-positive results. A false-negative result indicates that infection is absent when in fact, it is present; a false-positive result indicates that infection is present when in fact, it is not.

For a blood bank, false-positive results merely mean that healthy blood is sometimes needlessly discarded; for individuals, false-positive results are unacceptable. That is why confirmatory tests, which produce a very low rate of false-positive results, are used to verify all positive HIV results obtained through an ELISA test before such a result is reported to the individual being tested.

■ ELISA or EIA Antibody Technique

An ELISA, also known as the "enzyme immunoassay" (EIA), is used to screen for antibodies to HIV. It depends on the highly specific interaction of antibodies and antigens. Antibodies are proteins released into the blood by immune cells to help fight off infecting viruses and other pathogens; antigens are protein components of any microbial pathogen that stimulate the production of specific antibodies. When an antibody contacts its antigen, it attaches tightly to it—or binds with it, as scientists say. (For more on antigens and antibodies, see Chapter 16.)

How ELISAs Are Performed

The basic steps in preparing and performing an ELISA for HIV antibodies are as follows:

■ HIV is grown in infected lymphocytes in the laboratory. The lymphocytes are broken open—lysed—and the virus particles, or virions, are isolated. The virions are chemically disrupted and the proteins that make them up are collected.

■ The walls and floor of small test wells in a plastic plate (a microtiter plate) are coated with the HIV proteins. These proteins serve as antigen for the test. (These steps, which are depicted in the top half of Figure 2.1, are performed by the companies that manufacture ELISA test kits.)

■ The blood serum to be tested is added to the antigen-coated well (see bottom half of Figure 2.1). The serum was prepared in the testing laboratory by allowing a blood sample to clot; the clear fluid that remains—the serum—is then drawn off and used in the test. If antibodies against HIV are present in the serum, they bind tightly to the HIV antigens coating the well. The serum is then rinsed from the well.

■ A second antibody—a "detector" antibody—is added to the well. The detector antibody is produced by an animal, often a goat. It is made so as to bind to any human antibody, including the one in the microtiter plate well (which has become tightly bound to the HIV antigens). The detector antibody also carries an enzyme that has been chemically attached to it (see Figure 2.1). The excess anti-human antibody is rinsed from the well.

■ A chemical—referred to as a "substrate"—that reacts with the enzyme is added to the well. The substrate reacts with the enzyme on the anti-human antibody to produce a color, often yellow. The intensity of the color reflects the amount of detector antibody present, which, in turn, is proportional to the amount of antibody to HIV in the serum being tested.

■ Thus, if antibody to HIV is not present in the serum tested, none will bind to the HIV antigen, and when the substrate is added to the well, the solution in the well will remain clear. The solution is then said to be "nonreactive."

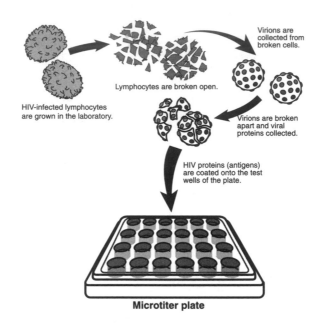

Virions are collected from broken cells.

Lymphocytes are broken open.

HIV-infected lymphocytes are grown in the laboratory.

Virions are broken apart and viral proteins collected.

HIV proteins (antigens) are coated onto the test wells of the plate.

Microtiter plate

Microtiter plate

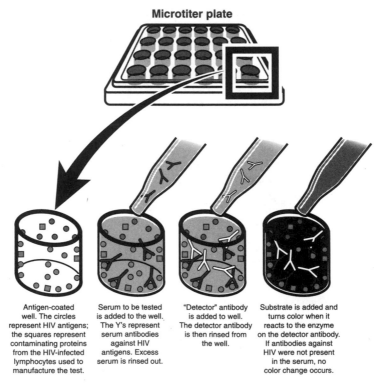

Antigen-coated well. The circles represent HIV antigens; the squares represent contaminating proteins from the HIV-infected lymphocytes used to manufacture the test.

Serum to be tested is added to the well. The Y's represent serum antibodies against HIV antigens. Excess serum is rinsed out.

"Detector" antibody is added to well. The detector antibody is then rinsed from the well.

Substrate is added and turns color when it reacts to the enzyme on the detector antibody. If antibodies against HIV were not present in the serum, no color change occurs.

Fig. 2.1 ▪ The ELISA test for HIV as performed in a microtiter plate. The top half of the diagram illustrates how the test's manufacturer prepares the plate. The bottom half shows how the test itself is performed.

ELISA is a procedure that has many applications. As applied to the detection of HIV antibodies, different testing kits have been developed by manufacturers to meet different situations. For example, instead of coating the microtiter wells with antigen, some manufacturers use plastic microspheres that are coated with viral antigen. A "dot blot" is a variety of ELISA in which small circles (i.e., dots) of antigen are placed on a paper-like material. A drop of blood or a serum sample is placed on the circle and anti-human antibody is added to produce a color. This technique is used in connection with home specimen-collection kits (see below).

Contaminating Proteins Produce False Positives

As described already, the antigens used in many HIV ELISAs are prepared by growing HIV in cultures of human white blood cells. When viral proteins are collected, it is difficult to separate them completely from the proteins of the human cells. These cellular proteins end up as contaminants of the viral antigens used in the test.

These contaminants can produce false-positive test results in serum samples from people who have been exposed to proteins from other humans in sufficient quantities to produce anti-human antibodies. False positives of this type are particularly prone to occur when testing women who have borne children, people who have received blood transfusions, or injection drug users.

Newer ELISA technology avoids this problem by using viral proteins produced by bacteria through recombinant DNA technology, or made synthetically, that is, assembled from amino acids by protein-synthesizing machines.

p24 Antigen Test

ELISA technology is also used to directly detect HIV antigen rather than antibody in serum. These tests reveal the presence of the capsid protein, p24, in serum (for more about p24 in HIV, see Chapter 18). Because the p24 antigen test detects HIV directly, rather than an antibody to the virus, it can detect HIV infection sooner in the window period, thereby reducing the number of false-negative results obtained with standard HIV ELISA tests.

In the p24 test, the walls of a microtiter plate or tiny plastic beads are coated with antibodies to p24. The serum to be tested is then incubated with these antibodies. If p24 is present in the serum, it binds tightly to the antibody. The excess serum is washed away. Another antibody to HIV, often a rabbit anti-HIV antibody, that also becomes bound to p24 is then added. Last, a goat antibody is used to detect the rabbit antibody. This produces a color as in the ELISA tests just described. As in the standard ELISA, a p24 test that reveals the presence of antigen in a serum sample is verified with a confirmatory test.

The p24 antigen test has been refined to the point that blood banks nationally use it along with combination HIV-1/HIV-2 antibody tests for screening donated blood, as mentioned already. This reduces to the extent possible the occurrence of false-negative results due to the window period. The rare remaining false negatives represent the only current risk of HIV infection acquired through blood transfusions (see Chapter 3).

■ OTHER TYPES OF SCREENING TESTS

■ Oral Fluid Tests

Sometimes called the "saliva test," the oral fluid test actually detects HIV antibodies found in "oral mucosal transudate." This is a fluid that is collected using an approved test pad that is placed between cheek and gum (after gently rubbing the cheek with the pad). The pad is left in place for two minutes. During that time, it absorbs a saliva-like fluid—the oral mucosal transudate—that is produced by the mucous membrane of the cheek and has higher levels of HIV antibodies than saliva itself. The sample is analyzed by a certified laboratory using an ELISA that is specifically licensed for testing oral fluid; the confirmatory test is a Western blot performed on the same oral fluid sample.

The oral fluid test is performed by a health-care professional. When done correctly, it is as accurate as the HIV serum antibody test. Nonetheless, the Centers for Disease Control and Prevention (CDC) recommend that all new diagnoses of HIV infection based on oral fluids be confirmed using a second, newly collected specimen.

■ Urine Tests

Low levels of anti-HIV antibodies are also present in urine, and an ELISA-type test has been developed for their detection. As with other HIV ELISA tests, positive results must be verified by a Western blot or other confirmatory test.

■ Home Specimen-Collection Kits

In 1996, the Food and Drug Administration (FDA) approved the marketing of two kits designed to allow the self-collection of blood samples, in the privacy of one's own home, to be mailed in for HIV testing under conditions that protect the user's anonymity. (Note that it is incorrect to refer to this procedure as "home testing" since the testing itself is still done by a laboratory; true home testing for HIV has never been approved by the FDA because it would deprive users of immediate competent counseling.)

As of this writing, two home specimen-collection kits are available over the counter (Confide, by Direct Access Diagnostics; and Home Access, by Home Access Health). Each kit carries a unique identification number. Use of the kits involves pricking a finger and placing drops of blood on three circles outlined on a piece of filter paper. The paper is then mailed to a designated licensed laboratory, where the blood is analyzed. If two of the drops produce a positive result, a confirmatory test is run on the third drop. Users are instructed to telephone the laboratory after about a week to learn the results, using the kit's unique number to identify themselves. Test results are given by trained counselors. (See Chapter 1 for an explanation of the purpose of counseling.)

■ CONFIRMATORY TESTS FOR HIV AND HOW THEY WORK

A large number of serum samples from people in the general population that are reactive on a first ELISA test are not reactive when the test is repeated. If a sample does test positive a second time, however, the result must be verified by a confirmatory test. A confirmatory test is designed to distinguish a false-positive ELISA result from a true positive. The most common confirmatory test is the Western blot.

■ Western Blot

Like an ELISA, a Western blot uses HIV proteins to capture anti-HIV antibodies in blood serum. A Western blot has a much lower false-positive rate, though, because it uses HIV proteins that are separated into distinct groups, or bands. Separating individual viral proteins in this way also separates them from many contaminating cellular proteins that are responsible for many false-positive ELISA results. It also reveals to which HIV proteins the antibodies in the serum sample react, and this is another important merit of this test. However, the Western blot is impractical for use as a screening test because it is labor-intensive and expensive, and has a higher rate of false-negative results.

A Western blot from start to finish can be thought of as occurring in two phases: obtaining and separating the HIV antigens, and testing the serum against the antigens. The presence of anti-HIV antibodies is detected by a color reaction, as in an ELISA test. The test works as follows:

- The antigens used in the test are prepared by manufacturers of Western blot kits as for an ELISA test kit (see above).

- The viral proteins in the mix are now separated by size using the technique of gel electrophoresis. This is done as follows: The mix of proteins is placed on the end of an upright rectangle of a plastic-like gel. An electrical current draws the protein mixture through the gel. Large proteins migrate through the gel slowly while small proteins migrate faster. When the current is turned off, proteins of different sizes occupy distinct and characteristic locations within the gel, each forming a band; larger proteins such as gp160 and gp120 are at one end and the smaller proteins such as p24 and p18 are at the other end, in that order.

- The bands in the gel are transferred—or blotted—onto a special paper (nitrocellulose paper). The paper is then cut into narrow strips. This completes the preparation of the antigen used in a Western blot. The paper strips with antigen bands in place are provided to testing laboratories as part of Western blot test kits.

The remaining steps of a Western blot follow those of the ELISA test.

- The paper strips are incubated with serum from the patient. If antibodies to HIV proteins are present in the serum, each kind of antibody attaches to the corresponding HIV protein; that is, it binds only with its particular antigen in one protein band. The serum is washed away.

- The strips are exposed to anti-human antibody. This second antibody is linked to the enzyme. If HIV antibody from the serum tested is present on any of the bands, the anti-human antibody binds with it. The excess enzyme is washed away.

- The strips are now exposed to substrate. If serum anti-HIV antibodies are present, a reaction occurs between the enzyme and the substrate to produce a color. As in ELISA tests, the intensity of the color is proportional to the amount of serum antibody.

Judging the Results of a Western Blot

The U.S. Public Health Service considers a Western blot positive for HIV if antibodies are present for two of the following proteins: p24, gp41, gp120, and gp160. If no bands are reactive, the result is negative. If only a single band is reactive or if the wrong combination of colored bands is present, the result is indeterminate. Causes of an indeterminate result include the following:

- The person is in the window period of HIV infection and not all antibodies that will become detectable are present yet. Such a person should be retested six weeks later.

- Very infrequently (0.3% to 0.5%) the Western blot test result is persistently indeterminate for some people, for reasons that remain poorly understood.

- The person is truly HIV negative.

■ Other Confirmatory Tests

Indirect Immunofluorescence Assay

Indirect immunofluorescence assays (IFAs) use a fluorescent dye to detect anti-HIV antibodies in serum. The test uses HIV-infected cells that are fixed to a microscope slide. The slide is incubated with the serum to be tested. Anti-HIV antibodies in the serum bind to the viral proteins on the surface of the cells. These bound human antibodies are in turn detected using anti-human antibody, again usually from goats. The goat antibodies are linked to a dye that fluoresces when exposed to ultraviolet light under a fluorescent microscope. The intensity of the fluorescence provides a measure of the amount of antibody in the serum. This test can detect the earliest antibodies produced against HIV during the acute stage of infection. IFAs are also labor-intensive and require a high degree of expertise.

Viral Culture Methods

Growing live HIV from infected cells was the first method used to detect HIV infection. This involves coculturing, that is, growing lymphocytes from the person to be tested along with lymphocytes from an uninfected donor. The cells are grown in a medium designed to encourage the growth of both lymphocytes and HIV. The test conditions can produce an explosive growth of virus.

A coculture is declared positive for HIV when increased levels of the viral enzyme reverse transcriptase (RT) or of the p24 protein are detected in the growth medium in at least two consecutive tests. The cocultured cells are also examined under a microscope for the presence of syncytia (giant cells with many nuclei that result from the coalescing of infected lymphocytes; see Chapter 18).

Coculture for the growth of HIV has a number of advantages over other tests. It produces virus that can be isolated, analyzed, and genetically characterized. It is also one method (in addition to the polymerase chain reaction described later) that permits the discovery of new types and subtypes of virus from individual patients. But viral culture methods are also expensive and time-consuming—cocultures must be studied for 14 days to 35 days, making them impractical as a basis for clinical decisions. The culture of HIV-infected cells also poses risks because it requires the handling of live virus. For these reasons, cell and viral culture methods are used primarily in research laboratories.

■ VIRAL GENOME TESTS FOR HIV AND HOW THEY WORK

Several clinical trials concluded in 1996 that measuring "viral load"—the amount of free virus in the blood—is an earlier and more reliable predictor of future clinical course than is a change in the number of CD4 cells. Measuring changes in viral load now also helps physicians and patients determine when antiretroviral drug treatment should begin or when viral resistance to anti-HIV treatment is beginning and the treatment should be changed. Methods that can detect virus in blood or lymphocytes include the polymerase chain reaction (PCR), quantitative competitive PCR (QC-PCR), and branched-chain DNA amplification (bDNA). The last two methods also measure viral load.

■ Polymerase Chain Reaction

PCR reveals the presence of specific segments of DNA in cells and other kinds of samples. The method is so sensitive that it can detect the presence of a single HIV provirus in 100,000 cells (the provirus is the DNA that HIV produces and inserts into the chromosomes of infected cells; see Chapter 18). PCR can also detect viral RNA (HIV's genetic material) from virions isolated from blood serum, although the RNA must first be transcribed into DNA in the laboratory using RT. For this reason, the use of PCR to measure viral RNA is also known as RT-PCR.

PCR works by creating a chain reaction in which a short length of target DNA (a gene or part of a gene, for example) is copied repeatedly by a polymerase enzyme, until millions of copies are produced over a period of several hours. This amplification process makes a DNA fragment readily detectable in the laboratory. (The same process can be used to produce quantities of any segment of DNA needed for laboratory studies.)

PCR is the basis for extremely sensitive tests. This is also its drawback: PCR-based tests must be done by scientists or experienced technicians using adequate controls and sterile technique. Otherwise, contamination with target DNA can easily produce false-positive results.

■ Quantitative Competitive PCR

While PCR is extraordinarily good at determining whether HIV is present in a sample of cells or plasma, it cannot be used in any practical sense to determine the *amount* of virus present. QC-PCR modifies the PCR technique in such a way as to do so. In QC-PCR, a DNA sequence is designed in the laboratory to be very close in structure to the segment of target DNA. This laboratory-produced DNA is known as "competitor DNA."

QC-PCR is conducted by doing PCR on a series of samples of HIV DNA (usually a portion of the *gag* gene) from the serum of a patient. QC-PCR differs from the PCR test in that a known quantity of the competitor DNA is also added to each sample. The competitor DNA is added in increasing, tenfold increments (i.e., 10 copies of the competitor DNA are added to one sample, 100 copies to the next sample, 1,000 copies to the third sample, and 10,000 copies to the fourth sample).

During the test, as the two kinds of DNA make many copies of themselves during the chain reaction, the laboratory-made DNA competes with the HIV DNA for building blocks, that is, the molecules needed to make DNA copies. These materials—DNA nucleotides—are provided in excess as part of the test.

The quantities of target DNA and competitor DNA that result are then measured by electrophoresis. The amount of viral DNA present at the beginning of the test is proportional to the amount of competitor DNA present at the end of the test. This makes it possible to calculate the amount of HIV present in the original serum sample.

■ Branched-Chain DNA Amplification

PCR and QC-PCR are tests that amplify target DNA. bDNA involves amplifying a signal that is attached to target viral RNA or DNA. In preparation for this test, virus particles are separated from plasma or cells. Key components of the test are two kinds of oligonucleotide probes ("oligonucleotide" refers to a short fragment of DNA; "probe" refers to DNA that is designed to pair and attach to—or hybridize with—a specific place on another DNA strand). These two sets of the oligonucleotide probes consist of "capture" probes and "label-extender" probes.

Capture probes are designed to attach to the viral genome and anchor it in place; label-extender probes also hybridize with the genome, but they resemble flag poles with many pennants flying along their length. These pennants also carry an enzyme. In the last step of the bDNA test, as in the last step of an ELISA test, a substrate that reacts with the enzyme is added. The reaction produces a luminescence that can be measured. The level of luminescence correlates with the amount of virus present.

As few as 50 to 100 copies of viral genome are needed per milliliter (ml) of sample for detection. In addition, bDNA can be done accurately, quickly, and on a large number of samples. It can also be done in clinical laboratories without the expensive quality-control measures needed for PCR. bDNA is currently being used to detect a variety of viruses, including HIV, cytomegalovirus (CMV), hepatitis B virus (HBV), and hepatitis C virus (HCV).

■ THE MEANING OF VIRAL-LOAD NUMBERS

Viral-load measurements are usually reported in terms of copies of HIV RNA per milliliter of blood. They can also be reported as a log copy number per milliliter of blood. A log is a factor of ten. A 1-log change is the same as a tenfold change. A viral load of 5 logs can also be written as 10^5 copies, which is the same as saying a person has 100,000 copies of HIV RNA per milliliter of blood. Someone with a viral load of 3.4 logs ($10^{3.4}$) has a viral level of 2,511 copies per milliliter, between 1,000 (10^3) and 10,000 (10^4) copies per milliliter.

Researchers often report drops in the level of HIV in the blood following a specific treatment in terms of log reductions. For example, someone with a pretreatment level of 100,000 HIV RNA copies per milliliter of blood might be reported as having a 2-log reduction in viral load. That would equal a 100-fold drop, leaving the person with a post-treatment level of 1,000 HIV RNA copies per milliliter of blood.

■ ACCURACY OF HIV TESTING

Clinical tests of any kind, including those for detecting HIV infection, will produce some false-negative and false-positive results. How many false results a given test is likely to produce depends on the test's sensitivity and specificity.

- Sensitivity is a measure of the number of false-negative results a test can be expected to produce.

- Specificity is a measure of the number of false-positive results a test will likely produce.

(To help remember what sensitivity and specificity refer to, note that "negative" and "sensitivity" both contain the letter n, while "positive" and "specificity" both contain the letter p.)

Screening tests are designed to have high sensitivity because they are intended to detect all cases of infection, even though this may produce a number of false-positive results. According to one study done in the late 1980s, the sensitivity for two successively reactive ELISA HIV tests at that time was 99.7%, or 3 false negatives per 1,000 test results; the specificity at that time was around 98.5%, or 15 false positives per 1,000 test results.

Subsequent improvements, such as using HIV antigens produced in the laboratory using recombinant DNA technology, have increased the sensitivity and specificity of ELISA tests for HIV. Another major change involved replacing the usual goat anti-human "detector" antibody with a second set of recombinant HIV antigens. The detector antigens are also linked to an enzyme that produces a color when substrate is added.

ELISAs that use antigens as the detector molecule take advantage of the molecular structure of antibodies. Antibody molecules are shaped like a Y. Each arm of the Y has a site that can bind with the antigen. During an ELISA, serum is added to a well that is coated with antigen. Using one arm of the Y, anti-HIV antibodies present in the serum sample bind with the antigen; the binding site on the second arm remains free. When the detector antigen that is used in the newer and more sensitive ELISAs is added to the well, the antigen binds with that second arm on the Y to reveal the presence of the antibody.

These improvements on these new ELISA tests provide a sensitivity of essentially 100% and a specificity of 99.9%. They are now used by the American Red Cross National Testing Laboratories for screening donated blood. Thanks to them, today the risk of getting HIV infection from donated blood is estimated at 1 in 700,000 (see also Chapter 3).

As a confirmatory test, the Western blot has very high specificity, which minimizes the number of false-positive results. Western blots have a sensitivity of about 95% (primarily because of indeterminate results) and a specificity of 100%.

■ THE IMPORTANCE OF DISEASE PREVALENCE IN HIV TESTING

Why not test everyone for HIV infection? Because all screening tests have a property known as positive predictive value—the probability that a positive test result is truly positive. Positive predictive value is greatly influenced by the prevalence of the disease or infection in the population being tested. Why this is so is shown by calculating the positive predictive value for the same test when applied to a population in which HIV infection is highly prevalent as compared to a population in which the prevalence is low.

Consider first the example of a high-prevalence population—injection drug users in a major city in which half the drug users are infected (i.e., the prevalence of HIV infection in the population is 50%). For convenience, the size of the population is said to be 100,000. That means 50,000 people will be infected and 50,000 uninfected. The test used in the example will have a specificity of 99.9%—it will yield 1 false positive per 1,000 people tested, or 50 false positives per 50,000 people tested. The positive predictive value is calculated as follows:

$$\text{Positive predictive value} = \frac{\text{True positives}}{\text{True positives} + \text{False positives}}$$

$$= \frac{49,950}{50,000} = 99.9\%$$

This result means that a positive test result has a 99.9% chance of being a true positive. But that probability changes when the same calculation is applied to a population with a low prevalence of infection. Take, for example, self-selected and previously tested blood donors from the general population. Here, the prevalence of infection might be 1 case per 100,000 people.

Thus, for every 100,000 people, 1 person is infected and 99,999 are uninfected. If the test has a specificity of 99.9%, it means 0.1%—about 100—of those test results will be false positives. Now calculate the positive predictive value:

$$\text{Positive predictive value} = \frac{\text{True positives}}{\text{True positives} + \text{False positives}}$$

$$= \frac{1}{101} = 1.0\%$$

This means that a positive test result in this population has only a 1% chance of being a true positive!

ENDNOTE

1. More precisely, about 50% of people infected with HIV have detectable antibodies three to four weeks after infection; 99% have them within six to nine months; and a fraction of people never develop them. This is one reason why blood banks now use the p24 antigen test as well as the HIV antibody test to detect HIV infection.

■ *Chapter 3*

TRANSMISSION OF HIV

Scientists identified the means by which HIV was transmitted in the early days of the epidemic, well before the virus itself was discovered (see Chapter 20). No new modes of transmission have been discovered since. Throughout the world, people can contract HIV infection in three possible ways:

- Through sexual contact, either homosexual or heterosexual. Heterosexual contact is the leading means of HIV transmission worldwide, and the fastest growing mode of HIV transmission in the nation.

- Through contact with blood or other body fluids, blood products, or tissues of an infected person. This usually occurs by inoculation of HIV through needle sharing among users of illicit drugs; much more rarely, by accidental needle stick or splashes of blood on mucous membranes; and extremely rarely, through sustained contact of infected blood with breaks in the skin.

- Through transfer of the virus from an infected mother to her infant before or during birth, or shortly after birth through breast-feeding. This mother-to-infant transfer is also known as "perinatal transmission." Perinatal transmission is in rapid decline in the United States.

■ 35

Transfer of a virus from mother to infant is also known as "vertical transmission," which refers to transfer of the virus from one generation to the next. This term, along with "horizontal transmission," is used often in the scientific literature. Horizontal transmission refers to transfer of the virus from one person to another in a population. Sexual transmission and blood-to-blood transmission are both examples of horizontal transmission.

Free HIV particles have been isolated from blood, semen, vaginal fluid, and breast milk. Other body fluids in which HIV is found include cerebrospinal fluid, which bathes the brain and spinal cord; synovial fluid, which bathes the surfaces of joints; pleural fluid, which occupies the narrow space between the lungs and the chest wall; and amniotic fluid, which surrounds the fetus. Researchers have also isolated HIV from saliva, tears, feces, and urine, in which it is sometimes present in very small amounts. No cases of HIV transmission through these fluids have been fully documented.

Table 3.1 ■ Percentage of AIDS Cases according to Mode of Transmission: From the Beginning of the Epidemic to December 31, 1996

Mode of Transmission	United States Rates[1]	Estimated World Rates[2]
Sex between men	50	5–10
Injection drug use	26	5–10
Men who have sex with men and who inject drugs	6	Not available
Heterosexual intercourse	9	>70
Exposure of hemophiliacs to infected blood products	1	Not available
Exposure to contaminated blood or blood products during a medical procedure	1	3–5
Risk factor undetermined*	7	Not available

*The "Risk factor undetermined" category includes persons whose cases are still under investigation; persons unwilling to disclose high-risk information or unaware of a clear-cut exposure; persons with possible occupational exposure; and persons who were incompletely investigated upon their death, or who were lost to follow-up or declined to be interviewed.

Table 3.1 shows percentage of AIDS cases in adults and adolescents according to the mode of transmission in the United States and worldwide, from the beginning of the epidemic to December 31, 1996. It is important to realize that the leading modes of HIV transmission in the United States—sex between men and injection drug use—are different from the leading mode of transmission worldwide, which is heterosexual intercourse. Moreover, HIV transmission through heterosexual intercourse is increasing in the United States. This becomes clear when the exposure categories for AIDS cases reported in the year 1985 in the United States are compared with cases reported in 1996 (Table 3.2).

Table 3.2. ■ *Modes of Transmission in 1985 Compared with 1996: Percentage of AIDS Cases in the United States*

Mode of Transmission	Cases Reported in 1985[3]	Cases Reported in 1996[4]
Sex between men	67	40
Injection drug use	17	25
Men who have sex with men and who inject drugs	8	4
Heterosexual intercourse	2	13
Exposure of hemophiliacs to infected blood products	1	<1
Exposure to contaminated blood or blood products during a medical procedure	2	1
Risk factor undetermined	3	17*

The "Undetermined" category for 1996 will decrease over time as investigations of these new AIDS cases are conducted.

■ SEXUAL TRANSMISSION

Sexual transmission of HIV is thought to account for 90% of AIDS cases worldwide. In the United States, Canada, and most of Europe, most cases of sexual transmission have occurred between men having sex with men, but cases due to heterosexual transmission increased more than sixfold from 1985 to 1996 (from 2% to 13%) in the United States, and that proportion will probably continue to grow. Heterosexual transmission of HIV in western Europe, for example, increased nine times from 1985 to 1990. Worldwide, vaginal intercourse has always been the predominant mode of HIV transmission.

The risk of transmission from an infected male to an uninfected female through unprotected vaginal intercourse is thought to be about 1 per 100 sexual contacts (i.e., out of 100 couples having one instance of vaginal intercourse in which the man is HIV positive and the woman HIV negative, 1 case of transmission will occur). The risk of transmission during anal intercourse is believed to be considerably higher, with an estimated transmission rate of 1 in 20 instances of unprotected anal intercourse.

The risk of female-to-male transmission is lower, with a rate estimated to be in the range of 1 per 1,000 infected women (i.e., out of 1,000 couples having vaginal intercourse in which the woman is HIV positive and the man HIV negative, 1 case of transmission will occur). The higher rate of male-to-female transmission is thought to be one reason why women outnumber men in cases of infection due to heterosexual transmission (see Chapter 11). The risk of female-to-female HIV transmission is lower yet.

These rates are highly variable, though, because many factors may alter an individual's susceptibility and HIV's infectiousness. These factors include the following:

- The presence of either acute HIV infection or advanced HIV disease (AIDS) in the infected partner increases the risk of sexual transmission. Although individuals with asymptomatic disease are also infectious to others, people recently infected temporarily have very high levels of virus in their blood and body fluids and secretions, as do people with advanced disease, which makes them relatively more infectious to their partners.

- The presence of genital tract infections in either partner increases the risk. The risk of transmission markedly increases if yeast infection or genital sores or ulcers are present. Such sores can be caused by ulcer-producing sexually transmitted diseases (STDs) such as syphilis, herpes, and chancroid. Sores or ulcers in the uninfected partner facilitate contact between that person's CD4 lymphocytes and macrophages and HIV from the infected partner; sores in the infected person provide additional avenues for release of HIV, exposing the uninfected partner to a greater dose of virus. Note, too, that genital ulcers in an HIV-infected person tend to increase in frequency, extent, and duration as the health of his or her immune system declines.

- STDs that do not produce ulcers, such as gonorrhea, chlamydia, and trichomoniasis, also increase the risk of acquiring HIV. This is thought to occur because these diseases cause inflammation of the mucous membranes of the genital tract. Inflammation is a normal immune response to infection or injury, but it activates and attracts large numbers of white blood cells including monocytes, macrophages, and T lymphocytes to the inflamed area. In the HIV-infected partner this increases the amount of free virus and the number of virus-infected cells in genital secretions. In the HIV-negative partner the risk of acquiring HIV infection is increased because the inflammation of the genital tract concentrates cells susceptible to HIV infection in the genital tissues.

- Anal intercourse and, probably, intercourse during menstruation also increase the risk of sexual transmission. The rectal lining is thin, much more so than the vaginal lining, and contains many lymphocytes, macrophages, and other cells that HIV can infect. Anal intercourse also easily causes tears in the rectal lining that result in direct contact between infected semen and the blood of the receptive partner.

- Number of instances of intercourse is also related to risk. The greater the number of exposures to infected semen or vaginal secretions, the higher the risk of HIV transmission.

- Genetic characteristics of the particular HIV strain to which a person is exposed, as well as genetic characteristics of the exposed person, affect the risk of HIV transmission. A very small percentage of individuals have remained uninfected despite repeated exposure to HIV. It is now believed that certain individuals have a genetically determined natural resistance to HIV (see "Long-Term Nonprogressors," Chapter 4). Some strains of HIV appear to be more infectious than others. It has even been speculated that some HIV subtypes might be more infectious than others through vaginal intercourse.

■ Some studies have suggested that the use of oral contraceptives, di-aphrams, cervical caps, or intrauterine devices (IUDs) increases the risk of HIV transmission. This is difficult to determine because people who use these modes of contraception may be less likely to also use condoms during intercourse.

■ A risk of HIV transmission exists even during safer sex; minimizing this risk requires that condoms be used consistently and correctly (see Chapter 9).

■ Oral Sex

The risk represented by oral sex is relatively low as compared to that of anal or vaginal sex. Data are not available to determine the probability of HIV transmission by oral-penile contact. As of 1996, however, there were ten reports involving 17 persons who were thought to have become HIV infected through oral-penile sex. Although oral sex poses a low risk of HIV transmission, the Centers for Disease Control and Prevention (CDC) guidelines have consistently recommended use of a condom during oral-penile contact and a barrier during oral-vaginal contact.

A recent study[5] in monkeys suggested that oral sex could hold a higher risk of infection than once thought. The study involved placing free simian immunodeficiency virus (SIV) particles on the back of the tongue of seven infant rhesus monkeys. Six of the monkeys became infected.

The implications of this for humans are unclear. Scientists commenting on the study pointed out that the conditions used in the experiment did not really mirror what happens in humans during oral sex. Human saliva is known to have an inhibitory effect on the infectiousness of HIV. In addition, the concentrations of the virus used in the monkey study were higher than those most humans would encounter during oral sex.

Whatever the implications of this study for the risk of HIV transmission during oral sex, it certainly in no way implies risk of transmission through casual contact. There is no evidence at all of transmission through kissing, the sharing of eating utensils, etc. (see "How HIV Is NOT Transmitted").

■ BLOOD AND BLOOD PRODUCTS

HIV is present in blood of both asymptomatic and symptomatic people as free virus particles and in infected cells. The number of free virus particles in the blood can rise to extremely high levels during the period of acute infection. Then, within weeks, viral levels decrease and the virus nearly disappears from the blood. As the disease progresses, however, the number of CD4 cells in the blood drops and the number of free virus particles progressively rises again (see Chapter 4). In advanced HIV disease (i.e., AIDS), there might be as many as a million free virus particles per milliliter of blood, as a large proportion of CD4 cells are infected, each of which can produce thousands of virus particles daily.

Transmission by blood and body fluids can occur very efficiently through the sharing of needles and other equipment used to inject drugs, or through transfusion of HIV-contaminated blood or blood products. Although such cases have been very rare, media reports have periodically raised the public's concern about HIV transmission from HIV-infected patients to health-care workers, and from HIV-infected health-care workers to patients (see below).

■ Needle Sharing and Drug Use

Transmission of HIV among injection drug users (IDUs) occurs when the blood of an HIV-infected drug user is transferred to an uninfected IDU through the sharing of needles and syringes (drug injection equipment is also known as "works," "gimmicks," and "sets"). Needle sharing by IDUs is the leading cause of HIV transmission by blood, and the second leading mode of HIV transmission in the United States, after sexual transmission. CDC figures for 1995 showed that HIV transmission among IDUs accounted for 24% of reported AIDS cases in men that year nationwide and 38% among women. HIV can spread rapidly and efficiently through needle sharing. In New York City, HIV infection among IDUs went from less than 10% to more than 50% in five years in some groups studied. In Edinburgh, Scotland, the number of HIV-infected IDUs in one group went from zero to more than 40% in one year.

Because a vast majority of IDUs are heterosexual, they are also a leading factor in the spread of HIV to the heterosexual population and in the rapid increase in the numbers of women with HIV disease and AIDS and, hence, also in the numbers of newborns with HIV disease.

Two drug-injection practices in particular set the stage for HIV transmission during needle sharing: the initial drawing of blood into the barrel of the syringe to verify that the needle is inserted into a vein, and the practice of refilling the syringe repeatedly with blood following drug injection to rinse out any remaining drug. IDUs can prevent HIV transmission by adhering to the practices described in Chapter 9.

Noninjection Drugs and HIV Transmission

The use of alcohol, crack cocaine, and other mind-altering drugs also increases the risk of acquiring or transmitting HIV infection. Mind-altering drugs affect judgment and increase the probability of unsafe behavior. Trading sex for crack or other drugs is a practice that usually involves unprotected sex. It is thought to be responsible for the significant increases in the incidence of syphilis and other STDs, as well as that of HIV infection. Because syphilis produces genital ulcers, an increase in syphilis incidence also means, for the people affected, a higher risk of acquiring HIV infection through sexual contact.

■ Transmission by Transfusion: Safety of the Blood Supply

There never has been—nor is there now—any risk at all of acquiring HIV through the process of *donating* blood. However, HIV can be transmitted by transfusion of whole blood, the cellular components of blood, plasma, and clotting factors derived from blood. In the early 1980s, virtually 100% of the people who received transfusions of HIV-contaminated blood became infected because of the high dose of virus that can be present in a single unit of blood. In all, an estimated 12,000 people became HIV infected by contaminated transfusions.

The self-disqualification as blood donors of individuals at high risk for HIV/AIDS, and the screening of all blood donations have, since 1985, virtually eliminated this mode of HIV transmission in the Western world.

In the United States, testing the blood supply for HIV began in early 1985. In early 1997, the risk of receiving a pint of blood infected with HIV was estimated to be about 1 in 700,000. Transfusion of infected blood, however, remains the third leading cause of HIV transmission in Africa and many other developing countries, after sexual transmission and mother-to-infant transmission.

Also prior to testing, many of the estimated 15,000 hemophiliacs in the United States became infected with HIV in the early years of the HIV epidemic after receiving contaminated clotting factors. Hemophilia is a disorder of the blood-clotting system that is corrected by administration of clotting factors. These are proteins derived from plasma that is obtained by pooling many units of donated blood. Prior to 1985, clotting factor preparation methods did not inactivate HIV. One unit of HIV-infected blood in the entire blood pool could infect all the clotting factor preparations derived from it.

As a result, in the early 1980s, between 80% and 90% of people with hemophilia A in the United States became infected with HIV, and so did between 35% and 45% of people with hemophilia B. (People with hemophilia B require less frequent infusions of clotting factors.)

The screening of all blood donations and the heat treatment of clotting factors during their preparation have virtually eliminated clotting factors as a source of HIV infection in the Western world.

■ Transmission from HIV-Positive Patients to Health-Care Workers

The transmission of HIV from an infected patient to an uninfected health-care worker is possible if the health-care worker accidentally cuts himself or herself during surgery or sticks himself or herself with a needle that contains infected blood from the patient. This kind of on-the-job exposure to HIV is known as "occupational exposure." It can also occur if a health-care worker has open wounds—even tiny ones—or skin abrasions that come in contact with an infected patient's blood or other virus-laden body fluids. Exposure to any infectious agent that involves a cut, abrasion, or break in the skin—including a break caused by a needle stick—is referred to as "percutaneous exposure."

Evidence indicates that the risk of acquiring HIV infection from percutaneous exposure is low. Several studies have estimated the risk of HIV infection from such exposure. A 1990 study[6] followed 2,200 health-care workers exposed to HIV following accidental needle sticks or other kinds of injuries. Of these, 8 workers later tested positive for HIV antibodies. This rate—8 infections per 2,200 exposure—yields a risk of 0.36 infection per 100 exposures. This falls into the range of 0.13 to 0.39 infection per 100 exposures found by other studies. By comparison, 12 to 17 infections occurred per 100 accidental needle sticks with needles that contained blood infected with hepatitis B virus.

Note that the risk of HIV transmission from accidental needle sticks is much lower than the risk of transmission from needle sharing by IDUs. The two types of exposures differ: An accidental needle stick is a one-time event and does not usually involve a deep or substantial injection. Exposure through needle sharing likely involves repeated injections of a larger dose of infectious material directly into a vein.

There is also a possible risk of transmission through exposure of the mucous membranes of a caregiver's eyes, nose, or mouth to a patient's HIV-infected blood or other body fluids. One study followed the outcome of 1,000 mucous membrane exposures and found no cases of HIV transmission.

Although the risk of acquiring HIV infection through percutaneous or mucous membrane exposure is slight, it is believed advisable that a person accidentally exposed to HIV should consider prompt treatment with a combination of antiretroviral drugs (see Chapter 9). Recent data strongly suggest that such treatment reduces the risk of infection.[7]

■ Transmission from HIV-Positive Health-Care Workers to Patients

In the United States, the only verified case of transmission from a health-care worker to patients involved a dentist who infected 6 of his patients. The mode of transmission in this unique case remains unknown. Testing of the dentist's 1,100 patients revealed 9 who were HIV infected. Infections in 3 of them proved to be unrelated to the dentist: Not only did all 3 have a history of recognized risk factors, but molecular analyses showed that the viral strains present in these 3 patients were only distantly genetically related to the viral strain present in the dentist. Viruses isolated from the remaining 6 patients, however, were closely related to the virus from the dentist.

Studies of more than 22,000 patients who were cared for by 63 HIV-positive physicians and dentists showed no other cases of HIV transmission to patients.

Perinatal Transmission

Perinatal transmission of HIV is thought to occur in 15% to 30% of births to HIV-positive women. The rate is lowest in developed countries and highest in developing countries. Worldwide, it is the second most common mode of HIV transmission after sexual transmission. Each year in the early 1990s, about 7,000 HIV-infected women in the United States gave birth to some 2,000 infected infants. Perinatal transmission may occur through a number of different pathways; it can happen before birth, during delivery, or during breast-feeding.

A seminal clinical trial concluded in 1994 found that azidothymidine (AZT) given orally to pregnant women for several weeks prior to delivery, intravenously during delivery, and orally to the newborns for six weeks could reduce perinatal transmission by two-thirds.[8] The study was a landmark because it was the first to show that a treatment for HIV could reduce the risk of virus transmission.

A strong correlation was later found between levels of free virus in the mother's blood (i.e., the mother's viral load) and perinatal transmission. A study found that high levels of free HIV in the mother's blood late in pregnancy or during delivery predicted risk of perinatal transmission.[9] The research also suggested that AZT helps prevent transmission by reducing the amount of free virus in the mother's blood prior to delivery. Other factors may also play a role, as some mothers with a low viral load did nevertheless transmit HIV to their infants. Some of these factors may be the following:

- The mother's immune status. A low CD4 count is also associated with an increased risk of perinatal transmission.

■ Exposure of the infant's mucosal membranes to maternal blood during delivery.

■ Prolonged period between the time the mother's water breaks and the time of delivery.

■ Presence of ulcerations in the mother caused by sexually transmitted infections.

■ Vaginal delivery. Some studies suggest that vaginal delivery increases the risk of transmission, but this has not been conclusively shown, and cesarean sections are not recommended as a means of reducing the risk of HIV transmission.

■ Vitamin A deficiency. In Africa, vitamin A deficiency in pregnant women appears to increase the risk of perinatal transmission. However, it is not known yet whether supplements of vitamin A reduce this risk.

Breast-feeding

Breast milk can also transmit HIV, which is found in both the cells present and the liquid portion of the milk. The risk of transmission is believed to be highest during periods of high viral load in the mother, that is, during acute HIV infection and during advanced HIV disease, or AIDS (see Chapter 4).

In the United States and other developed countries that have safe alternatives to breast milk, breast-feeding by HIV-positive mothers is discouraged. In developing countries that lack safe and affordable alternatives to breast milk, breast-feeding by HIV-positive mothers is regarded as holding less risk of disease for the infant than the available alternatives, at least in environments with poor sanitation. (As the incidence of HIV infection increases in developing countries, the earlier recommendation that all HIV-positive mothers in these countries should breast-feed rather than use formula is being re-evaluated. The decision now often depends on local sanitary conditions.)

▪ How HIV Is NOT Transmitted

If HIV were spread by insects, like the plague or malaria; by casual contact, like influenza; by sneezing, like a cold; or by water, like cholera, the pattern of the AIDS epidemic would be far different from what it is. Either entire households would be affected, or individuals would be affected randomly, or the epidemic's spread would be determined by climate, altitude, quality of water supply, and other such environmental factors. This is not the case for the epidemic of HIV/AIDS. It is spread in specific ways: sexual contact, blood-to-blood contact, and from mother to infant. These modes of transmission were established early in the epidemic and continuing surveillance over a period of 15 years has revealed no additional routes of HIV transmission.

In addition, reviews of some 14 epidemiological studies that involved a total of 757 individuals sharing households with HIV-positive people found no cases of casual transmission.[10] These included households of infected hemophiliacs, households with infected foster children, households with HIV-contaminated transfusion recipients, and other households of people with HIV/AIDS.

Members of these households shared such things as combs, towels, bed linens, eating utensils, plates, and drinking glasses. They touched and kissed. None of the studies produced any evidence of HIV transmission when unprotected sexual contact or needle sharing did *not* occur. Thus, there *is no evidence* that HIV is transmitted by any of the following:

- Talking, shaking hands, or other casual contact

- Hugging or ordinary kissing (there is a remote risk that deep kissing—French kissing or tongue kissing—could lead to infection, especially if open sores are present on the lips, tongue, or mouth)

- Sharing kitchens, lunchrooms, dishes, or eating utensils

- Touching floors, walls, door knobs, or toilet seats; or sharing offices, restrooms, computers, telephones, or writing utensils

- Being bitten by mosquitoes, fleas, bed bugs, and other insects

If precautions are taken to avoid blood-to-blood contact, there is no evidence that HIV transmission occurs in a nonsexual, non-needle-sharing relationship with a person who is HIV positive. ▪

ENDNOTES

1. Centers for Disease Control and Prevention. *HIV/AIDS Surveillance Report* 1996;8(2):10.

2. *UNAIDS and WHO Fact Sheet: HIV/AIDS: The Global Epidemic.* Geneva, Switzerland: World Health Organization, December 1996. (World Health Organization document based on the *Final Report: The Status and Trends of the Global HIV/AIDS Pandemic,* Vancouver, July 5–6, 1996.)

3. Unpublished CDC AIDS surveillance data for 1985, provided by the National Center for HIV, STD, and TB Prevention, Bethesda, MD.

4. Centers for Disease Control and Prevention. *HIV/AIDS Surveillance Report* 1996;8(2):10.

5. Baba TW, et al. Infection and AIDS in adult macaques after nontraumatic oral exposure to cell-free SIV. *Science* 1996; 272: 1486–1489.

6. Gershon RRM, Vlahov D, Nelson KE. The risk of transmission of HIV-1 through non-percutaneous, non-sexual modes—a review. *AIDS* 1990;4:645–650.

7. Centers for Disease Control and Prevention. Case-control study of HIV seroconversion in health-care workers after percutaneous exposure to HIV-infected blood—France, United Kingdom, and United States, January 1988–August 1994. *Morbidity and Mortality Weekly Report* 1995;44:929–933.

8. Conner HM, et al. Reduction of maternal–infant transmission of human immunodeficiency virus type 1 with zidovudine treatment. *New England Journal of Medicine* 1994;331:1173–1180.

9. Dickover RE, et al. Identification of levels of maternal HIV-1 RNA associated with risk of perinatal transmission: effect of maternal zidovudine treatment on viral load. *Journal of the American Medical Association* 1996;275:599–605.

10. Gershon RRM, Vlahov D, Nelson KE. The risk of transmission of HIV-1 through non-percutaneous, non-sexual modes—a review. *AIDS* 1990;4:645–650.

Chapter 4

HIV INFECTION AND THE
COURSE OF HIV DISEASE

HIV infection usually begins with transmission of the virus during un-safe sex or through exposure to contaminated blood, which most often occurs through the sharing of needles by injection drug users (see also Chapter 3). Children born to an HIV-infected mother can become infected during pregnancy, birth, or breast-feeding. (For a description of HIV infection in children, see Chapter 12.)

In the United States and other developed countries, the average time from the initial sexual infection to the development of advanced disease, or AIDS, is ten years in an untreated person. About 20% of infected individuals develop full-blown AIDS within five years; some—less than 5%—experience a period longer than ten years during which they manifest no, or few, symptoms and only a small and slow drop in CD4 lymphocyte numbers. These are "slow progressors."

A few others, 5% to 7%, show very low and steady levels of HIV in their blood, and normal or nearly normal CD4 cell counts for more than 10 to 15 years. These individuals are known as "long-term nonprogressors" (see below).

In most people, HIV infection progresses from the initial infection to

AIDS in four phases: acute infection; asymptomatic HIV disease; early HIV disease; and advanced HIV disease, or AIDS.

Disease progression involves an increasingly large number of free virions in the blood and increasing damage to the immune system, as revealed by decreases in the number of helper T lymphocytes in the blood. Helper T lymphocytes display the CD4 receptor molecule on their surface, earning them the designation of CD4 positive (CD4+), or simply CD4 lymphocytes. CD4 lymphocytes are key members of the immune system and are responsible for orchestrating critically important immune responses (see Chapter 16). They are also the primary target of HIV: The CD4 molecule (along with one or more co-receptors) is needed by HIV to infect cells, and it is the continued destruction of CD4 lymphocytes by HIV that is primarily responsible for the progression and development of HIV disease (for descriptions of the CD4 molecule and of CD4 lymphocytes, see Chapters 14 and 16).

Currently, CD4 lymphocyte counts—the number of CD4 lymphocytes per cubic millimeter (mm^3) of blood[1]—are routinely monitored in people with HIV infection. These counts play an important role in the management of HIV disease in the following ways:

- Trends in CD4 counts are presently the most commonly used indicator of a person's immune-system function; they are also a useful measure of disease progression. Trends in CD4 count are obtained by making multiple counts over time.

- Declining CD4 counts are closely correlated with an increasing risk of developing certain opportunistic infections and cancers (although some HIV-infected individuals with relatively high CD4 cell counts can sometimes develop opportunistic infections that are usually associated with much lower counts, while some individuals with extremely low counts can exhibit no signs of opportunistic infections).

- CD4 counts have been used to determine when to begin chemoprophylaxis, that is, the use of drugs to prevent certain opportunistic infections—*Pneumocystis carinii* pneumonia, or PCP, for example.

- CD4 cell counts are also key to the classification of HIV disease by the Centers for Disease Control and Prevention (CDC) and public-health officials. See Appendix 2.

Viral-load tests measure the amount of virions, or free virus particles, in blood plasma (i.e., viral load). Research has shown that changes in viral load are an earlier and more accurate indicator of both disease progression and response to therapy than are CD4 counts. Until recently, monitoring viral load was not technically possible. But new tests are available to physicians for this purpose (see Chapter 2). Today, viral-load testing is considered *essential* for determining the risk of disease progression in people with HIV, and for determining an individual's response to antiretroviral therapy (see Chapter 5).

■ THE FOUR STAGES OF HIV DISEASE

■ Acute Infection Stage: Normal CD4 Lymphocyte Count (500 to 1,200 Cells per mm³) at Onset

Acute infection, also known as "primary infection," begins immediately after HIV enters the body and starts multiplying in infected cells. Acute infection ends about two to six weeks later, following an initial drop in CD4 counts, seroconversion (see Chapter 2), and the return of CD4 counts to near-normal numbers.

Activity of HIV during Acute Infection
When HIV first enters the body, it appears unopposed by the immune system, which has never encountered this particular virus before. No one has preexisting immunity to HIV. The first week or two of HIV infection is a period of rapid viral multiplication, during which the virus spreads quickly through the body and reaches high levels in the blood in many individuals. High levels of HIV may also be present in semen and secretions of the cervix and vagina, making the individual highly infectious to any sexual partner. High viral levels may also occur at this time in the breast milk of a nursing mother, thereby increasing the risk of her transmitting HIV to her infant through breast-feeding.

In the course of acute infection, HIV infects several types of cells: Foremost are helper T lymphocytes, mentioned earlier, which die within one to two days of HIV infection.

HIV also infects monocytes and macrophages, which are immune-system cells that also display CD4 receptors and the CCR-5 chemokine receptor, a co-receptor for HIV. Monocytes are a type of white blood cell that can leave blood vessels to enter the tissues of the body to help fight infections. When this happens, monocytes become macrophages (for more on monocytes and macrophages, see Chapter 16). HIV-infected monocytes and macrophages are thought to serve as vehicles for transporting HIV to the brain and other tissues and to be reservoirs of infectious virus, because they are not killed by HIV as readily as are T lymphocytes.

The biological properties of the HIV particles present during acute infection tend to be different from those of virus present during advanced disease, or AIDS. The strains of HIV present during acute infection tend to use the CCR-5 co-receptor when infecting CD4 cells, to have slower rates of replication, and to be less deadly to CD4 cells than the strains of virus present during AIDS. During this late stage of disease, populations of HIV virions that are more deadly to the immune system arise in many patients. These virions use the CD4 molecule and the CXCR-4 chemokine receptor to enter and infect helper T cells and macrophages; it is these virions that promote the formation of syncytia among helper T cells in the laboratory, as described below.

Activity of the Immune System during Acute Infection

The immune system probably responds to HIV infection with both cell-mediated immunity and antibody-mediated immunity. Cell-mediated immunity mobilizes CD8 lymphocytes, which are also known as "cytotoxic T lymphocytes" (CTLs) or "killer T cells." CTLs destroy virus-infected cells. Antibody-mediated immunity, on the other hand, mobilizes B lymphocytes, which produce and release antibodies. (For more information on cell-mediated immunity and antibody-mediated immunity, see Chapter 16.)

Killer T cells probably respond to HIV infection first; then production of antibodies to mount an antibody immune response takes a few weeks (this is the "window period" during which HIV antibody testing produces false-negative results). In HIV infection, antibodies are produced against the viral envelope proteins gp160, gp120, and gp41; against the viral core protein p24; and sometimes against the polymerase enzyme p66/p51. (For information on the role of these proteins in HIV, see Chapter 18.)

These are the antibodies that are detected by standard ELISA antibody tests and confirmatory tests (see Chapter 2). They usually become detectable from 3 to 12 weeks following infection. Their presence in blood serum signifies that the person has seroconverted and now tests positive for HIV.

During acute infection, the number of CD4 cells in the blood decreases, as does the number of killer T lymphocytes. The drop in CD4 lymphocyte count probably results from the destruction of these cells by the rapid replication of HIV before a strong antibody response develops to fend off the virus. During this time, too, much virus is carried throughout the body by the blood and lymphatic systems. When the virions pass through lymph nodes, they are filtered out and effectively removed from the lymph fluid by special lymph-node cells known as "follicular dendritic cells," or FDCs.

FDCs are antigen-presenting cells; that is, they capture and display antigens to lymphocytes in the lymph nodes (see Chapter 16). Normally, antigens displayed by FDCs serve as a reminder to T and B lymphocytes that the antigen is still in the body. This keeps T and B lymphocytes activated, dividing, and in a state of vigorous defense until the infection is eliminated from the body.

For most infectious agents, this system works wonderfully, but in the case of HIV it tragically backfires. The capture of HIV by FDCs serves to concentrate the virus in the lymph nodes, spleen, and other lymphoid organs—where 95% of the body's lymphocytes reside—and it helps bring the virus into contact with large numbers of CD4 helper T cells. This contact enables HIV to infect large numbers of these cells. But it does even worse than that. Contact with the FDCs keeps the CD4 cells highly activated and dividing. And this, disastrously helps the virus because HIV can reproduce—replicate—only in activated helper T cells. Even antibody-coated HIV particles filtered by FDCs can infect CD4 cells that they contact. Ironically, then, a normally elegant mechanism for detecting antigen and activating the immune system becomes part of the catastrophic mechanism that ultimately destroys the immune system in the course of HIV disease.

Nevertheless, the immune system gains the upper hand during its first round of battle with HIV, perhaps through the efforts of CTLs. The number of free virus particles in the blood can reach peak levels of 100,000 to 1,000,000 particles per milliliter, but the immune system succeeds in reducing this enormous amount of free virus 100- to 1,000-fold. The number of CTLs now returns to normal, and the number of the CD4 cells increases, although temporarily and to below-normal levels. As this happens, symptoms of acute infection clear and the acute phase of HIV infection ends.

Opportunistic Infections and Cancers during Acute Infection

Occasionally, opportunistic infections characteristic of early HIV disease appear during acute infection. These can include oral candidiasis, esophageal candidiasis, or even PCP.

Symptoms of Acute Infection

Acute infection produces no noticeable symptoms in about half of the people affected. The others usually experience flulike symptoms such as low-grade fever, headache, fatigue, swollen lymph nodes (adenopathy), sore throat, rash, diarrhea, and muscle aches.

These symptoms can last from two weeks to two months, but only 20% to 30% of patients who experience them find it necessary to see a physician. Among those who do, HIV infection is often not suspected. Instead, many people attribute these symptoms to a low-grade viral infection, the flu, or mononucleosis.

There is evidence that the interaction between HIV and the immune system during the acute phase sometimes predicts how HIV infection is likely to progress in a person. Individuals with severe symptoms during acute infection are more likely to experience rapid disease progression; those who have few symptoms often experience slow disease progression.

Treatment during Acute Infection

Treatment is not usually sought during acute infection because its mild symptoms are typically not recognized for what they represent. But recent evidence has shown that taking multidrug antiretroviral therapy early, before HIV causes extensive damage to the immune system, can be highly effective in reducing viral load and slowing subsequent disease progression. The National Institutes of Health (NIH), therefore, recommends that the use of multidrug antiretroviral therapy during acute infection be carefully considered when the opportunity exists (see Chapter 5).

By the end of the acute infection stage of the disease, HIV is concentrated in the lymph nodes, spleen, and other lymphoid tissue. And in most people, the immune system has reduced the amount of free virus in the blood to low levels. Measurement of that level is highly predictive of the subsequent course of disease: The higher the viral load at this point, the earlier HIV disease is likely to progress.

■ Asymptomatic Stage: CD4 Lymphocyte Count above 500 Cells per mm³

This is the longest stage of HIV disease, lasting an average of 10 years, although in a few people it can be as short as 1 year or as long as 15 years.

During the asymptomatic stage, most HIV-infected individuals develop few symptoms of HIV disease. It is almost as if the virus has "gone underground." This is not, however, a state of latent infection: In more than 95% of all infected people, the virus is rapidly multiplying in lymphoid tissue and steadily destroying immune-system cells. The remaining 5% or less of people in the asymptomatic stage are either slow progressors or long-term nonprogressors, described below.

Activity of HIV

At one time, the asymptomatic stage of HIV disease was thought to be a period of latent infection; that is, HIV was believed to lie dormant in infected cells until, several years later, some event triggered its activation and disease progression. This was believed true because researchers could find little evidence of HIV in the blood, and because patients had relatively stable CD4 cell counts and few disease symptoms.

Today, scientists know that even though there are few or no disease symptoms during the asymptomatic stage, the virus is highly active in lymphoid tissues.

Each day during asymptomatic infection, billions of HIV particles are destroyed by the immune system's response to the virus, and an equal number are produced to take their place. Also each day, billions of CD4 lymphocytes are destroyed by HIV, only to be replaced with new cells produced by the immune system.

Following acute infection, the amount of free HIV in the blood fluctuates for six months or more, then it stabilizes at a baseline number that varies with the individual (this baseline level is also known as the "set point"). In most untreated individuals, baseline levels range from less than 1,000 to 100,000 copies of HIV per milliliter of plasma. A higher baseline is associated with a faster loss of CD4 lymphocytes, more rapid disease progression, and shorter survival.

The nature and progressive course of HIV infection are unprecedented among human viral infections. This transition by HIV from acute to chronic infection with persistent replication of virus is unique among viral infections in humans. Viral infections usually have one of three outcomes: They cause death within a short time, are eliminated from the body, or enter a true state of latency. HIV's ability to appear latent while multiplying and actively spreading throughout the body has created a new model for the course of a viral infection.

Activity of the Immune System

A gradual decline in the number of CD4 cells in the blood is usually seen during the asymptomatic phase of HIV disease. This probably reflects the immune system's diminishing ability to cope with the high rate of viral multiplication in the lymph nodes and the constant destruction of immune-system cells.

Another serious effect of HIV infection on the immune system is the loss of cytokine regulation. Cytokines are chemical messengers that are released by cells to influence the activity of other cells. Cytokines released by CD4 and other immune-system cells orchestrate—coordinate and control—immune responses. Examples of cytokines include the interleukins, the interferons, and tumor necrosis factor. Some cytokines stimulate immune-cell division, thereby triggering replication of HIV.

During HIV disease, the loss of cytokine regulation contributes to the destruction of the immune system in many ways:

- There is overproduction of some cytokines and underproduction of others, thereby disrupting the signals needed by immune-system cells to carry out effective immune responses.

- The ability of CTLs—CD8 cells—to destroy HIV-infected cells is inhibited.

- B lymphocytes, which produce antibodies, are caused to spontaneously proliferate and overproduce unneeded antibodies, a condition known as "hypergammaglobulinemia."

Opportunistic Infections

A few HIV-infected individuals develop early opportunistic infections during the asymptomatic stage. Aphthous ulcers—canker sores—occur in a small number of patients, as can cold sores caused by herpes simplex infection. Oral hairy leukoplakia, a condition that produces white patches on the tongue and elsewhere in the mouth, occasionally occurs, although it is more characteristic of more advanced HIV disease. HIV-infected women may develop recurrent vaginal candidiasis that may be resistant to treatment.

Symptoms

For the most part, HIV-infected individuals experience few outward signs or symptoms of immune-system impairment or HIV disease. Skin conditions sometimes arise, including psoriasis, itching of the hair follicles due to scabies, and bacterial or fungal infections. Exacerbation of ringworm or athlete's foot infections can also occur.

Treatment

Antiretroviral therapy is increasingly recommended for individuals with asymptomatic disease, particularly if the viral load is increasing. (See Chapter 5.)

■ Early HIV Disease: CD4 Lymphocyte Count of 200 to 500 Cells per mm³

Asymptomatic HIV disease gradually changes to early HIV disease during the slow drop in CD4 lymphocyte numbers usually seen during the asymptomatic phase. The change often becomes apparent with the development of one or more characteristic opportunistic infections (see below).

Activity of HIV

The rate of HIV multiplication in the lymph nodes and spleen remains high. At the same time, the internal structure of the lymphoid organs—thymus, bone marrow, spleen, and lymph nodes—gradually deteriorates, and partially as a result of this, the level of virus in the blood rises.

Activity of the Immune System

During early disease, about 1 out of 1,000 CD4 lymphocytes in the blood circulation is HIV infected. Delayed-type hypersensitivity skin tests, which test the responsiveness of T lymphocytes to common antigens, given during this phase of disease often show only a weak response. This is evidence of impaired cell-mediated immunity. The level of CD4 cells in the blood continues to drop.

Opportunistic Infections

Individuals with early HIV disease are at high risk of developing opportunistic infections characteristic of this stage. These are listed as category 'B' illnesses in the CDC's 1993 classification of HIV disease (see Appendix 2). Many HIV-infected individuals, however, remain asymptomatic. In the early years of the epidemic, persons who developed these disorders were described as having AIDS-related complex, or ARC.

Illnesses characteristic of early HIV disease include oral candidiasis, herpes simplex disease, shingles, and oral hairy leukoplakia. Bacterial infections that cause bronchitis, sinusitis, and pneumonia also often increase in frequency and duration.

Other Complications

The occurrence of opportunistic infections during early HIV disease stimulates the activity of the immune system, which works to overcome these infections. But each immune response triggers an additional round of cell division by CD4 cells, and these activated cells provide additional targets for HIV infection and replication. This is a reason for believing that the development of opportunistic infections accelerates the progression of HIV disease.

Symptoms

Skin conditions that appeared in the previous stage can worsen; seborrheic dermatitis, consisting of scaly dandruff-like eruptions, can develop. Symptoms can also include generalized lymphadenopathy, headache, fatigue, muscle pain, joint pain, intermittent fever, recurring diarrhea, and unexplained weight loss—wasting, or cachexia (see below).

Treatment

Most individuals in this phase of illness should receive combination antiretroviral therapy (see Chapter 5), treatment for opportunistic infections as they arise, and prophylaxis for PCP when their T lymphocyte counts reach 200 cells per mm^3.

■ Advanced HIV Disease (AIDS): CD4 Lymphocyte Count below 200 Cells per mm^3

Early HIV disease progresses to advanced HIV disease with the further decline of CD4 cell counts and the gradual appearance of serious opportunistic infections and cancers. Any HIV-infected individual with a CD4 count below 200 cells per mm^3 is considered to have AIDS according to the 1993 CDC system. These individuals are also at high risk of developing AIDS-defining clinical illnesses (category 'C' illnesses, see Appendix 2).

But even untreated persons with CD4 counts below 200 can survive for long periods free of opportunistic infections or other outward signs of AIDS.

Activity of HIV

Typically, the level of free virus particles in the blood can run between 100,000 and 1,000,000 virions per ml, mainly as a result of the complete deterioration of the interior structure of the lymph nodes, thymus, and bone marrow that occurs during advanced disease.

The populations of virions present in a person with advanced disease tend to be more virulent than those present during acute infection. Laboratory research has shown that more virulent strains of HIV tend to replicate faster than those present earlier in the disease, and that they tend to use the CXCR-4 chemokine receptor as a co-receptor when infecting CD4 lymphocytes. These populations of HIV also cause infected lymphocytes to fuse with uninfected ones. The result is the formation of syncytia, giant cells with many nuclei (the singular form of the word is "syncytium"). Lymphocytes cannot survive as syncytia, and these usually die within 48 hours. Syncytium-forming virus particles are particularly devastating to the immune system.

Laboratory research has also shown that HIV can enter cells not only as free virus particles, but also during direct contact between infected and uninfected cells. In cell culture dishes, researchers have observed HIV being transferred from infected macrophages to uninfected lymphocytes and from infected lymphocytes to uninfected epithelial cells, such as those lining the intestines or the genital tract. Such cell-to-cell transfer enables HIV to efficiently infect even cells that do not carry the CD4 molecule, while protecting HIV from attack by antibodies, which cannot enter cells and therefore can target only cell-free virus particles.

Activity of the Immune System

The level of CD4 cells in the blood falls rapidly over the course of advanced HIV disease. At this stage of disease, up to one out of ten CD4 lymphocytes in circulating blood is HIV infected. Malfunctions of the immune system include the following:

- Cells in the bone marrow that are precursors to new CD4 and other immune-system cells are weakened or destroyed in conjunction with deterioration of the marrow (the precursor cells themselves do not seem to be HIV infected).

- Cytokine production and release are profoundly disrupted.

- The number of B lymphocytes is relatively unaffected by HIV infection (HIV does not usually infect B lymphocytes), but the loss of cytokine regulation continues to result in overproduction of unneeded antibodies, or hypergammaglobulinemia.

- The immune system can become so impaired during advanced disease that it can no longer produce new antibodies upon immunization, or even to HIV itself. Paradoxically, some people with advanced disease may test negative for HIV antibodies.

- CD4 lymphocytes that are not infected by HIV respond weakly to antigens. The presence of influenza virus, for example, triggers only a weak reaction from lymphocytes uninfected by HIV. This impairment probably results from the lack of cytokine regulation, and it contributes to the development of opportunistic infections.

Opportunistic Infections and Cancers

Persons with advanced HIV disease are at high risk of developing AIDS-defining illnesses (see Appendix 2). These are severe opportunistic infections that can be viral, bacterial, protozoan, or fungal in origin (see also Chapter 7). Examples include the following:

- Viral infections result in shingles; cytomegalovirus (CMV) retinitis; and ulcerations around the mouth, anus, and genitals caused by a herpetic infection.

- Bacterial infections include tuberculosis, bacillary angiomatosis, and *Mycobacterium avium* complex (MAC).

- Fungal infections include PCP, esophageal candidiasis, and coccidioidomycosis.

- Protozoan infections include toxoplasmosis, cryptosporidiosis, and histoplasmosis.

- Cancers can include lymphoma, Kaposi's sarcoma, rectal cancer, and cervical cancer (see Chapter 8).

- Some AIDS-defining infections are more likely to occur when the CD4 count drops below 50 CD4 cells per mm^3. These include CMV esophagitis, MAC, cryptococcal meningitis, progressive multifocal leukoencephalopathy (PML), invasive aspergillosis, disseminated coccidioidomycosis, and disseminated histoplasmosis.

Other Complications and Symptoms

Gastrointestinal System

The gastrointestinal (GI) tract is an important target of HIV infection. About 60% of individuals with advanced disease experience problems relating to the GI tract. Weight loss is a frequent complication and contributor to the cause of death in individuals with HIV disease. There are two common causes:

Diarrhea or loose bowel movements are frequent symptoms of HIV disease, and have a variety of causes. Among the most common are opportunistic infections involving *Cryptosporidium, Microsporidium,* CMV, and *Mycobacterium avium-intracellulare* (MAC).

Loss of appetite can be a result of nausea, caused by either opportunistic infections or the side effects of medication.

Loss of appetite increases the risk of HIV-related wasting. Wasting, or cachexia, is the involuntary loss of more than 10% of baseline body weight with diarrhea (more than two stools a day) for more than 30 days. Wasting involves the loss of lean body mass—muscle mass—as well as fat, and it is most likely to occur when CD4 counts drop below 50 per mm^3. The cause of HIV-related wasting is poorly understood. For more information on wasting, see Chapter 13.

The liver and gallbladder—the hepatobiliary system—are frequent sites of complications and opportunistic infections during advanced HIV disease. Latent infections of the liver by hepatitis B and C viruses can be reactivated during HIV disease. Common opportunistic infections of the liver include mycobacterial infection, cryptosporidiosis, and CMV infection. Drugs taken to prevent PCP or to treat other opportunistic infections can also cause liver disease in people with advanced HIV disease.

Nervous System and AIDS-Related Dementia

About 30% to 50% of individuals with advanced HIV disease develop neurological problems. These can result from opportunistic infections, from malignancies, or directly from HIV itself.

The nervous system can be divided into two areas: the central nervous system (CNS), which consists of the brain and spinal cord, and the peripheral nervous system, which consists of the nerves that serve the body. Both the CNS and the peripheral nervous system are affected by complications and opportunistic infections that can occur during advanced HIV disease. They include the following:

- Headaches, which are common in people with advanced disease, may be a sign of meningitis, an inflammation of the membranes that surround the brain. The most common cause of meningitis in HIV disease is cryptococcosis, a fungal infection. A less common cause of meningitis is the bacterium responsible for tuberculosis, *Mycobacterium tuberculosis*. Meningitis that cannot be linked to an opportunistic infection is sometimes referred to as "aseptic" meningitis. It is thought to be caused by cytokines released in response to HIV infection of brain cells.

■ Cerebral toxoplasmosis, caused by a parasitic protozoan, is an opportunistic infection of the gray matter of the brain.

■ PML, caused by the JC virus (the initials are those of the patient from whom the virus was first isolated), is an opportunistic infection of the white matter of the brain.

■ CMV infection can also impair brain function, probably by infection and inflammation of brain tissue.

■ Cancers can occur in the brain during advanced disease. These include primary CNS lymphoma (see Chapter 8).

■ AIDS dementia complex, or HIV encephalopathy, is one of the most common neurological complications of advanced HIV disease. The cause is unknown, although scientists speculate that HIV-infected macrophages in the brain stimulate the release of cytokines and other compounds that damage healthy brain cells, causing a loss of brain tissue.

Signs of early AIDS dementia complex include loss of memory, reduced ability to concentrate, slowness of thinking, reduced coordination, changes in handwriting, loss of balance, unsteady gait, leg weakness, and frequent falls.

Advanced AIDS dementia complex can involve profound loss of memory (the individual can even become unaware of his or her illness), disorientation, inability to think, loss of speech, weakness, spasticity, and abnormal reflexes.

Antiretroviral therapy has reduced the incidence of AIDS dementia complex, and often slows its progress. See also Chapter 13.

■ Neuropathy—pain resulting from damage to peripheral nerves—is common during advanced HIV disease. Peripheral neuropathy usually occurs as pain or numbness in the extremities, especially in the feet and legs. It can produce burning pain in the soles of the feet or a severe aching of the feet that progresses up the leg. The condition is thought to be caused by nerve damage or inflammation of the nerves by HIV.

■ Some antiretroviral drugs, including ddI (didanosine), ddC (zalcitabine), and d4T (stavudine), also cause peripheral neuropathy. Prolonged use of AZT can produce a slowly progressing muscle wasting and weakness known as "AZT myopathy." This can be difficult to distinguish from myopathy that is HIV associated.

■ Psychological problems, particularly anxiety and depression, are common and usually treatable with counseling or antidepressants (see Chapter 13).

Treatment

■ Prophylaxis for PCP should begin when the level of CD4 lymphocytes drops below 200 cells per mm^3.

■ Prophylaxis for MAC is generally recommended for individuals with a CD4 lymphocyte count below 75 cells per mm^3.

■ Combination antiretroviral therapy is required to slow progression of the disease and preserve immune function (see Chapter 5).

■ Resistance to antiretroviral drugs, however, is also a characteristic of advanced disease.

■ Treatments are also needed to control opportunistic infections as they arise. Treatments that are successful must often be followed by lifelong suppressive therapy to prevent or reduce a recurrence of the disease (see Chapter 7).

■ LONG-TERM NONPROGRESSORS

A few HIV-infected individuals—the range is thought to be 5% to 7%—have survived for more than 10 or 15 years with normal CD4 counts and no signs of HIV disease. These people are known as long-term non-progressors.

The lymph nodes of long-term nonprogressors show little damage, even though lymphocytes within the nodes are infected by HIV. The nodes also tend to have lower numbers of infected CD4 cells than do the nodes of someone with progressing HIV disease.

What protects these individuals from developing HIV disease is still not well understood. Some scientists speculate that long-term nonprogressors are capable of producing an extraordinarily effective killer T-cell response against the virus. Another possibility is that some long-term nonprogressors are infected by a weak strain of HIV. And a few people might be infected by a weak strain of virus and mount a strong immune response.

A few individuals may also be genetically resistant to HIV infection. Recent research has shown that HIV uses receptors for chemokines, chemicals that play an important role in inflammation, along with the CD4 molecule to enter cells. The most important of these seem to be CCR-5 and CXCR-4, mentioned previously (for more information on chemokine receptors, see Chapters 14 and 18). It also appears that for genetic reasons some individuals either lack normal receptors or have them in very low numbers.

For example, most people are born with two good copies of the gene for the chemokine receptor CCR-5. But in about 1% of the Caucasian population (and in a much smaller proportion of African Americans), both copies of the CCR-5 gene are mutated and genetically defective. People who inherit two defective copies of the gene for CCR-5 (one copy from their mother and one from their father) are highly resistant to HIV infection. Those with one defective copy of the gene (about 15% of Caucasians and about 1% of African Americans) appear to have a slower progression of HIV disease.

■ CAUSE OF DEATH IN HIV DISEASE

The cause of death in most individuals with HIV disease is an HIV-associated cancer or opportunistic infection. Others die of heart disease or of wasting and severe weakness, which result from factors such as malnutrition, the cumulative effects of prior opportunistic infections, and the direct effects of HIV.

■ THE COURSE OF HIV DISEASE IS OFTEN ALTERED BY TREATMENT

Were it not for mention of treatments needed at each stage of HIV disease, this chapter could have been entitled "HIV Infection and the *Natural* Course of HIV Disease."

Indeed, for some 15 years after the emergence of the HIV/AIDS epidemic in the United States, the antiviral and other treatments available to people infected with HIV had minimal effect on the natural course of the disease. Its inexorable outcome was early death, with those who received state-of-the-art antiretroviral therapy surviving only a matter of months longer than those who received no antiviral treatment at all.

New antiretroviral therapies have been in use for only two years, a period too brief to assess their ultimate potential. But enough is known to state that their impact on the course of HIV disease will probably be profound for a majority of people with HIV/AIDS who live in developed countries. In those countries, at least, antiviral drug combinations represent new, potentially highly effective therapy that offers the possibility of new treatment strategies, and are rapidly changing the standards of medical care for HIV/AIDS.

Combination antiretroviral therapies are being used increasingly early in the course of disease—and should be considered as early as the acute phase of infection, when possible. Furthermore, continuing aggressive antiretroviral treatment with a succession of different drug combinations will prolong each phase of the disease and perhaps even stave off its most advanced stage, along with its many grave infections, cancers, and metabolic complications. Should this happen, the spectrum of life-threatening illnesses that now plagues people with AIDS should dramatically narrow. The occurrence of opportunistic diseases will then greatly recede in time, as will the need for prophylactic and therapeutic interventions now used to fight them.

It may therefore be predicted that a future description of "HIV Infection and the Course of HIV Disease" will be quite different from that presented in this chapter. It will not describe a generally relentless, progressive, and ultimately lethal breakdown of immune defenses, but a chronic, medically controllable infection that is not incompatible with a productive life and many years of well-being.

ENDNOTE

1. A cubic millimeter is also equivalent to a microliter (μl).

■ Chapter 5

TREATMENT OF HIV DISEASE

Antiretroviral drugs—drugs specifically targeted to HIV—are the primary treatment for HIV disease. This chapter describes the antiretroviral drugs that are currently available, explains why resistance to them can develop, and provides a summary of the scientific principles that underlie their use. It concludes with strategies under development. (Note: Optimal antiretroviral therapy varies with the individual, the stage of disease, and other factors. In addition, the field of antiretroviral therapy continues to evolve. For these reasons, specific HIV-treatment regimens are not presented in this book. For information on antiretroviral regimens call the HIV/AIDS Treatment Information Service or visit their Web site, or see the latest issue of AmFAR's *AIDS/HIV Treatment Directory* [See Appendix 1].)

In the past few years, potent new drugs have been developed to manage HIV infection, numerous advances have been made in the understanding of HIV and how it causes disease, and tests became available to measure the amount of HIV in the blood (i.e., viral load). This progress has redefined how HIV infection is treated and managed. The new drugs, for example, are combined in treatment regimens that as a group are known as "highly active antiretroviral therapy" (HAART), which in many people suppresses the reproduction (i.e., replication) of HIV to levels undetectable in blood by currently available tests and allows the body to at least partially replenish the number of CD4 lymphocytes in the blood. Physicians experienced in HIV disease also now have a much better idea of when antiretroviral therapy should begin (largely because of viral-load testing) and what drug combinations to use in particular patients.

The success of HAART has allowed many people with advanced HIV disease to return to an active life. It has also led some researchers to believe that a cure for the disease, at least at some stages, may be possible one day. At the same time, however, a great deal of uncertainty remains about HAART regimens. Researchers do not yet know how quickly HIV will develop resistance to combination therapy, or how well the human body will tolerate its long-term use. The development of cross-resistance—which occurs when viral resistance to one drug also results in resistance to other drugs of the same class—is also a concern. Scientists are also uncertain about how effectively the CD4 cells that arise during the use of HAART can fight infections. These questions are under investigation.

The cost of anti-HIV drugs also presents problems for many people who need them. A course of treatment for a single antiretroviral drug approved by the Food and Drug Administration (FDA) can range from $2,000 to $7,000 annually, and HAART regimens typically require taking three drugs simultaneously. Help with the cost of HIV treatment is available through private insurance, state Medicaid programs, and the Ryan White CARE Act, a federal assistance plan (provided under Title II of the AIDS Drugs Assistance Program [ADAP]). Individuals should ask their physician, social worker, or local AIDS service organization about the financial assistance programs for which they may qualify.

■ ANTIRETROVIRAL THERAPIES

Currently approved antiretroviral drugs work by inhibiting the action of one or the other of two viral enzymes that are essential for HIV replication, reverse transcriptase (RT) and protease. (HIV's replication cycle and the role of these enzymes in it are described in Chapter 18.) Conse-

quently, antiretroviral drugs are known as "reverse transcriptase inhibitors" (RTIs) and "protease inhibitors." Note that the use and side
effects of all anti-HIV drugs should be discussed with an experienced
physician before the drugs are taken.

■ Reverse Transcriptase Inhibitors

RTIs work by blocking the viral enzyme RT. This enzyme is used by HIV
to construct a DNA copy of its RNA genome shortly after the virus enters a host cell (see Chapter 18). RTIs are classified as either nucleoside
analogues or nonnucleoside analogues.

Nucleoside analogues

The nucleoside analogue RTIs (Table 5.1) work by mimicking nucleosides, molecules found in the cell that are needed for assembly of DNA
strands. Nucleosides are modified versions of the so-called bases that
form the cross pieces in the DNA double helix. The bases, named adenine, cytosine, guanine, and thymine, are first converted to nucleosides
before they can be incorporated into DNA. A nucleoside is produced
when a base is chemically linked to a sugar molecule; a nucleotide is produced when a phosphate group is linked to a nucleoside (see "The Bases
That Make Up DNA and RNA Exist in Three Chemical Forms in Cells,"
Chapter 15).

When RT is assembling a viral DNA strand in a newly infected cell, it
hijacks nucleotides made by the cell for the cell's own needs. When an
HIV-infected person takes a nucleoside analogue RTI such as AZT, cells
take up the drug and add a phosphate group to the molecules of AZT,
thereby converting them to their nucleotide form. RT will then add AZT
to the growing strand of viral DNA in place of the normal thymine nucleotide. Once this happens, however, AZT blocks any further assembly
of the viral DNA, thereby putting an early stop to that virus's replication
cycle.

A molecule with a structure that resembles that of another molecule
is known as an "analogue." Because all RTI drugs work by masquerading
as nucleosides, they are known as nucleoside analogue RTIs. Nucleoside
RTIs are the oldest class of anti-HIV drugs, and more are in development

(as are drugs that work as nucleotide analogues). Nucleoside RTIs in current use include the following:

- Abacavir (also known as 1592–U89) is an analogue of the nucleoside guanosine that is in phase III testing as of this writing.

- Didanosine (ddI) is an analogue of the nucleoside adenosine. It was the second drug to be approved for the treatment of HIV infection.

- Lamivudine (3TC) is an analogue of the nucleoside cytidine. The FDA announced the accelerated approval of 3TC in November 1995 for use in combination with AZT. It is noteworthy that 3TC has also been found to suppress the hepatitis B virus.

- Stavudine (d4T) is an analogue of thymidine. d4T was approved by the FDA in June 1994 for patients who were intolerant of zidovudine and didanosine, or whose disease was advancing while taking these treatments.

- Zalcitabine (ddC) is an analogue of the nucleoside cytidine.

- Zidovudine (ZDV), also known as azidothymidine, or AZT, is an analogue of the nucleoside thymidine. AZT was first synthesized as a potential anticancer agent in 1963. In 1986, during a phase II clinical trial, it became the first drug to show benefit to people with HIV disease by reducing the incidence of opportunistic disease or prolonging their lives. This finding greatly stimulated research to discover and test agents with similar or possibly better antiretroviral properties.

Nonnucleoside RTIs

Nonnucleoside RTIs (NNRTIs) (Table 5.2) work by binding to RT and stopping its action. NNRTIs are very specific for inhibiting HIV-1; they have no activity against HIV-2, a closely related retrovirus that also causes AIDS. Viral resistance (see below) to NNRTIs develops quickly, but the process is slowed when the drugs are used in combination with a nucleoside analogue RTI. One NNRTI, nevirapine, is also able to cross the blood-brain barrier. Clinical trials using NNRTIs are under way. Two of these drugs, nevirapine and delavirdine, have been approved by the FDA.

Table 5.1. ■ *Nucleoside Analogue Reverse Transcriptase Inhibitors*#*

Generic Name	Brand Name	Manufacturer	Development Stage	
			Adults	Children
abacavir	Ziagen	Glaxo-Wellcome	In clinical trials	
didanosine (ddI)	Videx	Bristol-Myers Squibb	Approved	Approved
lamivudine (3TC)	Epivir	Glaxo Wellcome	Approved	Approved
stavudine (d4T)	Zerit	Bristol-Myers Squibb	Approved	Approved
zalcitabine (ddC)	Hivid	Hoffman-LaRoche	Approved	
zidovudine (ZDV) (also known as AZT or azidothymidine)†	Retrovir	Glaxo-Wellcome	Approved	Approved
zidovudine & lamivudine	Combivir	Glaxo-Wellcome	Approved	

---

*FDA-approved drugs have at least three names: a generic name, a brand name, and a chemical name. The generic name is the name used when referring to the drug during clinical trials, in medical-research papers, and usually in the media; generic names are not capitalized. Brand names are given to a drug by its manufacturer for marketing purposes; brand names are registered and the initial letter is always capitalized. The chemical name of a drug is derived from its chemical structure. The chemical name for AZT, for example, is 3´-azido-3´-deoxythymidine (chemical names are not included in the tables in this chapter). In addition, during a drug's testing phase, pharmaceutical company may initially refer to it using a combination of letters and numbers.
†As of May 1997, AZT was the only antiretroviral drug approved for pregnant women.

■ **Protease Inhibitors**

Late in its replication, HIV produces an enzyme called protease (sometimes called proteinase). Its job is to cleave a large viral "polyprotein" as HIV buds from cells (see Chapter 18). If this large protein is not cleaved, the virus cannot assemble properly and only "defective" noninfectious virus particles are produced. Protease inhibitors (Table 5.3) work by blocking that essential cleavage reaction.

Table 5.2. ■ *Nonnucleoside Reverse Transcriptase Inhibitors#*

Generic Name	Brand Name	Manufacturer	Development Stage	
			Adults	Children
delavirdine (DLV)	Rescriptor	Pharmacia & Upjohn	Approved	
efavirenz	Sustiva	DuPont-Merck	In clinical trials	
nevirapine (NVP)	Viramune	Boehringer Ingelheim	Approved	

Table 5.3. ■ *Protease Inhibitors#*

Generic Name	Brand Name	Manufacturer	Development Stage	
			Adults	Children
indinavir	Crixivan	Merck	Approved	
nelfinavir	Viracept	Agouron Pharm.	Approved	Approved
ritonavir	Norvir	Abbott Laboratories	Approved	Approved
saquinavir	Fortovase and Invirase*	Hoffman-LaRoche	Approved	

*Invirase is the original hard-gel formulation of saquinavir, which is more poorly absorbed by the body than the newer Fortovase, which is a soft-gel preparation.
#Warning: Some of the antiretroviral drugs listed in Tables 5.1, 5.2, and 5.3 have similar names. As a result, pharmacies have been known to make serious mistakes when filling prescriptions, such as confusing ritonavir (a protease inhibitor) with Retrovir (a nucleoside analogue RTI), or Viramune (a nonnucleoside RTI) with Viracept (a protease inhibitor).

As a group, protease inhibitors are tolerated relatively well. However, they are metabolized in the liver by a group of cellular enzymes known as the "P450 enzyme system." These enzymes metabolize many other drugs as well. When a protease inhibitor is used in combination with such drugs, this can affect how quickly drugs (as well as the protease inhibitor itself) are cleared from the body, thereby possibly increasing their toxicity. Protease inhibitors also may not cross the blood-brain barrier in amounts sufficient to affect HIV-infected cells located in the brain. In addition, these drugs must be taken at specific times relative to meals; that is, some must be taken on a full stomach and others on an empty stomach.

A possible side-effect of protease-inhibitor use in combination ther-apy reported in a substantial fraction of patients—from 7% to over 60%—is the development of abnormal fat deposits in the abdomen (so-called "protease belly") and on the shoulders at the base of the neck ("buffalo hump"). This is accompanied by wasting of the face, arms, and legs (a condition known as "lipodystrophy"), along with elevations of certain lipids in the blood, particularly triglycerides. The cause of these deposits and blood abnormalities is presently unknown.

Although similar changes have occurred in HIV-positive individuals who were not taking any anti-HIV medications, it appears to be wors-ened or initiated by the use of protease inhibitors, and it can occur as early as four weeks after use of a protease inhibitor begins. All currently approved protease inhibitors have been associated with this condition, but the combination of ritonavir plus saquinavir may have the highest in-cidence. Its clinical significance is unknown. Further study of large num-bers of patients for longer periods is needed before any change in antiretroviral therapy or use of lipid-lowering drugs can be recom-mended.

Which protease inhibitor to use in a drug regimen depends on many factors, including the individual patient's medical profile and lifestyle. While research has established sound principles of HIV treatment (pre-sented below), all anti-HIV drugs have advantages and disadvantages, and there is still no standard way of combining and using them. The treatment of HIV disease remains in flux, and the use of HAART is still under study. For this reason, an individual seeking treatment for HIV dis-ease is best advised to rely on a physician experienced in this disease.

■ Drug Resistance and Antiretroviral Therapy

When AZT alone is used to treat HIV disease (that is, as monotherapy), it typically produces an increase in CD4 counts of 30 to 50 cells per mm^3, and it decreases the viral load by 60% to 70%. But after a few months, the viral load begins to increase again and the CD4 counts drop. A similar course is seen when many other antiretroviral drugs are used alone. The rebound in viral load and the renewed drop in CD4 cells occur because HIV quickly becomes resistant to single drugs.

It is generally believed that HIV develops drug resistance so effectively largely because of the high rate at which genetic mutations occur during its replication (see Chapter 18). These gene mutations occur because RT is prone to making errors when it copies HIV's RNA genes into DNA. Thus, when an HIV particle enters a cell and produces a provirus, it is the provirus that contains the gene mutations introduced by RT. When that provirus begins producing new virions, those virions will have genetic characteristics that are different from those of the virion that originally infected the cell (some proviruses end up with so many mutations that they cannot produce viable HIV particles at all).

This tendency of RT to make inexact copies of the virus's original RNA genes results in great genetic diversity (see Chapter 18) among the HIV particles infecting an individual. Thus, a person with HIV is soon infected with many genetically different populations of virions. Some of these populations consist of HIV particles that have relatively unmodified (or "wild-type") genes. These virions are sensitive to antiretroviral drugs and therefore cannot replicate in their presence. Other populations, however, consist of small numbers of HIV particles that, by chance, have mutations that make them resistant to one or more antiretroviral drugs. The growth of these mutated HIV particles is not slowed in the presence of these drugs. In fact, they then have a selective advantage over the wild-type HIV particles: The "drug-adapted" virions can infect cells and replicate, even as the wild-type virions are prevented from doing so, as long as the patient continues to be treated with those drugs to which the mutated virions are resistant. Some of these virion populations will have mutations that make them resistant to AZT, some will have mutations that make them resistant to ddI, others will be resistant to the nonnucleoside inhibitor nevirapine. Still others might have mutations that confer resistance to the protease inhibitors ritonavir or saquinavir. Quite possibly, virus populations might arise that are resistant to multiple drugs.[1]

Occasionally, chance produces mutations in HIV that confer resistance to one drug and reverse resistance to another drug. Take for example virions that have the most common mutation that confers resistance to AZT. If those mutant virions replicate and produce progeny virions that also have the most common mutation for resistance to ddI, this second mutation makes the virions again highly vulnerable to AZT.

The number of genetic mutations needed to make a virus resistant to any one drug can be very small. For example, a single mutation that causes a change of one amino acid in the structure of HIV's RT enzyme can produce a virus that is 1,000 times more resistant to the drug 3TC. It would take a dose of 3TC that is a thousand times stronger to block the replication of that mutated virus, a dose that would also be deadly to the individual.[2]

■ Compliance, Drug Resistance, and Antiretroviral Therapy

Compliance—the taking of drugs according to prescribed directions— plays an important role in preventing or slowing the development of drug resistance. Compliance is important for the effective use of all medications, but it is critical for antiretroviral regimens that are de- signed to suppress HIV. Skipping doses or reducing a drug's dosage even briefly allows the level of drug in the body to drop, giving HIV an op- portunity to replicate and develop genetic mutations that confer drug resistance. In the worst case, resistance to one drug can result in cross- resistance to all the drugs in the same class. Should this happen for pro- tease inhibitors, it would make all protease inhibitors, the most effective weapons against HIV currently available, ineffective thereafter for that individual.

Therefore, it is of the utmost importance to comply with the require- ments of HAART so as to suppress viral replication as completely as pos- sible, to prevent or forestall the development of drug resistance.

Sometimes, side effects or other problems might prevent patients from taking full doses of all their antiretroviral drugs. In such cases, it is bet- ter to either stop taking all these drugs altogether for a time, or to try a different combination of drugs, than to reduce the dosage.[3] In the ab- sence of any drugs, all virus populations replicate and compete with each other, although the wild-type virions replicate most effectively. The pres- ence of any antiretroviral drug at low levels, however, favors the replica- tion of the mutated drug-adapted, or drug-resistant, virions that then become the most numerous HIV particles in the body.

■ PRINCIPLES OF ANTIRETROVIRAL THERAPY FOR HIV

In 1997, the Office of AIDS Research of the National Institutes of Health (NIH) convened a panel of experts to assess the advances in basic research on HIV, treatment research, and testing in order to translate them into information useful to physicians and people with HIV. The result was the "Report of the NIH Panel to Define Principles of Therapy of HIV Infection."[4] The report presents 11 principles that guide current antiretroviral therapy. They are summarized here as follows:

> **1. HIV infection is always harmful, and true long-term survival without signifiant loss of immune function is unusual; continuous HIV replication damages the immune system and leads to AIDS.**

About 5% of people infected with HIV have survived for more than 10 or 12 years without treatment and with no signs of HIV disease. Presently, however, there is no way to identify at the time of diagnosis individuals who may be long-term slow progressors or nonprogressors. For this reason, all persons with HIV infection must be considered at risk for progressive disease.

The goal of HIV therapy is to prevent disease progression: that is, maintain immune function in a state as close to normal as possible, preserve quality of life, and prolong survival by effectively suppressing HIV replication. These goals can be accomplished only by initiating therapy, whenever possible, before significant damage has occurred to the immune system.

> **2. Regular, periodic viral-load tests and CD4 lymphocyte counts are necessary to determine when to initiate or modify antiretroviral therapy and to assess the risk of disease progression.**

Levels of HIV in the blood—viral load—are measured using HIV genome tests (see Chapter 2) and indicate the rate of HIV replicaton and suggest the rate of CD4 lymphocyte destruction; CD4 lymphocyte counts indicate the extent of HIV-induced immune damage already present.

As mentioned in Chapter 4, viral load first rises, then falls during the first six months after initial infection. After about six to nine months, it stabilizes and reaches a baseline level, or "set point." In many people with HIV infection, the baseline remains fairly constant from several months to several years, although it tends to rise over time. An increase in the baseline viral load is a predictor of disease progression. Two baseline measurements should be made one to two weeks apart by the same laboratory using the same assay to ensure that a true baseline viral load is obtained. Other important points about testing include the following:

- In individuals newly diagnosed with HIV, viral-load measurements should be performed during a period of clinical stability. Thereafter, testing should be done every three to four months to monitor risk of disease progression and to help determine when to initiate therapy.

- Measurements of viral load within six months after initial infection do not accurately predict the risk of disease progression because the level of HIV is probably still unstable.

- If the individual is experiencing symptoms of acute infection at the time of diagnosis, viral-load testing can be used to establish an HIV diagnosis even if the HIV antibody test result is negative or indeterminate.

- Viral-load testing should also be done before and after starting antiretroviral therapy as described under "When Therapy Is Initiated" under Principle 3.

- CD4 lymphocyte counts should be made at the time of diagnosis and generally every three to six months thereafter. CD4 cell counts are subject to significant variability, so treatment decisions must be based on trends in CD4 numbers over time, not on any one count.

- Prior to making treatment decisions, both viral load and CD4 cell counts should be determined at least on two occasions by the same laboratory using the same assay to ensure that the measurements are accurate.

- A threefold or greater (i.e., 0.5-log or more) change in viral load is considered significant; a drop of 30% or more in CD4 lymphocyte count from baseline is considered significant, as is a 3% or greater drop from baseline when CD4 lymphocytes are monitored as a percentage of total lymphocytes (this figure is used by some physicians instead of absolute numbers of CD4 lymphocytes; see Appendix 2).

3. The time to initiate anti-HIV therapy should be based on risk of disease progression and degree of immune deficiency, and these vary with individual patients.

All individuals with symptomatic HIV disease (i.e., thrush, wasting, unexplained fever, or AIDS) should be offered antiretroviral therapy. Determining when to initiate therapy in individuals who are asymptomatic or in the acute stage of HIV infection is more complicated (for acute infection, see "Considerations for Initiating Antiretroviral Therapy during Acute Infection").

■ Some of the Benefits and Risks of Early Antiretroviral Therapy in Asymptomatic Disease

Potential Benefits

- Control of viral replication and mutation, and reduction of viral load.
- Prevention of progressive immune deficiency.
- Potential preservation of a normal immune system.
- Delay in progression to AIDS and perhaps prolongation of life.
- Decrease of the risk that resistant HIV will emerge.
- Lessening of the risk of drug toxicity.

Potential Risks

- Reduced quality of life due to possible drug side effects.
- Earlier development of drug resistance.
- Limitations on future choices of antiretroviral agents.
- Risk of dissemination of drug-resistant HIV in the community.
- Long-term toxicity and treatment benefit of certain anti-HIV drugs are both still unpredictable. ■

There is no known threshold of HIV replication below which disease progression will not eventually occur. In theory, beginning antiretroviral therapy *before* the onset of disease progression as indicated by falling CD4 counts and rising viral load should have the greatest and most long-lasting effect on preserving health. But the benefits of initiating therapy in asymptomatic individuals must be weighed against the disadvantages (see "Some of the Benefits and Risks of Early Antiretroviral Therapy in Asymptomatic Disease").

In general, asymptomatic individuals with CD4 lymphocyte counts below 500 cells per mm^3 and viral loads greater than 10,000 by bDNA testing or 20,000 by RT-PCR testing should be offered therapy. The strength of the recommendation, however, should be based on an individual's readiness for treatment, and on the relative risk of disease progression. Disease progression, in turn, is based on *rates* of change in viral load and CD4 lymphocyte counts. (No data are available yet on the degree of benefit in starting antiretroviral therapy in individuals with CD4 counts above 500 cells per mm^3 and viral loads lower than those mentioned above; for pregnant women, see Principle 8.)

When Therapy Is Initiated

When the decision is made to initiate therapy in an asymptomatic person, the goal should be maximum suppression of HIV replication, preferably to undetectable levels (see Principle 4). Viral load and CD4 T-cell counts should be determined immediately before therapy begins and again four weeks later. After four weeks, the individual should experience a significant drop (tenfold or 1 log; see "The Meaning of Viral-Load Numbers," Chapter 2) in viral load; if such a drop is not seen, the physician should check for patient adherence to the treatment regimen or poor drug absorption. Viral-load testing should be repeated to verify the lack of response. At that point, the physician may recommend changing the treatment regimen. Viral load tends to reach a low (ideally, below the level of detection) within approximately eight weeks of HAART, although this can take up to 16 weeks in individuals with high initial viral loads.

The continued effectiveness of the treatment regimen should be monitored by viral-load testing every three to four months. By six months, the regimen should have reduced viral load to undetectable levels. If viral load remains detectable after six months, the viral-load test should be repeated to rule out the possibility of a temporary increase (this can happen, for example, when an immunization or concurrent infection activates the immune system, either of which can trigger a temporary increase in HIV replication and viral load). If the repeat viral-load test also shows a detectable viral load, a change in therapy should be considered (see "Considerations for Changing a Failing Antiretroviral Therapy").

When Therapy Is Postponed

When therapy is postponed in an asymptomatic person infected with HIV, viral-load measurements and CD4 counts should be performed (as described under Principle 2) at the time of diagnosis and then every three to four months thereafter. Note that these intervals can be flexible to meet the circumstances of individual cases.

> **4. The goal of therapy is to suppress HIV replication below levels detectable by viral-load tests.**

The emergence of drug-resistant forms of HIV is the major reason why antiretroviral therapy fails. The development of drug resistance can be delayed, and perhaps even prevented, through the use of combinations of antiretroviral drugs, the only regimens that can suppress HIV replication below levels detectable by current viral-load tests. As described earlier, suppressing HIV replication slows or suppresses the accumulation of viral mutations that give rise to drug-resistant virions. Furthermore, the extent and duration of viral suppression also predict the degree to which an individual will clinically benefit from antiretroviral treatment.

Suppression of HIV replication to undetectable levels does not mean that the infection has been eradicated or that virus replication has been stopped altogether. Virus replication may continue in certain tissues such as the lymph nodes or the central nervous system, and suppression may be temporary. For these reasons, viral-load monitoring should continue as described above.

If suppression of HIV replication to undetectable levels cannot be achieved, the goal of therapy should be to suppress viral replication as much as possible for as long as possible.

5. The antiretroviral drugs used in combination therapy must be carefully chosen and given simultaneously.

Effective suppression of HIV replication by combination therapy is not due simply to the number of drugs used; it also depends on which drugs are used. Careful drug selection is also important because the decision will affect the therapeutic options available to the individual in the future. The rational selection of drugs for combination antiretroviral therapy is based on the following:

■ The combination should not include antiretroviral drugs previously taken by the individual, or drugs that are cross-resistant with drugs previously taken by the individual.

■ The drugs should work together to show additive or synergistic activity against HIV.

■ None of the drugs should interfere with the anti-HIV activity of any of the other drugs in the combination.

■ When possible, it is best if the drugs used in a combination work together to delay the development of viral mutations that lead to drug resistance. That is, certain antiretroviral drugs when used in combination make it more difficult for viral resistance to develop. For example, there is evidence that it is difficult for HIV to simultaneously develop a certain mutation that leads to resistance to 3TC and mutations that lead to resistance to AZT. This phenomenon is known as molecular antagonism.

■ When possible, it is best to choose a drug combination that leaves as many future therapeutic options as possible, in case the regimen should fail (although it is most important to use a combination of drugs that a person can tolerate and that drives his or her viral load to undetectable levels).

Effective Regimens

Presently, the most effective combinations for suppressing HIV replication in individuals who have not previously taken antiretroviral therapy (i.e., antiretroviral "naive" persons) incorporate two nucleoside analogue RTIs plus a potent protease inhibitor. The use of two nucleoside analogue RTIs and an NNRTI is also reported to be effective in antiretroviral naive persons, but this combination needs further study and is not recommended at this time as a first-line therapy. This regimen is also less effective in persons previously treated with nucleoside analogue RTIs.

Antiretroviral drugs such as lamivudine (3TC) or the NNRTIs, which may be potent but to which HIV readily develops high-level resistance, should not be used in regimens that are expected to produce incomplete suppression of HIV replication (i.e., HIV levels in the blood are reduced, but remain detectable) because resistance is likely to develop quickly against them.

Use of Monotherapy

The NIH panel noted that no currently available single antiretroviral drug used by itself (i.e., as monotherapy)—not even the most potent protease inhibitor—can provide significant, long-lasting suppression of HIV replication. This is because drug resistance inevitably develops to any single drug. Even worse, cross-resistance may develop. For these reasons, monotherapy is not recommended for the treatment of HIV infection, with one exception: the temporary use of AZT by pregnant women to prevent perinatal HIV transmission (see Chapter 12).

Use of Two-Drug Combinations

Some physicians and HIV-infected individuals may consider using a two-drug combination, but they should recognize that no combination of two currently available nucleoside analogue RTIs has been shown to provide long-lasting suppression of HIV replication. An inability to profoundly suppress replication allows drug-resistant forms of HIV to develop. These may be cross-resistant to related drugs, thereby severely limiting future treatment options. The same is true of combinations consisting of one nucleoside analogue RTI and one NNRTI, or of two protease inhibitors. The latter combination has resulted in durable suppression of HIV replication in pilot studies, but this regimen needs further testing (a danger here is that if cross-resistance develops between protease inhibitors, it would eliminate this whole class of extremely potent antiretroviral drugs from future treatment options).

> **6. Each antiretroviral drug in a combination therapy regimen should always be used according to optimum schedules and dosages.**

As stated above, maximum suppression of HIV replication is the best approach to prevent development of drug-resistant variants of HIV. Ideally, the drugs used in combination therapy should be started within one or two days of each other; they should not be added in stages, as this may lead to temporary incomplete viral suppression during which the accumulation of viral mutations that lead to drug resistance may occur. Giving reduced doses or administering fewer than all the drugs of a combination at the same time should therefore be avoided. It is essential for physicians to educate and counsel patients about the goals and rationale for their HAART treatment, even if this means a short delay in initiating it.

Adherence to a Regimen Is Crucial to Its Success

Current combination therapy regimens require that individuals take multiple medications at specific times of day, and at specific intervals relative to meals. Deviating from prescribed intervals, or using one or all of the drugs only intermittently, greatly increases the risk for developing drug-resistant strains of HIV and failure of the treatment (as described earlier under "Compliance, Drug Resistance, and Antiretroviral Therapy"). For this reason, there should be an active collaboration between patient and physician once therapy is started. This should include a review of the drug-dosing intervals, the possibility of taking several medications at the same time, the relationship of drug dosing to meals and snacks, and concerns about the cost of therapy.[5]

Individuals who are homeless or who for other reasons have unstable living conditions or limited social-support mechanisms may find it particularly difficult to adhere to a combination therapy regimen. The NIH panel recommended that health-care providers work with HIV-infected individuals to assess their readiness and ability to commit to a HAART regimen. This assessment should be made on an individual basis; health-care workers should not assume that any specific group of people as a whole is unable to adhere to a particular regimen. No individual should be automatically excluded from consideration for antiretroviral therapy simply because he or she simply appears to exhibit characteristics judged by some to be predictable of noncompliance.

On the other hand, concern for the public health requires that if a patient does not respond to HAART because of a documented history of noncompliance with treatment requirements, and is not practicing safer sex, that individual's antiretroviral treatment may be discontinued. Under such circumstances, HAART is useless to the patient and may in fact lead to drug-resistant HIV mutants that are likely to be transmitted to his or her sexual partners.

7. Any change in antiretroviral therapy reduces future therapeutic options.

Any decision to change a therapeutic regimen is likely to limit an individual's future treatment options. It is therefore important not to abandon any regimen prematurely. During antiretroviral therapy, increases in viral load and in the rate at which they occur (which suggest higher HIV replication rates) indicate the urgency with which therapy should be altered.

A change in treatment regimen should be considered for any individual whose viral load steadily increases from an undetectable to a detectable level. A change in treatment is also usually considered for individuals who show evidence of drug toxicity or intolerance (sometimes these manifestations are temporary, and therapy may be safely continued along with patient counseling and continued evaluation).

To avoid making an unnecessary change in therapy, it is important, whenever possible, to determine why viral load is increasing. An individual may not adhere closely to his or her regimen because of a lack of understanding about the need for strict compliance. Such problems can be corrected. Also, a recent vaccination or concurrent infection could have stimulated immune responses that produce a temporary increase in HIV replication. Thus, clinicians should always perform two viral-load tests on separate occasions before changing therapy to rule out a transient increase in HIV replication.

Biological factors can also be responsible for rising viral loads. These include the emergence of drug-resistant variants of HIV, decreased absorption of antiretroviral drugs, and a change in the body's ability to metabolize the drugs. For more information, see "Considerations for Changing a Failing Antiretroviral Therapy."

8. Women should receive optimal antiretroviral therapy even when pregnant.

The preceding principles concerning the use and initiation of HAART therapy apply equally to men and women, both adult and adolescent. In general, the NIH panel recommended that the use of antiretroviral drugs and the initiation of treatment follow the same guidelines in pregnant HIV-infected women as in other adults. Thus, a pregnant woman's clinical condition, viral load, and CD4 lymphocyte counts should guide treatment decisions.

But the use of antiretroviral therapy in pregnant HIV-infected women also raises unique concerns. Two important considerations are the use of antiretroviral drugs to preserve the health of the mother, and the possible effect of these drugs in reducing the risk of HIV transmission to her child.

Use of Antiretroviral Drugs to Preserve the Health of the Mother
Determining whether to initiate HAART becomes more difficult if a woman is in the first trimester—weeks 1 to 14—of pregnancy (particularly the first 8 weeks). During this time, the embryo is most vulnerable to birth defects caused by chemicals in the body. Furthermore, no long-term studies have examined the safety of antiretroviral drug com-

binations during pregnancy. Therefore, pregnant women should discuss the potential advantages and hazards of such treatment with their physicians. Considerations include the stage of pregnancy; a woman's general state of health, viral load, and CD4 counts; and what is and is not known about the potential effects of antiretroviral drugs on the fetus.

The NIH panel advised that physicians consider delaying antiretroviral therapy until after 14 weeks of pregnancy (and particularly until after the first 8 weeks) when feasible.

Women who are already on a HAART regimen when pregnancy occurs should continue the therapy. However, if pregnancy is anticipated or diagnosed early in the first trimester (during the first 8–14 weeks), some women may choose to discontinue therapy until the end of the first trimester. It is not known if such a temporary discontinuation of therapy is harmful, although an increase in viral load should be expected and could increase the risk of disease progression in the mother and HIV transmission to the fetus. If therapy is temporarily stopped, all drugs should be discontinued simultaneously; when therapy is resumed, all drugs should be reintroduced simultaneously.

The antiretroviral regimen used for a pregnant woman should suppress HIV replication to undetectable levels; incomplete suppression increases the risk that drug-resistant forms of HIV will emerge, which will limit the woman's future treatment options. It may also limit the ability of the same drugs to decrease the risk of perinatal transmission.

Use of Antiretroviral Drugs to Reduce the Risk of Perinatal HIV Transmission

Transmission of HIV from mother to infant (perinatal transmission) can occur at all levels of viral load, although a high viral load is associated with a higher probability of transmission. AZT therapy effectively reduces perinatal HIV transmission regardless of the maternal viral load (see Chapter 12). Therefore, the use of AZT alone or in combination with other antiretroviral drugs should be offered to all HIV-infected pregnant women, regardless of viral load.

9. The principles of antiretroviral therapy presented above apply to both HIV-infected children and adults, although the treatment of HIV-infected children involves unique pharmacological, virological, and immunological considerations.

The data available on HIV infection in children support the principles of antiretroviral therapy as outlined for adults. Therefore, HIV-infected children should also be treated with combination antiretroviral therapy with the goal of long-term suppression of HIV replication to undetectable levels. Unfortunately, not all of the antiretroviral drugs used for HAART in adults are available in formulations (such as palatable liquid formulations) for infants and young children. In addition, studies on the action of many antiretroviral drugs in children have not been completed. Drugs for which this information is unavailable may produce undesirable side effects in children and should therefore be used only as part of a controlled clinical trial. For more on the treatment of HIV-infected children, see Chapter 12.

10. Persons with acute HIV infection may also benefit from combination antiretroviral therapy and suppression of virus replication to undetectable levels.

Theoretically, people in the acute stage of HIV infection should also benefit from combination therapy and suppression of virus replication to undetectable levels. Such therapy may curb the high levels of HIV replication that otherwise occur during acute infection, reduce HIV-related damage to the immune system, and produce a lower baseline (or setpoint) level of HIV replication during asymptomatic disease. Such effects would help preserve the function of the immune system and possibly improve the subsequent clinical course of the infection. It has also been suggested that the best opportunity to eradicate HIV infection may arise, in the future, during acute infection.

These benefits, however, are all theoretical. Preliminary data from small-scale studies support these predictions, but they have not yet been formally demonstrated to be valid. Therefore, the benefits of antiviral treatment during acute infection must be weighed against the risks; see "Considerations for Initiating Antiretroviral Therapy during Acute Infection."

> **11. All HIV-infected persons, including those with viral loads below detectable levels, should be considered infectious and should avoid sexual and drug-use behaviors associated with the transmission or acquisition of HIV and other infectious pathogens.**

It is not yet known whether HIV-infected individuals who are on therapy and have undetectable viral loads can transmit HIV infection to others through unsafe sex or needle sharing. For this reason, all HIV-infected individuals should continue to practice safer sex. Similarly, any HIV-infected person who injects drugs, whether illicit or medically prescribed, should not share injection equipment with others and use a sterile, disposable needle and syringe for each injection (see also Chapter 9).

Restored CD4 Lymphocyte Counts and Prophylaxis

Suppression of HIV replication to undetectable levels is often accompanied by increases in CD4 lymphocyte counts, often to levels above 200 cells per mm^3. Current research indicates that these new immune cells are unable to provide adequate protection against at least certain opportunistic infections. It is therefore important to continue the use of prophylactic therapy, even if CD4 counts return to levels above 200 cells per mm^3 (see Chapter 7).

■ CONSIDERATIONS FOR INITIATING ANTIRETROVIRAL THERAPY DURING ACUTE INFECTION

The acute phase of HIV infection produces no noticeable symptoms in about half of the people infected, and of those who do experience symptoms, only about 20% to 30% consult a physician because of them (the clinical symptoms of acute infection often resemble those of the "flu" or other common illnesses; see Chapter 4).

But many experts recommend antiretroviral therapy for individuals with laboratory evidence of acute HIV infection, including those in whom infection has been documented to have occurred within the previous six months (individuals who believe themselves recently infected but for whom the time of infection cannot be documented should be considered to be in the asymptomatic phase of infection).[6] The goal of therapy is suppression of viral load to undetectable levels; the DHHS guidelines note that any regimen that is not expected to achieve maximal suppression of viral replication is not appropriate for the treatment of acute HIV infection.

The use of antiretroviral therapy during acute infection, however, is based almost entirely on theoretical considerations—evidence of actual clinical benefit based on information from clinical trials is presently very limited. The theoretical rationale for the early use of HAART is based on four points:

- It should suppress the burst of viral replication that occurs during acute infection and decrease the number of virus particles dispersed throughout the body.

- It should decrease the severity of acute disease.

- It should decrease the initial baseline (or set-point) level of HIV, which is widely believed to affect disease progression.

- It should slow the rate of viral mutation by suppressing viral replication.

These potential benefits must be weighed against risks that are similar to those of HAART for individuals with asymptomatic disease and include the following:

- Drug toxicity and compliance with regimen of treatment might adversely affect the individual's quality of life.

- Should therapy fail to completely suppress viral replication, drug resistance may develop and limit future treatment options.

- Antiviral therapy may need to be continued indefinitely.

- It might blunt the development of an effective immune response. Triple-drug therapy taken within a few weeks following HIV infection may delay development of anti-HIV antibodies from months to more than a year, and it often prevents a CTL response. This occurs because the early use of HAART reduces the viral load to such low levels that not enough viral antigen is produced to provoke an immune response. Because of this, many scientists want to test the hypothesis that injections of recombinant HIV proteins should be combined with HAART when the latter is used soon after HIV infection.

To help define the optimal approach to the treatment of acute infection, the NIH panel recommended that newly diagnosed patients should be encouraged to enroll in clinical trials that study this question. If enrolling in a clinical trial is not feasible or desired, the panel recommended that combination antiretroviral therapy be given, with the goal of suppressing HIV replication to undetectable levels. Therapy should continue indefinitely until clinical trials provide data to establish its appropriate duration.

▪ If Therapy Is Initiated

If the decision is made to initiate antiretroviral therapy, viral load and CD4 counts should be determined as described already (at initiation of therapy, after four weeks,[7] and every three to four months thereafter). How long therapy should be continued is a matter of opinion. Many experts would continue to treat with antiretroviral therapy indefinitely because viremia is known to recur or increase when therapy is discontinued; others might be tempted to treat for a year, then discontinue therapy and evaluate the individual using CD4 cell counts and viral-load testing. In reality, the optimal treatment strategy in terms of what drugs to use and for how long is not yet known, although clinical trials are under way to help answer these questions.

▪ CONSIDERATIONS FOR INITIATING ANTIRETROVIRAL THERAPY DURING LATE-STAGE HIV DISEASE

Some people are first diagnosed with HIV infection only after advanced disease has developed (i.e., those diagnosed with any condition meeting the 1993 CDC definition of AIDS; see Appendix 2). HAART can slow disease progression and prolong life even in individuals with late-stage HIV disease (e.g., CD4 lymphocyte counts below 50 cells per mm^3). For this reason, and after possible complications are taken into consideration, all individuals with advanced HIV disease should be treated with antiretroviral drug combinations regardless of their viral load. If the decision is made to initiate HAART, the goal should again be to suppress the viral load to undetectable levels.

A number of factors complicate the use of antiretroviral therapy in individuals who are acutely ill, however. They include drug toxicity, drug interactions, and the ability of the individual to adhere to the therapeutic regimen.

The possibility of drug interactions is particularly a problem in persons being treated with multiple drugs, and it can influence the choice of drugs to be used in combination. For example, protease inhibitors affect the metabolism of the drug rifampin, which is sometimes given for active tuberculosis. At the same time, rifampin lowers the blood level of protease inhibitors, which can reduce their therapeutic effectiveness.

Medical complications of advanced disease also influence the use of combination antiretroviral therapy. Wasting and anorexia can prevent individuals from following the dietary requirements necessary for effective absorption of protease inhibitors. Protease inhibitors may also not be an option for individuals with HIV-related liver dysfunction. Because of the broad possibilities for detrimental drug interactions, individuals taking antiretroviral therapy should always discuss with their physician any new drugs they may consider taking, including over-the-counter and "alternative" medications.

■ CONSIDERATIONS WHEN INTERRUPTING ANTIRETROVIRAL THERAPY

Reasons for interrupting HAART may include intolerable side effects, drug interactions, the first trimester of pregnancy, and the unavailability of the drugs. If one antiretroviral drug must be discontinued, all other antiretroviral drugs that are part of the combination therapy being taken should be discontinued simultaneously, rather than continuing the use of only one or two of them. Discontinuing all drugs at once has the theoretical advantage of minimizing the emergence of drug-resistant viral strains (as described earlier in this chapter).

■ CONSIDERATIONS FOR CHANGING A FAILING ANTIRETROVIRAL THERAPY

The decision to change a failing regimen involves taking many complex factors into account. They include such things as the results of a physical examination and of clinical tests; remaining treatment options; viral load (measured on two separate occasions); the trend in CD4 counts; the stage of disease; and the individual's potential ability to tolerate a new regimen in terms of side effects, drug interactions, and dietary requirements.

The physician must distinguish between the need to change therapy due to drug failure versus drug toxicity. In the case of drug toxicity, the drug or drugs thought to be responsible for the toxicity should be replaced by alternatives of equal potency and from the same class as the agent being discontinued.

When a regimen is changed because of drug failure, the new regimen should incorporate drugs not previously taken by the individual. With triple-drug combinations, at least two, and preferably all three, agents should be changed to reduce the risk of drug resistance; changing only a single drug, even if it is a very potent one, is likely to result in viral resistance to the new drug.

In addition, the drugs chosen for a new regimen should not be cross-resistant to previously used antiretroviral drugs or induce similar patterns of viral mutations that are associated with resistance.[8] Specific criteria that should prompt considering a change in combination antiretroviral therapy include the following:

■ A less than tenfold (1.0-log) reduction in the viral load by four weeks following initiation of HAART.

■ Failure of the viral load to reach an undetectable level within four to six months of initiating HAART. (Although consideration should be given here to the viral load at the start of therapy. For example, an individual with 1 million virions per ml of plasma who then stabilizes after six months of therapy with a viral load that is detectable but below 10,000 virions per ml may not need an immediate change of therapy.)

■ Repeated detection of virus in plasma after it has been initially suppressed to undetectable levels. This occurrence suggests the development of drug resistance.

■ A threefold (i.e., 0.5-log) or greater increase in viral load from its stable low, as determined by repeated testing (to eliminate the possibility of a temporary increase in viral load due to simultaneous infection from another pathogen or vaccination, or to a spurious measurement due to the testing methodology).

■ Persistently declining CD4 lymphocyte counts, as measured on at least two separate occasions.

■ Clinical deterioration. A new AIDS-defining illness that develops after the initiation of HAART may or may not suggest a failure of that therapy. A poor antiviral response (e.g., a less than tenfold drop in viral load) does suggest such a failure. But if the individual was already severely immunocompromised when treatment began, and therapy produced a good antiviral response, the new opportunistic infection may reflect severely impaired immunity and not a failure of antiviral therapy.

Clearly, obtaining the expert advice of a physician very knowledgeable in the treatment of HIV disease—by referral or consultation, if necessary—is essential when considering a change in therapy. That expertise is also essential to those who require a change in antiretroviral therapy but who have exhausted their options among the currently approved drugs. These individuals should be referred for possible inclusion in an appropriate clinical trial.

▪ ANTIRETROVIRAL COMPOUNDS UNDER DEVELOPMENT

Research is under way to develop new, safer, and more effective RTIs and protease inhibitors, but other types of drugs and treatment strategies are also under investigation. The following compounds have shown activity against HIV in cell and animal studies and are in clinical trials. In most cases, there is little or no information as yet on their effectiveness, toxicity, or side effects in humans. For additional information on the treatments described below, as well as on new RTIs, protease inhibitors, and others, see the AmFAR *AIDS/HIV Treatment Directory* (which also lists the sites at which testing is being done).

▪ Integrase Inhibitors

Integrase is the third HIV enzyme necessary for the replication of HIV (along with RT and protease). After RT produces a DNA copy of HIV's RNA genome, the viral DNA travels to the cell nucleus where it is inserted into a chromosome of the host cell. The insertion of the viral DNA into the host DNA is accomplished (catalyzed) by the viral enzyme integrase. Zintevir (AR-177) is an experimental integrase inhibitor that is in early clinical testing.

▪ CI-1012, a Zinc Finger Inhibitor

Zinc fingers are structures present in some protein molecules that resemble narrow outpouchings (or "fingers"). These outpouchings enable these proteins to bind with DNA or RNA. HIV's nucleocapsid protein, which encapsulates HIV RNA inside the virion (see Chapter 18), is a protein that has zinc fingers. It is thought that the zinc fingers help stabilize HIV RNA when viral RT copies the viral RNA into DNA early in replication, and that they are also important during the assembly of new virions prior to budding. CI-1012 is a compound that disrupts zinc fingers of the nucleocapsid protein, probably by ejecting their zinc atoms. In this way, CI-1012 could block viral replication by interfering with both reverse transcription and virus assembly.

■ Hydroxyurea

Hydroxyurea is an oral anticancer drug used in the treatment of inoperable ovarian cancer and some leukemias. There is also laboratory evidence that hydroxyurea inhibits viral RT from copying viral RNA into DNA. In anti-HIV clinical testing, hydroxyurea has been used in combination therapy with a nucleoside analogue—AZT, ddI, or d4T.

■ Pentafuside

Pentafuside, or T-20, is a small, 36 amino acids long, peptide. It is derived from the HIV-1 gp41 protein. Pentafuside blocks the fusion of HIV with the cell membrane. This peptide has shown anti-HIV activity in the small number of patients who have received it, but human testing has been limited because presently there is no oral formulation of pentafuside, and it must be given intravenously.

■ Immune-Based Therapy

Immune-based therapies attempt to strengthen the immune system's response to HIV infection or to restore immune function. A number of immune-based strategies are undergoing testing in clinical trials, but to date none have been shown to be of clinical benefit. Immune-based therapies undergoing testing are described below.

Cytokines

Cytokines are compounds naturally produced by cells to regulate the activity and behavior of other cells (see Chapter 16). The following three cytokines are being tested for their ability to stimulate immune activity against HIV.

Interleukin-12

Interleukin (IL)-12 has a variety of effects on immune cells. One effect is to stimulate the activity of a subgroup of helper T cells known as helper T cells type 1, or TH1 cells. TH1 cells are important in activating the cell-mediated immune response, specifically cytotoxic T cells, which are believed to be important in fighting HIV.

Interleukin-2

IL-2 stimulates the proliferation of T lymphocytes and natural killer cells, as well as the proliferation of B lymphocytes and the production of antibodies by plasma cells. Several clinical trials have shown that IL-2 given along with combination antiretroviral therapy increases CD4 counts rather dramatically in some patients whose initial CD4 counts are over 200. It is not known how effective these new cells will be in fighting infections, and a larger controlled trial needs to be performed to determine IL-2's clinical benefit. IL-2 increases HIV replication because it activates the replication of T cells; it is therefore important to stress that IL-2 must be taken only by people who are receiving highly effective antiretroviral therapy, otherwise T-cell activation alone would stimulate HIV replication and increase viral load.

Interleukin-10

IL-10 has a number of effects on a variety of immune-system cells. For example, it promotes B-cell proliferation and antibody production. It also suppresses cell-mediated immunity, which is thought to be a major defense mechanism against HIV. However, at low doses it appears to have anti-HIV properties, although the mechanism of this effect is unclear.

Gene Transfer Therapy

Gene transfer therapy, or gene therapy, uses gene-splicing techniques (i.e., genetic engineering) to place one or more new or altered genes into cells. The new genes may be intended to replace faulty ones, augment the action of normal genes, or inactivate disease-causing genes. Foreign genes are delivered into target cells (which have been removed from the body) using a harmless virus such as an adenovirus or a mouse retrovirus. If all goes well, the genetically modified cells are returned to the body and the foreign gene(s) begins producing the desired protein. Other means of delivering foreign genes into cells include injecting, or "bombarding," genes directly into cells or encapsulating them in laboratory-produced, microscopic spheres of fat known as "liposomes," which cells take up.

Two major forms of anti-HIV gene therapy are known as "immunotherapeutics" and "intracellular immunization."

■ *Immunotherapeutics* is an approach that uses cells that are genetically engineered to overproduce HIV antigens to stimulate antibody and cellular immune responses (see Chapter 16) to HIV. One method that has undergone phase I testing in humans uses connective-tissue cells known as "fibroblasts." Fibroblasts are removed from an HIV-infected person and two HIV genes, *env* and *rev*, are transferred into them. The cells are then returned to the body, where they are intended to produce the viral envelope (Env) and Rev proteins (see Chapter 18) and so stimulate stronger immune responses to HIV.

■ *Intracellular immunization* encompasses one of three possibilities: Introducing an "antisense" gene that produces mRNAs that can bind to viral RNA and DNA and inactivate them; introducing genes that code for mutated HIV proteins that interfere with the function of normal HIV proteins; or introducing genes that code for anti-HIV antibodies, which can bind to and inactivate HIV proteins within the cell.

A third strategy, which may or may not use genetically engineered lymphocytes, is adoptive T-cell transfer. Thisn involves removing T lymphocytes from HIV-infected patients, selecting those with anti-HIV activity, growing them to large numbers, and returning them to the patient.

Therapeutic Vaccines

Therapeutic vaccines—as opposed to protective vaccines (see Chapter 10)—are designed to stimulate a more effective immune response to HIV in people who are already HIV infected. Most therapeutic vaccines tested have used the gp120 or gp160 envelope proteins produced by recombinant DNA technology. Using genetic engineering techniques, viral genes coding for these proteins were introduced into bacteria or other kinds of cells. These cells were then grown in large numbers and produced the viral recombinant proteins in large quantities for use as experimental vaccines.

An example of a therapeutic vaccine is the HIV-Immunogen vaccine, which uses whole inactivated HIV particles. During early testing, this vaccine was given to HIV-positive individuals with CD4 counts higher than 600 cells per mm³, and it produced significant increases in p24 antibody levels relative to the control group. Whether this can delay disease progression is being tested in two phase III trials. Enthusiasm for therapeutic vaccines, however, has waned over recent years because of disappointing results so far, particularly in the ability of such vaccines to stimulate cell-mediated immunity, believed to be important to an effective immune response to HIV. Nevertheless, trials are ongoing.

■ BUYERS' CLUBS

Unfortunately, even antiretroviral combinations that benefit many people do not work well for everyone. Some people experience side effects so severe that they are forced to discontinue using antiretroviral drugs. Others are able to tolerate them, but their viral load does not fall. This leaves these individuals with no effective anti-HIV treatment. Many of them, as well as others who are HIV positive, then often turn to buyers' clubs for drugs and other agents that might either slow the progression of their disease or alleviate its symptoms.

Through buyers' clubs, people can obtain some drugs that are approved in other countries but are either not, or not as yet, approved by the FDA for use in the United States. They may also obtain agents that are unproven and sometimes illegal. Some buyers' clubs, for example, specialize in medicinal marijuana, which may help treat AIDS wasting syndrome, appetite loss, nausea, and pain. Some clubs also provide alternative or complementary treatments, Chinese herbs, and nutritional and other supplements.

People who are considering the use of unapproved, experimental, untested, or alternative treatments should first carefully investigate any agent before using it. They should learn how effective the agent is purported to be, how it is administered, what its potential side effects are, whether it is toxic at certain levels, and whether it is thought to interact with other drugs. For suggestions on how to investigate alternative treatments, see "Complementary and Alternative Treatments," Chapter 13.

Anyone preparing to use a buyers' club should be sure to ask questions to learn if the club is reputable. The characteristics of a reputable buyers' club include the following:

- It is not-for-profit.

- It refrains from giving medical advice.

- It provides unbiased information.

- It minimizes the cost of its services and provides services to some who cannot afford them.

- It does its best to ensure that its products are truthfully labeled and free of contaminants.

- Its products meet the highest possible standards of purity and potency. Some buyers' clubs, for example, send samples to testing laboratories to check for purity. Nonetheless, buyers' clubs have limited control over the quality of their products.

- Also, ask if the club provides mail-order service, accepts major credit cards, or has an annual membership fee.

■ CONCLUSIONS

In research on antiretroviral therapy, as in all areas of HIV/AIDS research, much has been accomplished and much remains to be done. Combination antiretroviral therapies are now extending and improving the quality of the lives of many who take them, but formidable problems remain.

The treatment and care of people with HIV has become extremely complex. The success of HAART depends on a thorough understanding by physicians of how HIV causes disease and of how to optimally use the greater number of drugs now available to treat it. Physicians must also be willing to effectively educate their patients regarding the use of antiretroviral drugs: New and potent drugs are of little help to a person with HIV if the drugs are not used correctly, and this is the responsibility of both the physician and the patient. If the drugs are used incorrectly, this can reduce the effectiveness of other anti-HIV drugs that may be needed in the future.

Drug resistance remains a major problem. The best hope for people who have failed several drugs is new drugs that attack novel targets in

HIV or the same target in novel ways. In addition, the side effects of anti-HIV drugs taken over the long term are only beginning to emerge. Much more basic and clinical research remains to be done.

Individuals who respond well to HAART also experience an increase in CD4 lymphocyte counts. This has raised a new and vexing problem: Although the immune system in these individuals seems to have at least partially restored itself in terms of numbers of CD4 lymphocytes, the new cells appear unable to marshal effective immune responses. Thus, even people responding well to antiretroviral therapy must continue taking prophylaxis, at least for the time being, for protection from opportunistic infections. Overcoming this hurdle and fully restoring immune-system functions is a major challenge. If HIV/AIDS is to become a controllable chronic infection with which people can live without constant fears, research on immune reconstitution is essential.

The cumulative costs of HAART and prophylaxis for opportunistic infections, as well as both medical and laboratory monitoring, confront a growing number of people living with HIV disease, the federal and state governments, and community-based service organizations with difficult decisions related to the allocation of resources. Economic and socio-political issues indeed also limit the potential effectiveness of the new therapies.[9]

The use of costly, high-tech, antiretroviral regimens is a major problem globally: they will predictably remain largely unavailable to HIV-infected people in developing countries who make up 90% of people with HIV/AIDS worldwide. Even in the United States, a significant number of people cannot access, tolerate, or comply with the rigors of combination antiretroviral therapy; others do not respond to it.

The inescapable conclusion is that the epidemic of HIV/AIDS is far from over. Only through continued basic and clinical biomedical research dedicated to achieving a more complete knowledge of HIV; to finding ways of reconstituting immune-system functions damaged by HIV; and to understanding the correlates of anti-HIV immunity, which is necessary for the development of a protective HIV vaccine, can the epidemic come under control.

ENDNOTES

1. Note that drug resistance is never a matter of the HIV somehow "knowing" what drugs are present and deliberately adapting to them. The presence or absence of antiretroviral drugs only creates a set of conditions for the growth of HIV in the body. Because of the range of viral genetic variants present, some virions can survive and replicate in the presence of one or more given drugs and others cannot, just as the genetic makeup of some flies or mosquitoes allows them to survive an insecticide treatment while others are killed by it.

2. Genetic mutation is not the only way HIV acquires drug resistance. It can also happen when two genetically different HIV particles infect the same cell. Under these conditions, each virion can assemble part of its DNA strand using RNA from the other virion as well as from its own. The DNA strands and proviruses that will result will be mixtures of the genes from the two genetic variants. This type of genetic shuffling is known as "genetic recombination," and it can produce new and different populations of virus.

3. It is important to avoid unnecessary interruption of HAART, even when a drop in viral load is not seen. A recent study has shown that continuing to take a triple combination despite a persistently detectable viral load and documented resistance may still, by an unclear mechanism, preserve some T-cell function. See Kaufmann D, et al. CD4-cell count in HIV-1-infected individuals remaining viraemic with highly active antiretroviral therapy (HAART). *Lancet* 1998;351:723–24.

4. Centers for Disease Control and Prevention. Report of the NIH panel to define principles of therapy of HIV infection and guidelines for the use of antiretrovial agents in HIV-infected adults and adolescents. *MWWR* 1998;47(RR-5):1–83.

5. Cost is a major reason why some people do not take a medication as prescribed. Because of the risk of developing drug-resistant strains of HIV, it is a serious mistake to skip doses of antiretroviral therapy to make a prescription last longer or as a way of saving money. If the cost of a medication causes anxiety, by all means the problem should be discussed with one's physician or an AIDS service organization that can provide advice on possible financial assistance.

6. The NIH treatment guidelines recommend that with one exception, no individual be treated for HIV infection until the infection is documented by an ELISA and an accepted confirmatory test such as Western blot. The one exception is the treatment of individuals for postexposure prophylaxis (see Chapter 9).

7. Some experts believe testing at four weeks is not helpful in evaluating the response to therapy in acute infection because viral levels are typically decreasing at this time even in the absence of therapy.

8. Although assays are commercially available for determining the viral mutations in HIV that are associated with drug resistance, these methods have not yet been field tested to demonstrate their clinical usefulness, and they have not been approved by the FDA. Therefore, they are not recommended at present by the Department of Health and Human Services (DHHS) for routine use.

9. Several studies have shown that HAART therapy is cost effective as compared to the annual cost of treating a person with AIDS. In addition, a person responding to combination antiretroviral therapy can be a productive, taxpaying citizen.

Chapter 6

CLINICAL TRIALS AND DRUG DEVELOPMENT FOR HIV DISEASE

Clinical trials are the means by which researchers determine the safety and effectiveness of new drugs for the treatment of HIV and other diseases. They are also an important means for patients to receive the latest promising treatments even if these treatments are still experimental. At some point in their treatment, people with HIV disease are likely to face the decision of whether to join a clinical trial. This chapter explains what clinical trials are, why they are important, how they are done, and what things patients should consider before enrolling in one or more of them. Some of the problems and controversies that have arisen over clinical trials of potential HIV treatments are also reviewed.

For specific information about clinical trials under way for HIV disease and where they are being conducted, the reader can obtain the latest copy of the *AIDS/HIV Treatment Directory,* compiled and published by AmFAR. The treatment directory is available through AmFAR and through the National AIDS Clearinghouse. Other sources of information on clinical trials and new therapies are listed in Appendix 1. In addition to trials, "expanded-access" programs provide experimental drugs and treatments for people who for various reasons do not qualify for or do not have access to clinical trials. What these programs are is also described here. For a listing of specific programs, see AmFAR's *AIDS/HIV Treatment Directory.*

■ CLINICAL TRIALS ARE IMPORTANT TO MEDICAL SCIENCE

Clinical trials, sometimes known as drug trials, are studies by which doctors learn whether a new drug or a new treatment regimen is safe for patients, and whether it is more effective than an existing treatment. Carefully designed and controlled clinical trials are essential for continuing improvements in the standard of medical care for HIV disease and all other illnesses. People who participate in clinical studies always help improve the future treatment of illness for others and possibly for themselves as well.

Clinical trials are usually sponsored (i.e., proposed and paid for) by drug companies interested in bringing a drug they have developed to market. However, trials are always conducted by qualified medical researchers affiliated with university hospitals, medical-research centers, the National Institutes of Health (NIH), or community-based clinical research groups. The sponsors and investigators involved in a clinical trial can advertise for patients to participate or else they rely on referrals from physicians.

Many clinical trials testing new treatments for HIV disease are conducted under the auspices of the AIDS Clinical Trials Group (ACTG) of the NIH, supported by funds from the federal government. Others are supported and overseen by pharmaceutical companies and a few by AIDS-related nonprofit organizations such as AmFAR. All participating patients must be volunteers.

■ EXPERIMENTAL DRUGS ARE TESTED FIRST IN CELLS AND ANIMALS

Scientists try to learn as much as possible about a drug before giving it to humans in a clinical trial. Initial studies consist purely of laboratory work on the drug's chemical and physical properties. This phase of drug development is known as "preclinical research." It also involves testing the drug on healthy and diseased cells growing in laboratory cell-culture systems. Scientists seek to determine whether the agent under study is toxic to human cells and has the potential to control a disease condition or a disease-causing microbe. Work on living cells helps estimate the concentrations of drug needed to obtain the desired effect without killing the cells. Scientists then test a drug in laboratory animals, which gives researchers an idea of the drug's toxicity in an organism, how it is carried in blood, how it is absorbed by tissues, and how and how fast it is excreted.

But animal tests cannot reveal with certainty how the drug will act in humans—whether it will work and how safe it will be. These questions can be answered only by testing the drug in humans through a series of carefully designed and controlled clinical trials. For protection of the public, permission to conduct any trial in humans, in turn, requires the review and consent of experts with the Food and Drug Administration (FDA). For this purpose, the drug developer files an IND (For "Investigational New Drug") application with the FDA. The application involves sending the FDA information on everything known about the drug, starting with results of all cell and animal studies. An IND application also includes the proposed protocol, which is the document outlining precisely how the trial will be conducted. The FDA reviews that information and either denies the IND application or approves it with or without modifications. Approval means the trial can proceed.

■ HOW CLINICAL TRIALS ARE DONE

Clinical trials are usually performed in three phases, with each subsequent phase involving more patients and a longer period of time. Each phase requires separate FDA approval.

■ Phase I trials mark the first time a new agent is used in humans. Phase I trials involve a small number of usually healthy volunteers, and they last from a few weeks to less than a year. Because of their relatively high risk, phase I trials are often performed using volunteers who are admitted to a hospital so they can be observed around the clock by medical staff. The primary goal of a phase I trial is to determine to what extent a drug is safe for use in humans, and to establish its "maximum tolerated dose." This is done by first giving the drug at a very low dose, then gradually escalating it until undesirable side effects are clearly seen. During phase I testing, researchers learn such things as how well the drug is absorbed, metabolized, and excreted by the body; what side effects occur as the dosage is increased; what the maximum tolerated dose is; and how often the drug should be given. Many potential new drugs are dropped from further development during phase I trials because they make people too sick—they have too much toxicity—at doses still too low to be effective.

■ Phase II trials focus primarily on determining drug effectiveness. Drug safety and side effects are nevertheless still carefully monitored. Phase II studies can involve up to several hundred patients and can take a few months to two years to complete. Sometimes, phase II trials mark the first time the drug is used in patients with the disease the drug is intended to treat. The drug is given at the dose and frequency estimated to be optimal during the phase I trial, that is, a dose thought to be both safe for most people and effective against the disease.

Sometimes, phase I and phase II trials are combined to speed the development of a new drug. These studies involve a relatively small number of individuals with the disease the drug is intended to treat. They are designed to give, all at once, information on safety, dosage, and efficacy. Such studies are known as phase I/II trials.

■ Phase III trials test the safety and efficacy of a drug in several hundred to several thousand volunteers. They last from one to several years. Trials involving a large number of people are necessary to gain a broad understanding of the drug's safety and efficacy, its interactions with other drugs, its long-term toxicities and benefits, and its acceptability to the public.

■ THE IMPORTANCE OF RANDOMIZATION TO CLINICAL TRIALS

In phase III trials, and many phase II trials, participants who enroll in the trial are randomly assigned to one of at least two groups, or "arms," of the study. One group is known as the treatment arm; people in this group receive the experimental drug. The other arm is the comparison, or control arm; people in this group receive the standard treatment. Whether a particular patient is assigned to the treatment or to the control group is determined by lottery or by a computerized toss of the coin.

When a volunteer enters a two-arm randomized trial, he or she stands a 50-50 chance (or a 60-40, or 70-30 chance, depending on the protocol) of receiving the experimental treatment. Some individuals feel that if they are assigned to the control group, they will receive an inferior treatment (if the trial is also a "blinded" trial, neither the patient nor the investigator may know to which group he or she has been assigned; see below). But that is not necessarily the case. Members of the control group usually receive a treatment of known effectiveness (even if that effectiveness is not ideal), while the volunteers assigned to the experimental group receive a treatment of largely unknown effectiveness and safety. All that can be said of the experimental drug is that on the basis of earlier (phase I) studies, it is believed that the drug is tolerated by the body up to a certain dose over the short run, and that there is also a reason to believe—sometimes still mostly on theoretical grounds—that the drug may fight the volunteer's disease. Until the results of a phase II clinical trial are known, no one knows how effective the experimental treatment might be in humans, nor even, with any precision, what its spectrum of side effects might be. Members of a placebo control group may fare better than the treatment group because a strategy of watching, waiting, and treating symptoms of the disease as they occur may be more beneficial than experiencing the toxicity of the experimental drug. The results of a randomized clinical trial can show one of several possibilities:

1. The experimental treatment is more effective than the standard treatment; in this case, the experimental treatment could come to replace the standard treatment.

2. There is no detectable difference in safety or effectiveness between the experimental and standard treatments; in this case, the new treatment could serve as an alternative to the standard treatment.

3. The experimental treatment is less effective than the standard treatment but not ineffective; doctors under most circumstances would not use the new drug except in patients unable to tolerate the standard treatment.

4. The experimental treatment is as effective as the standard treatment, but makes patients sicker—it is more toxic—than the standard treatment.

5. The experimental treatment is less effective and has more undesirable side effects than the standard treatment.

If a phase III trial shows that the new drug is beneficial and safe, the sponsor of the drug will request that the FDA approve the drug for marketing to practicing physicians. This request is known as a "New Drug Application," or NDA. The FDA would certainly grant an NDA for a drug having the first outcome listed above, probably in the case of the second and third outcomes (depending on the agent), and perhaps even in the fourth because agents for the treatment of AIDS are so badly needed. On the other hand, because of marketing considerations, the sponsoring company may decide to produce the drug only if it achieves the first outcome.

Experimental drugs in phase III trials rarely produce results that are strikingly different from those of phase II trials, or, for that matter, reveal striking improvements over standard treatments. Usually differences in effectiveness are small. For this reason, large numbers of patients are needed in each group of a randomized clinical trial. Only by comparing large groups will differences in the various aspects studied in phase III trials become clear.

■ RANDOMIZATION HELPS REDUCE BIAS

Understandably, everyone involved in the testing of a new experimental drug wants to see it succeed. Patients who volunteer for the trial want to be helped by the new treatment; the physicians treating those volunteers want to see their patients improve and, therefore, the new treatment succeed. This desire to help and be helped is so strong that it can introduce the problem of bias into clinical trials.

Bias is the conscious or unconscious influence of emotions, or personal beliefs or interests on someone's judgment. Without randomization, a physician might unconsciously tend to assign healthier patient-volunteers to the experimental group because he or she believes that those patients have a better chance to be helped by the new drug. In such cases, the trial might show that the experimental treatment is better than the standard control treatment, although in reality that result occurred because the patients receiving the experimental drug were healthier at the start.

Randomization avoids this real and serious problem. It ensures that all the patients within the groups being compared in a trial have, on average, similar characteristics.

Sometimes patients wonder if randomization is ethical. Randomization *is* ethical when the researchers themselves *truly* do not know whether the experimental or the standard treatment is better in terms of safety and effectiveness.

■ ADDITIONAL MEANS OF REDUCING BIAS

■ Blind Trials

Blinding a trial is another method used to reduce bias. A blinded trial is one in which the patient-volunteers of a randomized trial do not know if they are receiving the experimental drug or the standard treatment. In a double-blind trial, neither the patients nor the researchers know whether a given patient has been assigned to the experimental or the control group.

Blinding ensures that any improvement that occurs as a result of merely participating in the trial is not mistakenly attributed to the experimental drug. Such a response in a patient is sometimes called the "placebo effect" because it also occurs in patients assigned to the control group who have not been given the medicine. Because of the placebo effect, clinical studies that are designed to simply enroll and treat patients without also using a control group will often produce misleading results. In certain cases, a blinded trial is impossible to carry out because some treatments have characteristic side effects that reveal the nature of the treatment. Trials that are not blinded are referred to as "open-label" studies.

■ Placebo-Control Trials

Blinded or double-blind trials can compare an experimental treatment to a standard treatment. If no standard treatment exists, then the experimental treatment has to be compared to a placebo. A placebo is a formulation of an inactive ingredient that looks and tastes like the experimental drug. Placebo trials compare the benefit of a new treatment to the benefit that can occur in people when they believe they are taking a drug.

Fortunately, placebo-control trials have become rare in HIV research. Most trials compare a new treatment with the best treatment currently available. Placebo trials are ethical only when no effective treatment is known for a certain condition (which is still the case for certain opportunistic diseases), or when there is no immediate danger in temporarily withholding treatment.

■ Protocols

A protocol is the book of rules and guidelines describing how a trial is to be conducted. The protocol describes such things as which patients are eligible for the trial, how and when patients are scheduled to receive treatment, what laboratory tests are to be ordered, and how the outcome of the treatment is to be measured. Which patients are eligible for a trial is determined by the trial's "inclusion and exclusion criteria."

Inclusion criteria might specify, for example, that patients entering the trial must have CD4 lymphocyte counts of 100 to 500 cells per mm^3, a count of 75,000 platelets or higher, a granulocyte (a type of white blood cell) count of 1,000 or more cells per mm^3, and a Karnovsky score (a way of assessing a patient's general health status) of 60 or higher and that they must be 13 years or older.

Exclusion criteria might include such things as having peripheral neuropathy, prior use of certain antiretroviral drugs, and the presence of systemic cancer. Inclusion and exclusion criteria are different for each trial.

It is essential for every clinical trial to have a detailed protocol that is closely followed by investigators. This ensures that all volunteers in the trial are medically managed in the same way, except for the differences in their treatment. A protocol is even more important in a multisite trial, one that is conducted simultaneously at several medical-research institutions. Because the data collected at all the sites will be pooled before being analyzed, it is critical that each site follow the same protocol very closely.

■ CLINICAL TRIALS INVOLVE BENEFITS, RISKS, AND OBLIGATIONS

Participating as a patient-volunteer in a clinical trial has certain benefits. Clinical trials are conducted in the best institutions by experienced professionals who provide state-of-the-art medical care to trial participants. In addition, most, if not all, of the medical care necessitated by the trial is provided at no cost to the volunteers (medical care for conditions unrelated to the trial is not provided).

There are also risks involved in clinical trials, including the following:

- An experimental drug can have unexpected or harmful side effects in humans. The three-phase clinical trial process is designed to minimize this risk, yet it remains true that the drug being tested could well be less safe than the standard treatment.

- The experimental treatment could be less effective than the standard treatment—or even worse than no treatment at all.

- While the experimental treatment might work for some people or at one stage of disease, it might not work for all or at all stages of disease.

- The new treatment might help patients for only a short time.

It is also important for patient-volunteers to realize that they are active participants in a scientific study that will benefit others and may benefit them, and that they are necessary allies with the physician-investigator. Volunteers who enroll in a trial, therefore, must assume the responsibility to abide by the requirements of the protocol. These can include frequent medical appointments and reliably following their treatment regimen even when it is inconvenient, for example. The responsibilities to be assumed by trial volunteers are described during the informed consent process, which is described below.

■ RIGHTS AND PROTECTIONS FOR PATIENTS IN CLINICAL TRIALS

While clinical trials do pose certain risks to patients, they also incorporate many safeguards designed to protect them. The following are required for clinical trials conducted in the United States:

■ Institutional Review Board

The Institutional Review Board (IRB) is a group of physicians, clergy, ethicists, patient advocates, and community representatives. An IRB exists at each hospital involved in clinical trials. The IRB ensures that the rights of trial participants will be protected, that the trial asks a valid question, and that the trial is ethical and as safe as possible. Every clinical trial in the United States must be approved by an IRB before it can begin.

■ Informed Consent

It is illegal to give any experimental drug to a patient without his or her consent. And this must be *informed* consent. Informed consent means that prior to enrollment, a volunteer must understand such things as the purpose of the study; the nature of the new drug and of the standard treatment used as the control; the study's possible risks and benefits to himself or herself; and the number, frequency, and kind of clinic visits and tests that will be required during the study.

This information is contained in an informed consent form that volunteers must sign and date before enrolling in a trial. Each point on the consent form must be explained by the physician or, more typically, by a protocol nurse.

■ Data Safety Monitoring Board

This is a group of physicians and other trained professionals (such as statisticians and ethicists) who are not otherwise involved in the trial, but who periodically review the data being collected in the course of the trial. If evidence arises that patients are being harmed, the safety monitoring board can order the sponsor to stop the trial. On the other hand, if one treatment proves clearly superior to the other before the trial is finished, the monitoring board can stop it so that all participants can be offered the superior treatment.

■ WHAT PATIENTS SHOULD KNOW ABOUT PARTICIPATING IN CLINICAL TRIALS

- No one can require or force a patient to join a clinical trial.

- If a patient is considering joining a clinical trial and does not understand something on the informed consent form, he or she should ask for an explanation. The patient is entitled to all the information he or she needs to arrive at an informed decision.

- An informed consent form is *not* a contract. Signing it does not bind the patient to remain in a clinical trial. He or she can drop out of the trial at any time, and for any reason, though this should not be done lightly. For example, if the patient feels that the treatment is harmful, that the trial is bad for his or her health, or that he or she is being mistreated, the patient should talk to the doctor or the protocol nurse. If not reassured, the patient should feel free to leave the trial.

- If a patient declines to enroll in a trial or drops out of it, this will not affect his or her relationship with the physician, and the patient will continue to receive the quality of medical care the physician can provide according to the patient's personal medical and economic circumstances.

- The patient should be highly suspicious of any clinical trial for which he or she is charged money, or that people claim will provide a miracle cure, or one that forces the patient to do something he or she does not want to do.

- Certain clinical trials cause very little inconvenience to participants. Others might require many medical tests and clinic visits. If the patient thinks it will be difficult to comply with some of the requirements of a trial he or she is interested in, the patient should tell the physician and ask for assistance.

- If the patient is participating in a trial and wishes to deviate from what is required by the protocol—he or she may want to take additional drugs or alternative treatments, for example—these concerns and intentions should be discussed honestly with the physician.

- If the tests and restrictions required by a protocol seem to make little sense or seem like a lot of trouble, it is important to remember that many of them are designed to protect *the patient* from possible side effects and to get reliable scientific information about a drug that has promise; otherwise it would not have reached clinical-trial testing at all.

■ EXPANDED-ACCESS PROGRAMS

People who are unable to enroll in a clinical trial and who have no other treatment options may be able to obtain promising experimental drugs through what has become known as "expanded-access programs." They include the following:

- A "treatment IND" allows pharmaceutical companies to provide experimental drugs that early clinical testing has shown to be probably safe and effective for the treatment of patients with serious illness who have exhausted FDA-approved treatments or for whom no approved treatment exists. Requests for drugs must be made by the physician to the drug manufacturer, and they are reviewed on a case-by-case basis. Drugs obtained under a treatment IND are purchased from the manufacturer, although at a cost below future market price.

- Open-label trials (sometimes called "parallel track testing") allow patients who do not qualify for controlled clinical trials and who have no therapeutic alternatives to receive a promising experimental treatment even if it is in very early clinical testing (e.g., early phase II trial). Very little may be known, in this case, about the safety and efficacy of these drugs.

- Compassionate-use INDs make experimental drugs available at no cost to very sick patients who have no other treatment options. Physicians must submit a written request to the drug manufacturer and must report the drug's effects on their patients. Requests are considered on a case-by-case basis. (Before 1992, the compassionate-use IND was the only way to gain access to experimental drugs for people with life-threatening diseases and no other treatment options.)

■ CONTROVERSIES RELATED TO CLINICAL TRIALS FOR HIV/AIDS

From the beginning, clinical trials for HIV disease have engendered controversy. Initially, the clinical-trial and drug-approval system was criticized (justly, many would say) for taking too long—typically, eight to ten years before a drug was approved for marketing. (However, the first anti-HIV drug, AZT, was tested in 1985 and 1986 and approved early in 1987, just two months after the submission of an NDA by its sponsor.) Expanded-access and accelerated-approval programs were instituted in 1992 by the FDA to hasten the review of drugs for life-threatening diseases.

The accelerated-approval process allows the FDA to approve a drug for marketing on the basis of one or more "surrogate" markers (as measured through laboratory tests rather than observation of real clinical benefits such as improvements in patients' health or their longer survival—see below). Sponsors who ask the FDA for accelerated approval are expected to continue testing the drug in clinical trials even after approval for marketing. The antiretroviral drugs ddI, ddC, 3TC, and saquinavir were all approved and made commercially available through an accelerated-approval process. But by late 1994, many people became concerned that drugs that had been insufficiently tested for their true effectiveness were entering the market.

It is a major drawback to both accelerated-approval and expanded-access programs that while they make new drugs available earlier to people with life-threatening diseases, less is known about the drugs' safety, effectiveness, and proper use at the time they reach the market. Drugs marketed on the basis of preliminary and incomplete data present a greater risk of unforeseen side effects, and even the risk that they are, in fact, clinically inactive. Many see this as a modest risk outweighed by the advantage of having new drugs available sooner for people with serious illnesses. Others justifiably worry that physicians are put into a position of prescribing drugs approved through the accelerated approval process, knowing very little about appropriate dosage, possible drug interactions, long-term toxicity, and even true effectiveness.

The FDA has also been criticized for not enforcing the requirement that drug companies conduct follow-up, postapproval, phase III clinical trials. The problem here is that the FDA has no enforcement powers once approval is granted.

Expanded-access and accelerated-approval programs have created another problem: Because the first makes experimental drugs widely available, and the other puts them rapidly on the market, patients have less motivation to enroll in randomized controlled clinical trials. As a result, whether complete data will ever be collected on drugs for life-threatening diseases through the clinical trial process is uncertain.

The FDA has used two strategies to accelerate the clinical trial process: telescoped trials and the use of surrogate markers.

■ Telescoped Trials

These are clinical trials that combine phase I and phase II trials to obtain data on drug safety, and preliminary evidence of efficacy and dosage. Telescoped trials involve more patients than typical phase I trials, and they are randomized. Telescoped trials may not provide adequate information on the optimal dosage for a drug. As a result, patients might end up taking a dose that is higher than necessary, which can mean more severe side effects and higher drug cost.

■ Surrogate Markers

In clinical trials of antiretroviral drugs, the best indicators to show that a drug is effective are clinical outcomes such as longer survival time and fewer occurrences of opportunistic infections. But for the slowly progressing disease caused by HIV infection, completing a study using such clinical end points could take months or years. So researchers began using laboratory, or surrogate, markers instead. Surrogate markers are changes in some disease sign or symptom that signal a response to treatment.

An example of a surrogate marker for HIV disease is the number of CD4 lymphocytes, the white blood cells that are destroyed by HIV. CD4 counts are used as a measure of the health of an HIV patient's immune system. If CD4 counts are stabilized or increased by a certain treatment, this is considered a sign that disease is not progressing or that the treatment is helping the patient; whether it also means the treatment will extend the patient's life, however, remains unknown.

Another surrogate marker is viral load, the amount of free virus in the blood. Recent research has shown that a consistently low viral load does extend survival, but it cannot be automatically assumed that because a new antiretroviral agent lowers viral load, the agent will also prolong survival in those using it; the agent could reduce viral load, for example, but have side effects that actually shorten survival time.

For such reasons, the effectiveness of drugs approved on the basis of CD4 counts, changes in viral load, or other surrogate markers must be verified through a clinical trial. That trial is usually under way at the time the drug is approved, and the FDA has the authority to rescind approval if the trial does not verify the drug's efficacy.

The drawbacks to using surrogate markers include the following:

- An experimental therapy that is effective—that extends life—could go undetected because it works in a way unrelated to the surrogate marker.

- Toxic side effects—especially longer-term side effects—that outweigh short-term benefits can be missed.

- A surrogate marker that proves to be associated with improved survival during the testing of one drug may or may not be applicable to a different drug.

- An experimental drug might seem efficacious in terms of the surrogate marker but in reality is toxic or clinically ineffective.

Thus, relying on surrogate markers for drug efficacy involves risks. The challenge is to find markers that are reliably correlated with survival and drugs that have few side effects.

■ CLINICAL TRIALS FOR HIV DISEASE LOSE PARTICIPANTS

For a clinical trial to produce results that are scientifically useful, that is, that reliably show whether a new drug is effective, the trial must involve a certain number of patients in each of the groups being compared to each other. The size of the groups is determined statistically.

The smaller the expected difference between treatments, the larger the number of participants will be required, and vice versa. A major problem that confronts clinical researchers is that too many patients initially volunteer but later drop out of drug trials.

An example of the problem was reported in a September 1995 issue of the journal *Science.* It involved ACTG Protocol 175, which compared the effectiveness of AZT to the effectiveness of AZT plus ddC, AZT plus ddI, and ddI alone. The trial involved patients previously treated with AZT ("AZT-experienced patients") and patients never treated with AZT ("AZT-naive patients"). The trial showed that AZT-experienced patients with midstage disease who continued to take AZT had death rates of about 10% during the trial. But in patients who took ddI alone or AZT plus ddI, the death rate dropped to 5% to 6%—a significant increase in survival rate.

The researchers felt fortunate to have detected such a difference because more than half—53%—of the study's 2,467 patients had discontinued their assigned treatment prematurely and had dropped out of this important trial. This is one example of the problems that many researchers say are creating a crisis in the development of drugs for HIV disease.

Progression of HIV disease can often be slowed by antiretroviral treatments and by the prevention and treatment of opportunistic infections. Unfortunately, many of the drugs that have been available for HIV disease have had only limited effectiveness. As a result, patients often became desperate, and their despair has manifested itself in ways that have undermined the accuracy of clinical trials in the following ways:

- Some patients have lied about their medical history to meet protocol entry criteria.

- Once enrolled in a trial, some patients have used drugs that were not permitted by the protocol, particularly if they thought they were randomized into the control group.

- Patients dropped out of a trial early—sometimes after only a few weeks—to enlist in a different trial or to put together their own treatment regimen.

To detect the sometimes subtle differences between a new drug and a standard treatment, clinical trials must be scientifically sound: They must be strictly randomized, they must involve a sufficiently large number of patients, and the patients must adhere to the requirements of the protocol. But to succeed, clinical trials must also be acceptable to patients. To induce patients to comply with protocols, some experts recommend the following:

- Allow patients to enroll in more than one clinical trial at a time, as long as the trials do not conflict with one another.

- Allow patients in a trial testing a sequence of drugs to change to the next series of drugs should their symptoms worsen, rather than allowing such a change only according to an arbitrary timetable.

- Always use standard-of-care controls.

- Patients receiving the experimental treatment should receive the standard of care plus the test drug. This allows all patients to receive the best available treatment.

■ How to Join a Clinical Trial

If you are a person with HIV disease, your doctor may at some point suggest that you join a clinical trial. Alternatively, you may want to investigate for yourself what clinical trials are available for people at your stage of disease. Sources of information on clinical trials are listed in Appendix 1.

If you cannot decide whether to enter a clinical trial, discuss the decision with people you trust such as your HIV/AIDS expert physician. When you agree to enter a trial, keep in mind that the requirements of the trial may affect, in addition to yourself, other people in your life—you may need transportation to a clinic on a regular basis, for example. Be sure these people understand how important the trial is to you. If you have trouble arranging transportation or meeting some other requirement of the trial, discuss the problem with the protocol nurse or the physician conducting the trial.

The following is a list of questions you should ask him or her:

- Is the trial a phase I, phase II, or phase III study?

- Is it randomized?

- How will I be protected from possible side effects?

- What aspects of care will be provided at no cost, and what costs might I become responsible for?

- If the drug produces favorable results, will I be given a free supply until it is approved and available for purchase?

- What will happen if the trial is stopped or if I am removed from the trial?

- What if the drug doesn't work for most people but it works for me? Can I continue taking it?

- If I am in the control group and get worse, will I be given the experimental drug? Or vice versa, if the experimental drug makes me feel worse, can I be switched to the control group receiving the standard treatment? ■

Chapter 7

OPPORTUNISTIC INFECTIONS AND HIV DISEASE

The primary effect of HIV on the body is the gradual destruction of key immune-system cells, particularly helper T lymphocytes. Helper T cells, also known as the CD4 lymphocytes, play a key role in initiating and coordinating immune responses (see Chapter 16). The loss of CD4 lymphocytes and other cells with the CD4 receptor, especially monocytes/macrophages, causes a progressive weakening of the immune system. This in turn gives microbes that are normally kept in check by the immune system an opportunity to flourish and cause disease. For this reason, the diseases induced by these microbes are known as "opportunistic infections." (The progressive dysfunction of the immune system is also linked to the development of a number of cancers in HIV-infected patients; see Chapter 8.)

Opportunistic infections are directly responsible for up to 90% of the deaths associated with HIV disease. They develop primarily from two sources. Some, such as toxoplasmosis, occur through the reactivation of an infection acquired by many people earlier in life, often during childhood. An infection such as this is kept under control and harmless by a fully functional immune system. As the immune system becomes progressively dysfunctional during HIV disease, the infection then redevelops and causes disease.

Other opportunistic infections represent pathogens that are newly acquired from the environment. Many arrive in the body when inhaled into the lungs as either free spores or spores associated with dust and dirt; others are ingested with water or raw foods. Again, a normal immune system prevents them from causing disease, but the damaged immune system of people with advanced HIV disease is no match for them. *Mycobacterium avium* is a microbe acquired from the environment that is dangerous only to people with profound immune impairment.

Some microbes, such as the fungi responsible for athlete's foot and candidiasis, are so common in both the environment and the human body that they are simply considered always present from birth. They cause serious disease only in cases of immune impairment. In the case of *Pneumocystis carinii,* scientists now believe the pneumonia (PCP) it causes in people with HIV disease results mainly from newly acquired *Pneumocystis* infections.

Opportunistic infections also occur in people whose immune system is severely depressed following organ transplantation or chemotherapy for some types of cancer (chemotherapeutic drugs damage cells in the bone marrow that give rise to immune-system cells). Thus, research on the prevention of opportunistic infections in people with HIV disease is helping to prevent opportunistic infections in other immune-suppressed patients as well.

As described in Chapter 4, "HIV Infection and the Course of HIV Disease," HIV disease progresses from one phase to the next as the number of CD4 lymphocytes declines and viral load increases. The loss of CD4 cells signals the gradual decrease in immune function, and the growing risk of various opportunistic infections—although all the opportunistic infections that occur during early HIV disease can also occur during later stages of disease.

Opportunistic infections can be caused by any of four types of microbial life:

- Bacteria. These are the most primitive types of cells, and they are capable of independent life in the environment. Bacterial infections are usually treated with antibiotics.

■ Viruses. Viruses are not capable of independent life but must be inside of cells in order to reproduce, or replicate. Viral infections are usually unaffected by antibiotics and must be treated with antiviral drugs. (See also Chapter 17.)

■ Fungi. These are primitive plant-like organisms. In people with HIV disease, fungal infections can occur on the surface of the skin, as in athlete's foot or ringworm; on mucous membranes of the mouth, throat, and vagina, as in candidiasis; or as an infection that spreads (disseminates) throughout the body, as in disseminated coccidioidomycosis. Systemic fungal infections tend to be more resistant to treatment than are bacterial infections, and a longer course of treatment is often necessary. Note that yeasts are also fungi.

■ Protozoan parasites. These are one-cell animals that invade human cells and live in them as parasites. Many of these organisms also enter the body during a spore-like phase in their life cycle. Cryptosporidiosis and toxoplasmosis are examples of protozoan infections.

■ PREVENTION, MANAGEMENT, AND TREATMENT OF OPPORTUNISTIC INFECTIONS

While a broad range of infections is known to arise in people with HIV disease, it is very unlikely that any one person will experience all the opportunistic infections possible. The kinds of infections that do arise can vary in different parts of the country and the world because the organisms that cause them are found more abundantly in some areas than others.

Whenever possible, it is essential to prevent opportunistic infections. For PCP, *Mycobacterium avium* complex (MAC), and toxoplasmosis, this is done through prophylaxis, that is, the use of drugs to prevent primary infection or reactivation. (Prophylaxis comes from a Greek word meaning "to guard before.")

A strong immune system is the first line of defense against opportunistic infections. Thus, the early use of combination antiretroviral therapy (see Chapter 5) can help preserve immune function and prevent opportunistic infection. Diet and rest are also important in helping to maintain the health of the immune system (see Chapter 13).

The management of opportunistic infections is divided into three phases:

- Primary prophylaxis, or preventing an initial infection. Preventing opportunistic infections from ever occurring is important whenever possible because once the disease arises, the drugs used to treat it will usually not eliminate the disease-causing organism from the body. This means that when treatment stops, there is a good chance the infection will return. CD4 counts determine when primary prophylaxis should begin.

- Treatment of an active infection.

- Secondary prophylaxis. This is used to prevent an infection from recurring, and it must usually be taken for life. It is also known as suppressive, or maintenance, therapy.

The use of prophylaxis is often essential to the survival of someone with HIV disease. Before prophylaxis was used, PCP was the most common opportunistic infection to appear in people with AIDS, and the leading cause of their death. Because of prophylaxis, however, the incidence of PCP and frequency of deaths from PCP is now much lower.

As HIV infection progresses to advanced and late-stage disease, however, there may be cases in which the advantages and disadvantages of prophylactic or suppressive drugs for some opportunistic infections should be discussed with a physician. The advantages of prophylactic therapy include the following:

- Prevention of disease

- Decreased severity of disease

- Decreased risk of and necessity for hospitalization

- Probable decrease in the number of sick days and lost wages

- Potential psychological benefits

- Preservation of health insurance benefits by staying healthier

The disadvantages of prophylactic or suppressive therapy for some infections can include the following:

- Additional drug side effects

- The risk of harmful drug interactions, which becomes a growing consideration as the number of drugs taken increases

- The possibility that use of the drug will produce drug-resistant forms of the pathogen, which is of particular concern with fungal infections

- The psychological effect on the patient of adding another drug to those already being taken, which may discourage the patient from following his or her prescribed antiretroviral treatment

- Cost of the therapy

■ Combination Therapy and Prophylaxis for Opportunistic Infections

In many HIV-positive individuals, highly active antiretroviral therapy (HAART) reduces the viral load to undetectable levels and leads to an increase in CD4 cell counts to above 200 cells per mm^3, the level at which PCP prophylaxis begins. When this happens, can prophylaxis be discontinued? No. Although the number of CD4 cells may rise to above 200 cells per mm^3, the new lymphocytes are thought to be immature and unable to respond to antigens (i.e., they are "antigen naive"). Antigen-naive lymphocytes are unable to generate effective immune responses and suppress opportunistic infections.

For this reason, the U.S. Public Health Service/Infectious Diseases Society of America (USPHS/IDSA) guidelines for the prevention of opportunistic infections[1] recommend that people on combination antiretroviral therapy who have CD4 cell counts that rise above 200 cells per mm^3 continue prophylaxis *based on their lowest CD4 count.*

Research is under way to determine whether HAART started early in HIV disease will preserve the function of CD4 lymphocytes and the immune system. The hope is that if combination antiretroviral therapy is started early and HIV is suppressed before it does significant damage to the immune system, it may be possible to avoid many, perhaps most, of the opportunistic infections and cancers associated with HIV disease. It is therefore important for anyone who thinks he or she has been exposed to HIV to seek testing and, if found to be HIV positive, to begin anti-retroviral treatment as early as possible (see Chapter 5).

■ OPPORTUNISTIC INFECTIONS DESCRIBED IN THIS CHAPTER

For a listing of the opportunistic infections and cancers used by the Centers for Disease Control and Prevention (CDC) to define and classify HIV/AIDS, see Appendix 2.

This chapter describes the most common opportunistic infections that can occur during HIV disease. They are listed alphabetically under the following headings:

- Bacillary angiomatosis

- Candidiasis—oral, esophageal, vaginal

- Coccidioidomycosis

- Cryptococcosis

- Cryptosporidiosis

- Cytomegalovirus (CMV)—retinitis, esophagitis, colitis

- Herpes simplex infection

- Histoplasmosis

- Microsporidiosis

- *Mycobacterium avium* complex (MAC)

- Oral hairy leukoplakia

- *Pneumocystis carinii* pneumonia (PCP)

- Shingles (varicella-zoster virus [VZV])

- Toxoplasmosis

- Tuberculosis (TB)

Caution: The drugs mentioned for prophylaxis, treatment, and suppression of the opportunistic infections described here are given for information only. They can have different degrees of effectiveness and severe side effects, and some are not well tolerated and do not apply to children and pregnant women. People with HIV disease should always discuss treatment options with a physician experienced in the treatment of HIV disease.[2]

■ BACILLARY ANGIOMATOSIS

Bacillary angiomatosis is an infection that is caused by species of the bacterium *Bartonella* (which is also responsible for cat-scratch disease in the general population).

Bacillary angiomatosis occurs most often in men and during advanced HIV disease, when the number of CD4 lymphocytes falls below 100 cells per mm³. The infection can affect the skin and internal organs. It can also produce bacteremia—infection of the blood, which can produce fever, chills, and weight loss.

The most common signs of infection are reddish-purple papules, nodules, or plaques on the skin. These swellings range in size from one-eighth of an inch to larger than one inch. They can occur singly or number up to 100 or more. The nodules often bleed easily and are sometimes painful to the touch. Nonpigmented nodules can also occur deeper in the skin. These can be painful to the touch and may affect underlying bone.

Bacillary angiomatosis can also produce ulcerous nodules on the mucous membranes of the mouth, nose, stomach, intestines, and anus. In the respiratory tract, the disease causes sores on the larynx, trachea, and bronchi. When bone infection occurs, it usually arises in the lower part of the arm or leg and can be painful. Infection of the liver causes abdominal pain and fever. Other sites of infection can include bone marrow, lymph nodes, heart and spleen, and (rarely) the brain.

Recognition and diagnosis of bacillary angiomatosis is sometimes delayed in people infected with HIV because the skin manifestations often resemble Kaposi's sarcoma and other infections of advanced HIV disease.

A definitive diagnosis often requires microscopic examination of biopsied tissue or culturing the infectious organism from blood or an affected site.

■ Reducing Risk of Exposure

People with HIV disease, particularly those who are severely immunocompromised, are at unusually high risk of developing relatively severe disease due to infection by *Bartonella* species. It is unclear how the bacteria responsible for bacillary angiomatosis are transmitted, but cat bites and scratches are strong risk factors. For this reason, people with HIV disease should consider the potential risks of cat ownership. The USPHS/IDSA guidelines recommend the following:

- Those who decide to acquire a cat should adopt or purchase an animal that is more than one year old and is in good health.

- Declawing a cat is not generally advised, but HIV-infected individuals should avoid rough play with cats and situations in which scratches or bites are likely. Wash any cat-associated wound promptly. Cats should not be allowed to lick an open cut or wound of an HIV-infected person.

- Care of cats should include flea control (*Bartonella* has been isolated from cat fleas, but it remains unknown whether the fleas actually transmit the infection to humans or other animals).

- There is no evidence that routine testing of a pet cat for *Bartonella* reduces the risk of infection.

■ Prevention of Disease

There is no evidence to support the use of a drug for prophylaxis of bacillary angiomatosis.

■ Treatment

Bacillary angiomatosis is reported to respond well to the antibiotics erythromycin and doxycycline or other macrolides or tetracyclines.

■ Prevention of Recurrence

Relapse of bacillary angiomatosis often occurs even after prolonged antibiotic therapy. USPHS/IDSA guidelines make no firm recommendation for suppressive therapy to prevent the recurrence of bacillary angiomatosis, but long-term suppression of infection with erythromycin or doxycycline should be considered.

■ CANDIDIASIS

Candidiasis is an infection of mucous membranes by the yeast (fungus) *Candida albicans,* normally a harmless member of the flora of the gastrointestinal tract. About 80% of healthy people harbor the fungus. Under certain conditions—such as suppression of the immune system—*Candida albicans* proliferates and causes disease. Occasionally, other species of *Candida* will produce candidiasis, but this usually occurs in patients with advanced HIV disease who have been taking therapy to prevent recurrence of *Candida albicans.*

Candidiasis commonly occurs in the mouth and throat (oral candidiasis), in the vagina (vaginal candidiasis), and in the esophagus (esophageal candidiasis).

■ Oral Candidiasis (Thrush)

Thrush, or candidiasis of the mouth and throat (also known as "oropharyngeal candidiasis"), is one of the earliest and most common opportunistic infections of HIV disease. It often occurs when the number of CD4 lymphocytes drops below 300 cells per mm^3. Its occurrence generally signals progression from asymptomatic HIV infection to early symptomatic HIV disease. In HIV disease, oral candidiasis can occur months or years before the onset of more serious opportunistic infections.

Oral candidiasis can take several forms. The most common form—pseudomembranous candidiasis—produces painless white spots or patches on the tongue, gums, palate, lining of the cheeks, or throat. These spots, or plaques, range in size from fractions of an inch to large patches. They consist of dead skin cells, and yeast cells and other components of the fungus. The plaques are easily scraped away. Removal of the patches leaves the skin surface red or slightly bleeding.

A second form of oral candidiasis, erythematous candidiasis, produces smooth red patches, usually on the palate, tongue, and lining of the cheeks. These can be difficult to see. This form of candidiasis can also be a harbinger of advancing HIV disease.

A third form of candidiasis—angular cheilitis—is less common in HIV-infected patients. It produces cracks or fissures at the corners of the mouth.

In rare cases, oral candidiasis extends into the bronchial airways and the lungs, a condition that requires prompt antifungal treatment.

Definitive identification of candidiasis can be obtained by culturing scrapings from the mouth and by microscopic examination of scrapings. Conditions that can be visually mistaken for oral candidiasis include the following:

- Aphthous ulcers or herpesvirus infection can produce whitish sores in the mouth, but they tend to be more painful than oral candidiasis.

- Oral hairy leukoplakia produces thick white patches on or along the sides of the tongue. The patches often have folds or vertical corrugations and a rough, hair-like texture. Unlike oral candidiasis, oral hairy leukoplakia cannot be scraped away.

■ Vaginal Candidiasis

Vaginal candidiasis is a common infection in up to one-third of healthy women. It can be an early and persistent opportunistic infection in women with HIV infection. Symptoms can begin when the level of CD4 lymphocytes is as high as 500 cells per mm^3. Vaginal candidiasis produces a creamy white discharge from the vagina or removable white plaques on the vulva. It also causes itching, burning pain, and pain during intercourse.

■ Esophageal Candidiasis

Candidiasis of the esophagus is the most common gastrointestinal infection in persons with AIDS. It can make swallowing difficult and cause pain on swallowing. Oral candidiasis with difficulty in swallowing is often a good indicator of esophageal candidiasis, though that symptom does not always occur. (Other causes of painful swallowing include CMV or herpesvirus infection, or an ulcer.)

■ Reducing Risk of Exposure

Candida is commonly found on the skin and on mucous membranes. No measures are available to reduce exposure to this and related fungi.

■ Prevention of Disease

The USPHS/IDSA guidelines do not recommend routine primary prophylaxis for candidiasis for the following reasons: Treatment of the disease is highly effective; most forms of candidiasis are not associated with mortality; prophylaxis could lead to the development of drug-resistant forms of *Candida;* continuous prophylactic treatment would increase the possibility of drug interactions; and prophylactic treatment is expensive. There is evidence, however, that fluconazole can reduce the risk of oral, esophageal, and vaginal candidiasis (and cryptococcosis) in individuals with advanced HIV disease.

■ Treatment

Initial treatment of oral candidiasis usually involves the use of topical therapies such as a clotrimazole lozenge or other antifungal medication (i.e., a suspension). A number of topical over-the-counter treatments for vaginal candidiasis are also available. For severe or recurrent candidiasis, the treatment of choice is an azole drug such as ketoconazole, fluconazole, or itraconazole.

■ Prevention of Recurrence

Suppressive therapy is usually not recommended for the reasons given previously. But if recurrences are frequent or severe, the USPHS recommends that patients use a topical treatment with nystatin or clotrimazole, or take orally ketoconazole, fluconazole, or itraconazole. Adults and adolescents with a documented history of esophageal candidiasis, particularly multiple episodes, should be considered candidates for chronic suppressive therapy with fluconazole.

■ COCCIDIOIDOMYCOSIS

Coccidioidomycosis (kok sid e oy´ do mycosis) is an infection of the lungs caused by a fungus that normally lives in soil. Coccidioidomycosis tends to occur when the number of CD4 cells drops below 250 cells per mm³.

General symptoms often resemble those of a lower respiratory tract infection. They can include fever, cough, shortness of breath, loss of appetite, and weight loss. In people with HIV disease, coccidioidomycosis often disseminates to other areas of the body. Disseminated disease often occurs in the membranes surrounding the brain (i.e., the meninges); the bones of the skull, hands, feet, and joints; skin; and the soft tissues. Depending on the location of the disease outside the lungs, symptoms of disseminated coccidioidomycosis can include swollen lymph nodes (generalized lymphadenopathy), skin nodules or ulcers, and headache.

Coccidioidomycosis is caused by the fungus *Coccidioides immitis,* which is common in the soils of the southwestern United States, particularly in California, Arizona, and Texas. Its range also extends to Mexico and Central and South America. The risk of developing coccidioidomycosis is 10% or more for people with HIV infection who live in areas where the fungus is found. The number of cases of the disease tend to increase following dust storms, heavy construction, and other events that disturb soil inhabited by the fungus.

Infection occurs when spores from the fungus are inhaled into the lung. There, they can cause inflammation. In most people with an intact immune system, the infection usually produces no symptoms or the symptoms of a simple upper respiratory tract infection.

■ Reducing Risk of Exposure

People living in or visiting areas in which *Coccidioides immitis* occurs cannot completely avoid exposure to the organism. Whenever possible, though, they should avoid exposure to activities associated with increased risk (i.e., exposure to farm fields during plowing, dust storms, and building excavation sites).

■ Prevention of Disease

USPHS/IDSA guidelines make no recommendation for routine chemoprophylaxis of coccidioidomycosis.

■ Treatment

Itraconazole or fluconazole is the preferred treatment. Alternative drugs include amphotericin B (which is a very active drug against this disease, but also the most toxic of the group).

■ Prevention of Recurrence

Individuals treated for coccidioidomycosis require lifelong suppressive therapy. Fluconazole is the preferred agent; alternative drugs include itraconazole and amphotericin B.

■ CRYPTOCOCCOSIS

Cryptococcosis is the most common cause of meningitis in people with AIDS. It is caused by the yeast *Cryptococcus neoformans.* Development of cryptococcosis usually requires significant impairment of the immune system and generally does not occur until the CD4 count drops below 100 cells per mm^3.

Symptoms of cryptococcosis include headache, fever, lethargy, nausea, and vomiting. Patients often experience intermittent symptomatic and asymptomatic periods.

The infection can occur in the brain itself, where it can mimic the appearance of a brain tumor in diagnostic images produced by computed tomography (CT) and magnetic resonance imaging (MRI). Other sites of infection include the lungs, liver, heart, skin, lymph nodes, adrenal glands, and genitourinary tract. Diagnosis of cryptococcal meningitis is important because early treatment of the disease can be very effective. There are also other causes of meningitis in HIV-infected patients.

They include the bacterium that causes TB, and possibly HIV itself.

Cryptococcosis has been a significant cause of death in people with HIV disease. The mental status of the person when cryptococcosis is diagnosed is an important indicator of the person's prognosis. A patient who is confused, is lethargic, or has otherwise impaired mental status usually has a poor prognosis.

Cryptococcus neoformans is found in soil and in the droppings of pigeons and other birds. The source of infection is thought to be inhaled fungal spores. The fungus is then carried by the blood to other parts of the body. The most common site of infection is the meninges, the membranes that surround the brain, which become inflamed and cause cryptococcal meningitis. An estimated 6% to 10% of people with HIV disease develop cryptococcal meningitis.

■ Reducing Risk of Exposure

HIV-infected persons cannot completely avoid exposure to *Cryptococcus neoformans,* but avoiding sites likely to be heavily contaminated with the fungus (e.g., areas heavily contaminated with pigeon droppings) may reduce the risk of infection.

■ Prevention of Disease

The USPHS/IDSA guidelines indicate that the drugs fluconazole and itraconazole can reduce the frequency of cryptococcal disease in patients with advanced HIV disease. Prophylaxis should be considered for patients with a CD4 lymphocyte count lower than 50 cells per mm^3. Prophylaxis is not recommended for routine use, however, because of a lack of proven survival benefits, the possibility of drug interactions, the possibility that it will give rise to drug-resistant strains of *Candida* and *Cryptococcus,* and its cost.

■ Treatment and Suppressive Therapy

Amphotericin B is given initially as the preferred treatment. Fluconazole is given to complete the treatment and for lifelong suppressive therapy.

■ CRYPTOSPORIDIOSIS

Cryptosporidiosis is a common cause of diarrhea in persons with HIV disease. The infection is caused by *Cryptosporidium parvum,* a protozoan parasite that infects cells lining the digestive tract. Chronic cryptosporidiosis that lasts more than 30 days is also an AIDS-defining condition.

Symptoms of cryptosporidiosis include severe diarrhea, weight loss, abdominal cramps, nausea, and vomiting. There is usually no fever. In patients with a CD4 lymphocyte count above 300 cells per mm^3, cryptosporidiosis can clear up on its own. In persons with a lower CD4 count, it can become a chronic illness with many recurrences and remissions. In late-stage HIV disease, cryptosporidiosis can be unremitting and contribute to the cause of death.

Cryptosporidium also sometimes infects cells lining the airways and lungs. Symptoms resemble those of a general respiratory infection. They can include coughing, wheezing, shortness of breath, hoarseness, and croup.

Cryptosporidium infection begins with ingestion of the spore-like oocysts, which are produced by the protozoan. The parasite passes through a many-staged life cycle that ends with the production of more oocysts. These are released into the intestine to reinfect the same host or pass out in the feces to infect new hosts.

The oocysts are very resistant to destruction. They remain viable in the environment for many months, and they remain infectious even after being exposed to many common disinfectants, including the chlorine in tap water. Oocysts are destroyed by boiling.

■ Reducing Risk of Exposure

Sources of infection include humans of all ages, dogs, cats, and farm and laboratory animals. Oocysts can be passed from person to person, probably from hand to mouth after contact with items such as diapers from infected children. Cryptosporidiosis is also transferred between sexual partners. Unprotected anal intercourse and oral-anal contact increase the risk of infection. The USPHS/IDSA guidelines recommend the following to reduce exposure to cryptosporidiosis:

■ Avoid contact with human and animal feces. Wash hands after contact with human feces during diaper changing, after handling pets, and after gardening or having other contacts with soil. Avoid sexual practices such as unprotected anal intercourse and oral-anal contact that may result in exposure to feces.

■ Newborn and very young pets may pose a small threat of exposure to *Cryptosporidium*, but it is not necessary to destroy or give away healthy pets. Persons acquiring a new pet should avoid bringing any animal with diarrhea into the household and should avoid obtaining a dog or cat less than six months old (individuals willing to accept the small risk of acquiring a puppy or kitten less than six months old should have the animal's stool examined for *Cryptosporidium* by a veterinarian before they have contact with the animal). They should not adopt stray pets.

■ Avoid exposure to calves and lambs, and to areas where these animals are raised.

■ Avoid drinking water directly from lakes, streams, or rivers. Cryptosporidiosis can also be contracted from water accidentally swallowed while swimming in lakes, reservoirs, rivers, or public swimming pools.

■ Outbreaks of cryptosporidiosis sometimes occur in municipal water supplies. To learn if *Cryptosporidium* occurs in a local water system, contact the water safety board or health department. During *Cryptosporidium* outbreaks, boiling water for one minute will eliminate the risk of cryptosporidiosis.

Special water filters will also reduce the risk of contracting cryptosporidiosis from tap water. These filters are known as "submicron filters." Use only those filters that operate by reverse osmosis, those that are labeled "absolute" 1-micron (1-μm) filters, or those that meet National Sanitation Foundation (NSF) standard no. 53 for "cyst removal." Avoid "nominal" 1-μm filters, as they may not remove all oocysts.

One can also drink bottled water to reduce the risk of cryptosporidiosis, but one should not presume that all brands are free of *Cryptosporidium*. Water from wells and springs is less likely to be contaminated with *Cryptosporidium* oocysts than is water from rivers or lakes.

Distilled water or water treated by reverse osmosis is safe, as is water passed through the filters just recommended.

■ The risk of exposure to cryptosporidiosis from ordinary municipal tap water is uncertain. In the case of cryptosporidiosis outbreaks, tap water can be filtered or bottled water used as just described. A physician should be consulted for advice as to whether either is necessary, as those who pursue these options often encounter difficulties in selecting and using them consistently.

■ Other important sources of *Cryptosporidium* infection include ice made from contaminated tap water and fountain beverages served in restaurants, bars, and theaters (these drinks and the ice they contain are made from tap water). Beverages safe to drink are nationally distributed bottled or canned carbonated soft drinks, and noncarbonated soft drinks and fruit juices that do not require refrigeration until opened. Nationally distributed brands of frozen fruit juice concentrate are safe if reconstituted with water from a safe source. Fruit juices that must be kept refrigerated can be either fresh (unpasteurized) or heat treated (pasteurized); only those juices labeled "pasteurized" should be considered free of *Cryptosporidium*.

■ Prevention of Primary Infection and Recurrence

No drug is available for the prevention of primary or recurrent cryptosporidiosis.

■ Treatment

There is no good treatment for cryptosporidiosis. Many agents have been tested, but research is hampered by lack of a simple system for culturing *Cryptosporidium* in the laboratory and by lack of a good animal model in which to test prospective drugs.

■ Primary therapy is supportive care, with intravenous administration of fluids, electrolytes, and nutrients, supplemented by liquids taken by mouth.

■ Antiretroviral therapy that results in improved immune-system function sometimes improves symptoms.

■ CYTOMEGALOVIRUS DISEASE

CMV is a herpesvirus that causes disease in up to 40% of people with advanced HIV disease. The virus can affect a variety of organs, but symptomatic CMV disease most often occurs in the eyes, producing CMV retinitis; the esophagus, producing CMV esophagitis; and the intestines, producing CMV colitis.

CMV disease usually arises through the activation of a CMV infection acquired earlier in life that persisted as a latent infection. Activation of the virus usually occurs during late-stage HIV disease, when CD4 lymphocyte counts have dropped below 100 cells per mm³.

General symptoms of CMV infection include fever, muscle pain (myalgia), a drop in white blood cell count, and weight loss. Specific symptoms depend on the organ affected.

■ CMV Retinitis

CMV retinitis is seen in up to 40% of people with advanced HIV disease. The virus causes loss of sight by producing swelling of cells in the retina, the light-sensitive lining of the eye, and by causing its detachment and killing its cells. Loss of sight due to retinal detachment or due to the death of retinal cells is irreversible; loss of sight due to swelling is reversible. Antiviral treatment (see below) can halt progression of CMV retinitis; left untreated, the condition progresses to blindness.

■ CMV Esophagitis

About 10% of HIV-infected people with CMV disease develop CMV esophagitis, an inflammation of the lower esophagus. It produces large, shallow ulcers in the region of the esophagus that joins the stomach. CMV esophagitis more typically occurs in patients with a CD4 count below 50 cells per mm³. After candidiasis of the esophagus, CMV esophagitis is probably the second most common cause of pain on swallowing.

■ CMV Colitis

CMV colitis, or infection of the intestines by CMV, produces fever, weight loss, anorexia, malaise, abdominal pain, and severe diarrhea. It can also produce hemorrhaging and perforation of the intestine, both of which are life-threatening conditions.

Similar symptoms of gastrointestinal inflammation, however, are produced by other infectious agents found in individuals with advanced HIV disease. These include *Cryptosporidium,* microsporidia, *Giardia* protozoa, and *Salmonella* bacteria. Similar symptoms can also be produced by gastrointestinal lymphoma and Kaposi's sarcoma. CMV colitis occurs in less than 10% of people with both advanced HIV disease and CMV disease.

■ Reducing Risk of Exposure

USPHS/IDSA guidelines recommend the following for reducing exposure to CMV:

- HIV-infected persons at low risk for CMV infection but who anticipate possible exposure to CMV (such as through blood transfusion or employment in child care, where the virus can be readily acquired through contact with an infected child) should be tested for antibody to CMV. People at low risk for CMV infection include those who have not had male homosexual contact and who are not injection drug users. Those who test negative for CMV (and who therefore are uninfected) should avoid situations that place them at risk for acquiring CMV infection.

- Latex condoms should be worn during sexual activity because CMV is shed into semen, cervical secretions, and saliva.

- HIV-infected adults and children are at increased risk of acquiring CMV infection at child-care facilities. Good hygienic practices such as hand washing are important to reduce the risk of exposure.

- HIV-infected individuals who are seronegative for CMV and require a blood transfusion should receive only CMV antibody–negative or leukocyte-reduced cellular blood products in nonemergency situations.

■ Prevention of CMV Disease

USPHS/IDSA guidelines recommend the following:

- The best protection against severe CMV retinitis is early recognition of the disease. An important warning sign is an increase in the number of "floaters" (vague objects that float across the field of view within the eye). Individuals should also assess their visual acuity through the simple test of trying to read a newspaper. Some experts recommend that individuals with CD4 lymphocyte counts below 100 cells per mm^3 receive regular eye exams that use a funduscope, a device used to examine the interior of the eye through the pupil. If evidence of CMV retinitis is found, treatment must be sought promptly.

- Oral ganciclovir has been shown to delay the onset of CMV retinitis, but use of the drug remains controversial. Its use may be considered in patients with a CD4 lymphocyte count below 50 cells per mm^3, but side effects, limited efficacy, lack of improved survival, and cost should be considered before implementing the use of this drug.

■ Treatment

The drugs ganciclovir and foscarnet comprise the standard treatment for CMV disease. Foscarnet also seems to slow HIV replication in some patients. Both drugs work by blocking the viral enzyme DNA polymerase, which is required for viral replication. Cidofovir is a third drug approved for the treatment of CMV retinitis. The major side effect of cidofovir is kidney damage, so the drug is given with a second drug, probenecid, and plenty of fluids to help protect the kidneys.

The antiviral drugs used to treat CMV disease block the virus from spreading, but they do not eliminate it from the body. Thus, lifelong suppressive therapy is necessary. Effective regimens include intravenous or oral ganciclovir, intravenous foscarnet, intravenous ganciclovir plus foscarnet, and intravenous cidofovir. CMV retinitis is also treated by surgically implanting a 4-mm-diameter device—a vitreal implant—in the eye. The implant slowly releases ganciclovir into the eye, thereby placing a high concentration of drug near the site of infection. The implant does not provide protection for the person's other eye or for other organs of the body. The implant must also be replaced periodically for effective maintenance therapy.

■ HERPES SIMPLEX VIRUS INFECTION

Herpes simplex virus (HSV) infection is one of the most common of viral infections in the U.S. population. There are two types of human herpes simplex viruses. HSV type 1 (HSV-1) is primarily responsible for cold sores or fever blisters that develop around the mouth and nose. HSV type 2 (HSV-2) is the primary cause of genital herpes, which produces cold sore–like outbreaks on and around the anus and genitals. Both viruses, however, can cause sores at either site—HSV-1 is responsible for genital sores in 15% of cases.

In HIV disease, an initial HSV-1 infection can produce painful vesicles along the lips, tongue, mouth, and throat. The vesicles often merge and erupt to produce large ulcerous sores that are covered by a pale-yellow film. Recurrences in some HIV-infected patients are more frequent than in non-HIV-infected people; other HIV-infected patients experience mild, infrequent, and self-healing recurrences. Recurrences tend to become more frequent and to last longer as the immune system weakens, particularly when the number of CD4 lymphocytes falls below 50 cells per mm^3. If severe HSV sores are left untreated, they can persist for weeks.

HSV infection of the genitals begins as fluid-filled vesicles that quickly ulcerate, producing painful sores. The period of sore formation can be prolonged in HIV-infected individuals, with continued virus shedding and local pain. In some individuals—even those not infected with HIV—shedding of virus, during which the virus can be transmitted to others, can occur even in the absence of sores. Other symptoms can include swelling and tenderness of groin lymph nodes and difficulty urinating.

Other sites of HSV infection in people with HIV disease include the following:

- Perianal region. HSV infection often produces ulcerated itchy and painful sores around the anus that can extend upward between the buttocks or internally in the rectum. Rectal sores make defecation painful and difficult. Symptoms of rectal HSV sores can include constipation, fever, impotence, and impaired bladder function.

- Esophagus. Infection of the esophagus by HSV can make swallowing painful and difficult and can interfere with eating. Similar symptoms can be caused by esophageal candidiasis or CMV infections.

- Brain. Infection of the brain by HSV is rare in HIV-positive patients, but when it occurs, it is a life-threatening condition. Symptoms can include fever, headache, nausea, lethargy, and personality change. Definitive diagnosis can be difficult because cryptococcal infection and toxoplasmosis produce similar symptoms.

About 70% of Americans are infected with HSV-1, while 16% are estimated to be infected with HSV-2. HSV-2 infection tends to be more common in women than in men, but the highest known frequency occurs in HIV-infected homosexual and bisexual males, 68% to 77% of whom tend to be infected (other HIV-infected populations have yet to be studied well).

Both types of HSV are transmitted through direct contact of a healthy mucous membrane with an infected, virus-laden one. When a person is initially infected with HSV, the immune system, using both antibodies and cytotoxic T lymphocytes (see Chapter 16), works to clear the infection at the site of contact. But before this happens, HSV particles enter nearby sensory nerves and travel up their length to the body of the nerve cell, which lies in the dorsal ganglion near the spinal cord. There the virus resides as a latent infection.

Reactivation of a latent HSV infection can be triggered by events such as stress, fever, exposure of the face to sunlight, menstruation, nerve injury, or a weakening of the immune system. The virus particles then travel down the length of the nerve and cause eruptions and sores in the area of skin served by the nerve. Release of the virus from the skin—viral shedding—occurs whether sores are present or not.

■ Reducing Risk of Exposure

Herpes simplex is transmitted through direct contact of mucous membranes. It is therefore important to use latex condoms during every act of sexual intercourse to prevent HSV transmission, and to avoid all sexual contact—including oral sex—when genital sores are present.

■ Prevention of Disease

Prophylaxis is not recommended to prevent initial herpes infection.

■ Treatment

Acyclovir is the drug of choice for the treatment of herpes simplex infections. Foscarnet is an effective treatment in most cases of acyclovir-resistant HSV, which occurs in a small percentage of people with HIV disease.

Because episodes of active HSV infection respond well to treatment, secondary prophylaxis (suppressive therapy) is not usually necessary. Individuals who experience frequent and severe recurrences, however, can be given oral acyclovir as suppressive therapy. Intravenous foscarnet or cidofovir can be used to treat infections resistant to acyclovir (such infections tend to resist ganciclovir as well). Topical preparations of foscarnet and cidofovir are also available.

■ HISTOPLASMOSIS

Histoplasmosis is a disease caused by the fungus *Histoplasma capsulatum*. It primarily affects the lungs, although it can disseminate to other areas of the body in individuals with a weakened immune system. In HIV disease, histoplasmosis usually starts occurring when the CD4 lymphocyte count drops below 200 cells per mm³, becoming more common with CD4 counts below 100 cells per mm³.

In individuals with advanced HIV disease, histoplasmosis can cause a respiratory illness accompanied by fever and weight loss. By the time of diagnosis, the disease has often spread to other areas of the body. This can produce enlarged lymph nodes (local or generalized lymphadenopathy), enlargement of the liver and spleen (hepatosplenomegaly), and sores in the colon. In a small number of patients, disseminated histoplasmosis also causes meningitis and ulcerated sores on the skin and in the mouth. On rare occasions, it will infect the retina, the pancreas, the prostate, and the membranes surrounding the heart and lungs.

Histoplasma capsulatum lives in soil enriched with bird and bat guano. It is found worldwide, but in the United States it is common in the Mississippi and Ohio river valleys, particularly in the states of Illinois, Indiana, Kentucky, Ohio, and Tennessee. Infection can result when fungal spores are inhaled into the lungs.

■ Reducing the Risk of Exposure

Avoid activities that increase the risk of infection, such as cleaning chicken coops, disturbing soil beneath bird roosting sites, and exploring caves.

■ Prevention of Disease

Itraconazole can reduce the frequency of histoplasmosis in people with advanced HIV disease (e.g., CD4 lymphocyte counts below 100 cells per mm^3) and who live in areas where *Histoplasma capsulatum* is endemic. However, in deciding whether prophylaxis is necessary, physicians should consider the possibility of drug interactions, drug toxicity, development of resistance, cost, and the need for prophylaxis or suppressive therapy for other fungal infections (e.g., cryptococcosis, candidiasis).

■ Treatment and Suppressive Therapy

Amphotericin B is the recommended treatment of severe histoplasmosis; itraconazole is effective for milder cases.

The USPHS/IDSA guidelines recommend use of itraconazole as lifelong suppressive therapy.

■ MICROSPORIDIOSIS

Microsporidiosis is thought to be a cause of diarrhea in many HIV-infected patients, although the disease is poorly understood. The infection is caused by a group of very small parasitic protozoa that live within cells that line the digestive tract. The protozoan *Enterocytozoon bieneusi* is chiefly responsible for the disease, although related species can also be involved.

Microsporidiosis produces a profuse, watery diarrhea, profound weight loss, and abdominal pain. Fever is absent. A definitive diagnosis is often difficult.

■ Reducing Risk of Exposure

Careful attention to hand washing and personal hygiene generally is the only precaution available to reduce the risk of exposure.

■ Prevention of Disease

No prophylactic drug is known to effectively prevent microsporidiosis.

■ Treatment

No effective treatment for microsporidiosis is known at this time. The most promising agent is albendazole.

■ *MYCOBACTERIUM AVIUM* COMPLEX

MAC is the most common bacterial opportunistic infection in people with advanced HIV disease. It is also one of the last opportunistic infections to develop in the course of HIV disease progression: Generally, it becomes apparent when the CD4 lymphocyte count drops below 50 cells per mm^3, and cell counts as low as 10 cells per mm^3 are common at the time of MAC diagnosis.

Symptoms of MAC infection include fever, malaise, weight loss, chronic diarrhea, and abdominal pain. The infection can interfere with the absorption of food and nutrients from the intestines, thereby contributing to malnutrition and wasting during late-stage disease.

Disseminated MAC infection affects a variety of organs, including the lungs, liver, spleen, lymph nodes, bone marrow, intestines, and blood. MAC infection is found almost exclusively in people with HIV disease; it rarely occurs in people who are immune suppressed for other reasons.

Two species of bacteria are responsible for MAC infections, *Mycobacterium avium* and *Mycobacterium intracellulare,* collectively referred to as *Mycobacterium avium* complex. Both are closely related to *Mycobacterium tuberculosis,* the bacterium that causes TB. MAC bacteria are found commonly in nature and probably enter the body by the inhalation of dust and during the consumption of food and water. The infection is not transmitted from person to person, so patients with MAC infection need not be isolated, as must HIV-infected patients with active TB.

MAC infection is thought to begin in the intestines. The bacteria then spread from there to the lymph nodes, blood, and other organs of the body.

■ Reducing Risk of Exposure

The bacteria responsible for MAC are commonly found in food, water, and the environment. There are no recommendations for avoiding exposure.

■ Prevention of Disease

USPHS/IDSA guidelines recommend the following:

- Clarithromycin or azithromycin is recommended for prophylaxis when the CD4 lymphocyte count drops below 50 cells per mm^3. Individuals who cannot tolerate clarithromycin or azithromycin can be given rifabutin.

- The presence of disseminated MAC should be ruled out before prophylaxis is started. If disease is present, multidrug therapy is used to treat it, whereas prophylaxis requires only one drug. If only one drug is given to treat the disease, drug resistance may develop. Similarly, TB should be ruled out in individuals receiving rifabutin for MAC, as resistance to rifabutin can result in cross-resistance to rifampin and make treatment of TB much more difficult.

■ Treatment and Suppressive Therapy

Aggressive treatment of MAC can relieve symptoms, but treatment does not eliminate the bacteria from the body, and recurrence is probable.

The recommended treatment is clarithromycin plus ethambutol. Azithromycin is an alternative to clarithromycin, but its effectiveness is uncertain.

Patients treated for disseminated MAC infections should continue to receive full therapeutic doses for life.

■ ORAL HAIRY LEUKOPLAKIA

Oral hairy leukoplakia produces white patches typically on the sides and surface of the tongue, but sometimes also on other areas of the mouth such as the soft palate, the lining of the cheeks and throat, and the floor of the mouth. It is a benign condition that occurs in about 20% of HIV-infected individuals with asymptomatic disease and a CD4 lymphocyte count above 500 cells per mm^3. It is, however, an indicator of progression from asymptomatic infection to symptomatic disease. The infection is relatively harmless, although it can be uncomfortable.

The white patches of oral hairy leukoplakia have a rough texture and a corrugated surface. They can vary in size from fractions of an inch to patches that cover the surface of the tongue. Oral hairy leukoplakia also occurs, but rarely, in immune-suppressed transplant recipients and during certain chemotherapy treatments for cancer.

Oral hairy leukoplakia results from a thickening of the outer cell layers of the oral mucous membrane. The thickening is produced by cells in the mucous membrane that are infected with Epstein-Barr virus (EBV), a type of herpesvirus.

Oral hairy leukoplakia can resemble oral candidiasis (thrush), but unlike oral candidiasis the surface of oral hairy leukoplakia cannot be scraped away. Physicians can diagnose oral hairy leukoplakia by microscopic examination of tissue from the affected area.

■ Prevention of Disease

There are no means available to prevent or suppress oral hairy leuko-plakia. (While EBV is transmissible by kissing, there is no evidence that oral hairy leukoplakia is transmitted this way.)

■ Treatment

Treatment of oral hairy leukoplakia is sometimes desired to improve appearance or to relieve discomfort. Oral acyclovir sometimes improves the condition, but when treatment stops, the condition recurs. Antifungal therapy can be used to control simultaneous candidiasis (see "Candidiasis," above).

■ *PNEUMOCYSTIS CARINII* PNEUMONIA

PCP is the most common HIV-associated pneumonia. Historically, prior to the use of prophylaxis, more than 80% of those with advanced HIV disease (AIDS) had at least one attack of PCP, and this opportunistic disease has been the leading cause of death among people with AIDS. Often, it was the first AIDS-defining illness to occur in people infected with HIV, usually developing in adults when the CD4 lymphocyte count dropped to 200 to 300 cells per mm^3.

Today, despite the existence of PCP prophylaxis, many people with HIV infection still develop PCP. In many cases, these are people who did not seek testing and consequently were unaware of their positive HIV status until PCP developed. Others develop PCP because they do not receive PCP prophylaxis. This can happen because they cannot tolerate the treatment, because of limited access to competent health care, or because it is their choice. A few develop PCP because prophylactic treatment is ineffective for them.

Generally, nonspecific signs of PCP can occur days to months before respiratory problems arise. These include fatigue, unexplained fever, and weight loss. (Oral candidiasis, another indicator of immune suppression, may also have occurred by this time.) Respiratory symptoms of

PCP include fever; shortness of breath, or dyspnea; and an unproductive cough, a cough that does not produce sputum.

PCP is caused by *Pneumocystis carinii*, a microbe that can be acquired during childhood and resides in the body as a latent infection. When acquired, *Pneumocystis carinii* infection remains asymptomatic until suppression of the immune system permits its activation and the development of disease.

PCP is a life-threatening condition that damages lung tissue, allowing fluid to enter the lungs. This produces dyspnea and reduces the amount of oxygen entering the blood. Left untreated, PCP causes the brain and heart to receive insufficient oxygen and death occurs. *Pneumocystis carinii* sometimes infects tissues other than the lungs. In fact, it can infect all major organs, including the brain, heart, and kidneys.

■ Reducing Risk of Exposure

Some authorities recommend that HIV-infected persons at risk for PCP not share a hospital room with a patient who has PCP. This would make sense, but information is insufficient to support this recommendation as standard practice.

■ Prevention of Disease

USPHS/IDSA guidelines recommend the following for prophylaxis of PCP:

- HIV-infected adults and adolescents, including pregnant women, should receive prophylaxis for PCP if they have a CD4 lymphocyte count below 200 cells per mm^3, an unexplained fever above 100°F for two weeks or longer, or a history of oral candidiasis.

- Trimethoprim-sulfamethoxazole (TMP-SMX) is the preferred drug for PCP prophylaxis. TMP-SMX can also provide cross-protection for toxoplasmosis and many bacterial infections.

- Patients who experience adverse side effects with TMP-SMX should persevere, if at all possible, in using this highly effective and inexpensive protective treatment. For those who have stopped TMP-SMX prophylaxis because of its side effects, the drug can be reintroduced starting with a lower dose and gradually increasing it. This is a desensitizing regimen.

■ Patients who cannot tolerate TMP-SMX can also try dapsone alone; or dapsone plus pyrimethamine plus leucovorin; or aerosolized pentamidine administered by the Respirgard II nebulizer (Marquest, Englewood, Colorado). Regimens that include dapsone plus pyrimethamine also protect against toxoplasmosis but not against bacterial infections.

■ For the time being, the following treatments for PCP prophylaxis should be considered only in unusual situations in which the above-mentioned agents cannot be used: aerosolized pentamidine administered by other nebulizer devices available in the United States, intermittently administered parenteral pentamidine, oral pyrimethamine-sulfadoxine, oral clindamycin plus primaquine, oral atovaquone, and intravenous trimetrexate. The efficacy of these agents for PCP prophylaxis has not been established through controlled clinical trials.

■ Treatment

TMP-SMX given orally or intravenously is the treatment of choice for mild, moderate, or severe PCP. TMP-SMX, however, is poorly tolerated by about 20% to 30% of patients. Dapsone-trimethoprim and clindamycin-primaquine are alternative therapies for the treatment of mild PCP in people who cannot tolerate TMP-SMX.

Intravenous pentamidine is the treatment of choice for severe PCP in people who cannot tolerate TMP-SMX. (Aerosol pentamidine has produced poor results as a form of PCP treatment.)

Prednisone can be used as adjuvant therapy in people with moderate to severe PCP and low oxygen levels in their blood. Prednisone has been clearly shown to reduce mortality in these individuals.

■ Prevention of Recurrence

USPHS/IDSA guidelines recommend that to prevent recurrence, adults and adolescents with a history of PCP should receive for life one of the prophylactic regimens just described.

■ SHINGLES

Shingles is caused by reactivated VZV (varicella-zoster virus), the herpes-type virus that causes chickenpox during childhood.

Symptoms of shingles include severe pain along the path of one or more infected nerves and a localized or segmented red rash. Papules develop on the skin of the affected body area. They become fluid-filled vesicles that can coalesce with neighboring vesicles to form larger blister-like swellings.

In patients with HIV disease, VZV infection can spread to areas of the skin beyond the rash, and it can also disseminate to internal organs such as the liver; the lungs, where it can produce pneumonia; or the brain, where it causes inflammation (i.e., encephalitis). These can be life-threatening conditions. If VZV reactivation occurs along certain nerves of the face, it can result in infection of the cornea. This condition often also includes vesicles on the tip of the nose. Postherpetic neuralgia—pain that persists after skin blisters have healed—can also occur. Recurrent episodes of shingles are common in people with HIV disease.

During a childhood case of chickenpox, varicella-zoster virions invade sensory nerves and travel up their length to the main body of the nerve cell, or neuron. The body of these neurons lies in the dorsal root ganglia, bundles of nerve cells located near the spinal cord. The VZV then quietly resides there as a latent lifelong infection. As the immune system weakens either with old age or with an acquired or induced immune deficiency, this virus becomes reactivated. It travels back down the length of the sensory nerve to cause shingles in the area of skin served by this nerve.

■ Reducing Risk of Exposure

HIV-infected children or adults who have not had childhood chickenpox, or who tested seronegative for VZV, are susceptible to infection by this virus and should avoid exposure to it through contact with people with either chickenpox or shingles.

■ Prevention of Disease

The USPHS/IDSA guidelines recommend that HIV-infected children and adults who are susceptible to VZV be given zoster immune globulin within 96 hours of contact with someone who has chickenpox or shingles. (The guidelines note that acyclovir would be a logical drug for the prevention of chickenpox in susceptible HIV-infected adults and children, but that data are lacking on the effectiveness of this approach.)

No measures are available to prevent shingles.

■ Treatment

Acyclovir is the treatment of choice for shingles. Foscarnet is recommended for the treatment of acyclovir-resistant VZV.

■ TOXOPLASMOSIS

Toxoplasmosis is an opportunistic infection caused by the protozoan *Toxoplasma gondii*. This protozoan lives in cats and other animals, and it is transmitted by contact with feces and by the eating of raw or undercooked meat.

Toxoplasmosis in people with HIV disease nearly always results from the reactivation of a latent *Toxoplasma gondii* infection acquired in childhood. About 75% of the people in the United States have antibodies to *Toxoplasma gondii*. Women with active toxoplasmosis infection during pregnancy can transmit the infection to their fetus (see Chapter 12).

Toxoplasmosis tends to cause three types of disease:

- Cerebral toxoplasmosis, or toxoplasmic encephalitis, results from toxoplasmic infection of the gray matter of the brain. This is the most common form of toxoplasmosis, occurring in 5% to 15% of people with HIV disease whose CD4 lymphocyte count has dropped below 100 cells per mm^3.

  Early symptoms of toxoplasmic encephalitis can include headache, confusion, lethargy, and low-grade fever. Later symptoms can include weakness, tremors, vision loss, speech disturbances, loss of coordination, sensory loss, and seizures. Personality changes including anxiety, agitation, paranoia, and dementia can occur. Infection of the spinal cord can produce sensory and coordination disturbances in one or more limbs, and loss of bladder or bowel control. Symptoms of life-threatening disease include seizures, coma, and cerebral hemorrhage.

■ Ocular toxoplasmosis, or toxoplasmic retinochoroiditis, is a relatively infrequent infection of the retina of the eye, less common than CMV retinitis (see "Cytomegalovirus Disease," above).

■ Pulmonary toxoplasmosis, or toxoplasmic pneumonitis, occurs in rare instances with infection of the lungs. Its symptoms are very similar to those caused by PCP; they include fever, cough, and difficulty breathing.

A definitive diagnosis of toxoplasmosis can be difficult to make. Antibody tests for identifying a reactivated infection have limited usefulness. In addition, the images of cerebral toxoplasmosis produced by CT and MRI often resemble those produced by central nervous system (CNS) lymphoma, progressive multifocal leukoencephalopathy (PML), CMV and HSV infection of the brain, and Kaposi's sarcoma.

For these reasons, patients suspected of toxoplasmosis are often treated for this infection and observed for improvement in their symptoms and a clearing of the lesions previously seen on CT and MRI scans.

■ Reducing Risk of Exposure

All HIV-infected individuals should be aware of the possible sources of toxoplasmosis. This is particularly important for those who lack antibodies to *Toxoplasma*.

Toxoplasmosis is acquired through contact with fecal material from infected cats; through the consumption of raw or undercooked infected meat, especially pork, lamb, and venison (beef is infected less often); or through drinking water contaminated with *Toxoplasma*. To reduce the risk of exposure, the USPHS/IDSA guidelines recommend that HIV-infected individuals take the following precautions:

■ Never eat raw or undercooked meat, particularly undercooked pork, lamb, or venison. Meat should be cooked to an internal temperature of 150°F; meat cooked until it is no longer pink inside generally has reached an internal temperature of 165°F and therefore satisfies this requirement.

- Wash hands after contact with raw meat and after gardening or having other contacts with soil.

- Wash fruits and vegetables well before eating them raw.

- HIV-infected individuals need not part with a pet cat, and they need not have the cat tested for toxoplasmosis.

- The encysted stage of *Toxoplasma gondii*, which can be present in the feces of infected cats, can remain viable for up to 18 months in moist soil. Change a cat's litter box daily. This is best done by an HIV-negative person who is not pregnant. An HIV-infected individual who changes a litter box should wear gloves and wash his or her hands thoroughly afterward.

- A pet cat should be kept indoors and fed only canned or dried commercial food or well-cooked table food, not raw or undercooked meats.

- HIV-infected people should not adopt or handle stray cats.

■ Prevention of Disease

HIV-infected individuals should be tested for antibody to *Toxoplasma* soon after the result of their blood test for HIV is known. Those who test positive to antibody for *Toxoplasma* should be considered at risk for developing toxoplasmosis.

The USPHS/IDSA recommends the following:

- HIV-infected individuals with a CD4 lymphocyte count below 100 cells per mm^3 and who have antibodies to *Toxoplasma* should receive prophylaxis against toxoplasmosis.

- TMP-SMX given to prevent PCP also appears to prevent cerebral toxoplasmosis. (Pentamidine does not seem to offer similar protection.)

- People who cannot tolerate TMP-SMX should try dapsone plus pyrimethamine.

■ Treatment

The combination of pyrimethamine plus leucovorin (to reduce marrow toxicity) plus sulfadiazine is standard therapy for toxoplasmosis. Up to nine out of ten patients respond to this treatment, but 20% to 40% of patients experience side effects, usually to the sulfadiazine. Clindamycin can be substituted for sulfadiazine in these patients.

■ Prevention of Recurrence

Drug regimens for toxoplasmosis are ineffective against the encysted form of the parasite, so discontinuing the therapy results in a relapse in 40% to 80% of patients. For this reason, suppressive therapy must be taken for life.

Pyrimethamine plus leucovorin plus sulfadiazine given at a dose lower than the treatment dose is highly effective. Clindamycin is commonly substituted for patients who cannot tolerate sulfadiazine. However, only the combination of pyrimethamine plus leucovorin plus sulfadiazine also protects against PCP.

■ TUBERCULOSIS

People with HIV infection are at high risk of developing TB, which tends to occur when the CD4 count drops to 300 to 400 cells per mm^3, somewhat earlier than other AIDS-defining opportunistic infections. TB is, however, preventable and curable if detected early in HIV-positive people.

Symptoms can include fever, night sweats, weight loss, cough, and coughing up blood (hemoptysis). The variety of symptoms can vary, however, depending on the site of infection.

TB is caused by the bacterium *Mycobacterium tuberculosis*. This bacterium can be present in the body as a latent infection, effectively suppressed by the immune system, or it can be present as active TB. It can affect any organ, although the primary site of infection is usually the lungs. The infection can spread to other areas of the body through the lymphatic and blood systems.

Active TB is highly contagious for people with a weakened immune system. Pulmonary TB is acquired by inhaling droplets produced when an infected person coughs or sneezes. Blood coughed up by a person with TB is also infectious.

When a person with a strong immune system becomes infected by TB bacteria, his or her immune system does not eliminate the bacteria from the body. Rather, it surrounds them with a capsule that includes large numbers of immune-system cells, primarily macrophages. The capsule and the cells it contains is known as a "granuloma." The granuloma provides a barrier that prevents the bacteria from multiplying, spreading in the body, and producing disease. This barrier breaks down in people with a weakened immune system, such as people with HIV disease. This is why it is important that TB infection be detected early in them, that prophylactic treatment be initiated promptly, and that immunodeficient people with active TB be given multidrug treatment for the disease. They should also be tested to determine if they carry drug-resistant strains of *Mycobacterium tuberculosis*.

■ Diagnosis

A tuberculin skin test is a standard screening test for TB that is given to HIV-positive individuals during their initial examination. The skin test, or PPD test (for purified protein derivative), reveals whether the person has been infected by TB bacteria. The PPD test involves injecting under the skin a small amount of protein derived from dead TB bacteria. A positive test result indicates that the bacteria are present in the body. The test does not reveal, however, whether the infection is latent and contained by the immune system, or active and causing disease.

The culturing of *Mycobacterium tuberculosis* from sputum (coughed-up mucus) is the gold standard for the diagnosis of active pulmonary TB. Sputum cultures also determine whether an individual is infected with drug-resistant forms of *Mycobacterium tuberculosis*. Culturing the bacteria, however, takes several weeks, which is too long to help determine which drugs should be used for initial treatment of active TB.

HIV-infected persons who have a positive PPD test result should receive a chest X-ray and clinical examination for TB. If active disease is present, the individual should begin treatment immediately; if active disease is not present, he or she should begin prophylaxis.

■ Reducing Risk of Exposure

The possibility of exposure to TB is increased for people who work in health-care facilities, correctional institutions, homeless shelters, and similar settings. An HIV-infected individual employed in one of these settings should discuss the risk of TB exposure with his or her physician. The discussion should consider the person's duties, the prevalence of TB in that setting, and the precautions being taken to prevent TB transmission within the facility.

■ Prevention of Active TB

Prophylactic treatment is recommended for HIV-positive persons in whom a PPD test result is positive at the time they are found to be positive for HIV or in whom a positive PPD test result was found earlier in life; it is also recommended if they had recent contact with someone who has active TB. Risk of past exposure to TB is higher in someone with a history of homelessness, imprisonment, alcoholism, or use of illicit substances.

- Isoniazid (INH) taken for 12 months is the preferred regimen to reduce the risk of active TB in individuals with *Mycobacterium tuberculosis* infection. To reduce the risk of peripheral neuropathy, those receiving INH should also receive pyridoxine. (Note: Acetaminophen should not be taken when using isoniazid, as the combination can cause liver damage.)

- Rifampin taken for 6 to 12 months is recommended for patients unable to take isoniazid.

- HIV-infected individuals exposed to multidrug-resistant forms of TB should receive high-dose ethambutol and pyrazinamide, plus a fluoroquinolone such as ofloxacin or ciprofloxacin. Ofloxacin or ciprofloxacin is recommended, as many strains of *Mycobacterium tuberculosis* are resistant to ethambutol and pyrazinamide. **Prophylactic treatment of drug-resistant TB should extend for at least one year.**

■ Treatment

The emergence and rapid spread of drug-resistant strains of *Mycobacterium tuberculosis* has changed the way in which active TB infection is treated in HIV-positive individuals. Because current tests cannot determine for as long as six weeks whether a person is infected with multidrug-resistant TB, treatment now routinely begins with the use of four to six drugs. The Centers for Disease Control and Prevention recommends a four-drug regimen that consists of isoniazid, rifampin, pyrazinamide, and ethambutol or streptomycin.

This treatment should be modified for people who likely were exposed to multidrug-resistant TB and for people who live or work in areas where it is common. The treatment regimen for TB should then include at least two more drugs to which local strains of *Mycobacterium tuberculosis* are known to be susceptible.

Take Medicine Exactly as Prescribed to Prevent Emergence of Dangerous New Strains of TB

The existence of multidrug-resistant strains of TB is a relatively recent event. Twenty years ago, two drugs, isoniazid and rifampin, were needed to cure TB. But because people often stopped taking the drugs too soon, isoniazid- and rifampin-resistant strains arose, and this led to the development of multidrug-resistant strains of TB.

The emergence of multidrug-resistant TB comes with tremendous cost to society: illness or death in people infected with the bacteria, the obvious cost of developing new drugs, and the less obvious costs of expensive prevention measures such as improving the ventilation systems in hospitals, homeless shelters, and soup kitchens to reduce the risk of TB transmission. Today, taking the full course of treatment for TB is regarded as so important that many cities assign social workers to watch people with active disease take their medicine. This "observed compliance" is done to ensure that individuals take their full course of treatment.

The point cannot be overemphasized: To avoid the emergence of still newer and more highly drug-resistant strains of TB, anyone treated for active TB must complete his or her drug regimen exactly as prescribed.

■ Prevention of Recurrence

Suppressive therapy is not needed after a recommended treatment for TB is successfully completed.

ENDNOTES

1. Centers for Disease Control and Prevention. 1997 USPHS/IDSA guide-lines for the prevention of opportunistic infections in persons infected with human immuno-deficiency virus. *MMWR* 1997;46(No. RR-12).

2. For more complete information on the prevention of these opportunis-tic infections in adults, children, and pregnant women, see the 1997 USPHS/IDSA guidelines. *Ibid.* The guidelines are also available through the CDC's site on the World Wide Web; see Appendix 1.

■ *Chapter 8*

CANCER AND HIV

Cancer, along with opportunistic infections, has been a hallmark of HIV disease from the beginning of the AIDS epidemic. It was the sudden appearance of a rare form of pneumonia, *Pneumocystis carinii* pneumonia (PCP), and a rare form of cancer—Kaposi's sarcoma (KS)—in gay men that heralded the emergence of AIDS in 1981.

Three types of cancer—KS, lymphoma, and cervical cancer—are seen much more frequently in patients with immunodeficiency than in the general population. For this reason, the Centers for Disease Control and Prevention (CDC) includes these cancers as AIDS-defining illnesses in people who are HIV positive (see Appendix 2). Other forms of cancer, however, can occur in people with HIV disease but no more frequently than they do in the non-HIV-infected population.

Unfortunately, cancer in people with HIV disease can be particularly difficult to treat. The immune deficiency caused by HIV, along with the drop in production of white blood cells in the bone marrow that accompanies HIV infection, makes the treatment of cancer more complex. People with HIV disease also tend to have cancers that are diagnosed at an advanced stage, that progress more rapidly, and that respond less well to treatment than the same malignancies in people without HIV disease.

Today, improvements in antiretroviral treatment for HIV disease is allowing many people with the disease to live longer. How these advances in treatment will affect future cancer rates in people infected with HIV is unknown. It could mean that because people with HIV disease are living longer, their incidence of cancer will rise. On the other hand, if antiretroviral therapy preserves or restores the function of the immune system, the rate of cancer in people with HIV disease could drop.

■ THE CAUSES OF CANCER

The fundamental causes of cancer involve mutations that damage genes responsible for the control of cell division, cell differentiation, and the natural process of programmed cell death or self-destruction (apoptosis). These mutations can occur from exposure to cancer-causing chemicals and from exposure to ionizing radiation and ultraviolet light. Many people also inherit genetic mutations that predispose them to cancer. Thus, cancer often arises because of genetic mutations that people are born with, plus genetic mutations that are acquired by exposure to cancer-causing agents.

Viruses have also been linked to some cancers, including those cancers listed as AIDS-defining illnesses. A newly discovered herpesvirus, known as KS-associated herpesvirus (KSHV) or human herpesvirus-8 (HHV-8), has been implicated in the development of KS. Epstein-Barr virus (EBV) is associated with many forms of non-Hodgkin's lymphoma, as well as Hodgkin's disease and Burkitt's lymphoma. Human papillomavirus types 16 and 18 have been linked to oral and cervical cancer and other anogenital cancers, and hepatitis B and C viruses are associated with liver cancer. Finally, the retrovirus human T-cell lymphotropic virus type I (HTLV-I) is associated with adult T-cell leukemia/lymphoma. HIV, which is also a retrovirus, has not been shown to directly cause cancer.

■ TYPES OF CANCER

Cancer is the name given to many different diseases that arise when cells grow out of control and invade other tissues. A cancerous tumor is often referred to as a "malignant neoplasm." "Neoplasm" means new growth, and it refers to the tumor. "Malignant" refers to the ability of a cancerous tumor to invade and destroy neighboring tissues and to spread, or metastasize, to other areas of the body. A benign tumor, on the other hand, does not spread to other tissues; it continues to grow, but it remains localized.

Tumors are referred to as "primary," or "secondary" or metastatic. A primary tumor is a tumor that originated in the tissue in which it is located; a secondary or metastatic tumor is a tumor that originated elsewhere in the body and spread to lymph nodes or to more distant sites in the body.

In general, the various types of cancer fall into two overall groups: cancers of the blood and lymphoid system, which include the leukemias and lymphomas; and cancers that arise in other tissues and form solid tumors.

■ Cancers of the Blood and Lymphatic Systems

Malignancies of the blood and lymphatic system are also known as "hematopoietic malignancies." "Hematopoietic" refers to the formation of blood cells. These malignancies consist of immature, nonfunctioning blood cells.

- *Leukemias* are malignancies of white blood cells found in bone marrow, the blood, the spleen, and other organs. There are several types of leukemias, depending on the origin and the degree of immaturity of the cells involved.

- *Lymphomas* are malignancies primarily of T and B lymphocytes. Most lymphomas fall into two overall categories: Hodgkin's disease (or Hodgkin's lymphoma) and non-Hodgkin's lymphoma (NHL). NHL, in turn, includes many different types of lymphoma. Rarer forms of NHL include Burkitt's lymphoma. NHLs constitute the second most common type of malignancy occurring in people with HIV disease, and they are described further below.

- *Myelomas* are lymphoma-like malignancies that arise mostly from white blood cells that are involved in antibody production (mature B lymphocytes known as plasma cells).

■ Solid Tumors

- *Carcinomas* are cancers that arise in cells that form epithelial tissue, the tissue that covers or lines organs of the body. An epithelium can be one cell thick, as it is in the intestines, or many cells thick, as it is in the skin. Cervical carcinoma is a malignancy of the epithelium that covers and lines the cervix ("cervix" is the name given to the opening of the uterus).

- *Sarcomas* are malignancies that arise in muscle, connective tissue, and bone. Sarcomas also occur in the liver, lungs, spleen, kidneys, bladder, and tissues that make up the blood vessels. KS is a cancer of the lining of certain blood vessels.

■ THE IMMUNE SYSTEM AND CANCER

In 1968, doctors began noticing that the incidence of lymphoma was higher in patients whose immune system was suppressed following kidney transplantation (suppression of the immune system is necessary prior to and following organ transplantation to prevent the body from rejecting the transplanted organ).

The incidence of some lymphomas is now known to be 30 to 50 times higher in transplant recipients than in the general population. Children born with certain immune deficiencies face a manyfold greater risk of lymphoma than do immunologically normal children. Transplant recipients also have higher rates of KS and squamous cell carcinoma of the skin.

These findings are evidence of the role played by the immune system in controlling cancer. Certain immune cells—among them natural killer cells (see Chapter 16)—patrol the body hunting for malignant cells and early tumors and are capable of destroying them.

This activity of immune-system cells has been known as "immune surveillance." Immune surveillance may actually protect against the viruses that have been closely associated with AIDS-related cancers. Damage to the immune system during HIV disease results in a loss of immune surveillance, and that in turn may allow the virus-associated cancers to develop in people with AIDS. For this reason, these malignancies are sometimes referred to as "opportunistic cancers."

■ TREATMENT OF CANCER

Cancer is traditionally treated through the use of surgery, radiation therapy, or chemotherapy. Newer forms of treatment include the use of biological response modifiers, which are cytokines and other substances that stimulate immune or other responses against tumor cells. Treatments for cancer can be local or systemic. A local treatment is a treatment that is restricted to the tumor itself and the area immediately surrounding it. Surgery is an example of a local treatment. A systemic treatment is a treatment that is delivered throughout the body. Chemotherapy is a systemic treatment because it is infused into a vein and carried throughout the body.

■ Surgery

Surgery is the oldest means of treating solid tumors. The surgical treatment of cancer involves the removal of the tumor along with a margin of healthy tissue and sometimes lymph nodes that drain the area of the tumor. Removal of small tumors or precancerous tissue is sometimes done using lasers (laser surgery), using cold (cryosurgery), or using heat or electricity (electrocautery).

■ Chemotherapy

Chemotherapy is the use of drugs to treat cancer. It is often used following tumor surgery as a means of killing cancer cells that may have spread to other areas of the body. Most chemotherapy drugs work by damaging cells that are undergoing cell division. Leukemia and lymphoma cells often divide particularly rapidly, and chemotherapy is a very effective treatment for these malignancies.

Most chemotherapy drugs also damage healthy cells that are dividing, including those in the bone marrow that produce new white blood cells and blood platelets (which are important for clotting). The loss of these white blood cells, all of which are components of the immune system, represents a form of immune suppression that weakens a patient's resistance to infections. In people with AIDS, this chemotherapy-induced immune suppression occurs in addition to the immune suppression caused by HIV. This limits and complicates the use of chemotherapy to treat cancer in HIV patients.

Chemotherapy also damages the actively dividing cells in the hair follicles, and cells that line the mouth and intestines. This results in hair loss and other side effects of chemotherapy. Nausea and vomiting can occur because of the effects many of these drugs have on the central nervous system (CNS) and on the vomiting center in the brain. Antinausea drugs are now available and often control the nausea and vomiting caused by chemotherapy.

Chemotherapy is usually administered by infusing one or more drugs into the body as a systemic treatment. For solid tumors, chemotherapy is sometimes given with or after surgery or radiation therapy. This use of chemotherapy as follow-up to surgery or radiation is known as "adjuvant therapy." It is intended to kill tumor cells that may have spread to other areas of the body. Occasionally, chemotherapy is injected directly into a solid tumor as a form of local treatment, as is sometimes done in the treatment of individual KS lesions.

■ Radiation Therapy

Radiation therapy uses ionizing radiation such as gamma rays or strong X-rays to kill tumor cells. Sometimes, radiation therapy is used before surgery to shrink the size of a tumor. Radiation therapy also often weakens the immune system through the destruction of bone marrow cells.

■ Biological Response Modifiers

These are natural and synthetic substances that stimulate or inhibit the activity of cells, including immune cells. Biological response modifiers include interferons, which have antiviral and antitumor effects; interleukins, which influence the growth and activity of white blood cells; and growth factors such as granulocyte colony-stimulating factor (G-CSF), which stimulate the development of blood cells. Interferon is an important drug in the treatment of KS.

■ HIV-ASSOCIATED MALIGNANCIES

■ Kaposi's Sarcoma

KS is a proliferation of cells that make up the walls of small blood vessels. HIV-associated KS (also called "epidemic KS") produces from one to many purple, pink, or red spots, patches, or nodules visible through the skin. The lesions usually occur on the face, neck, chest, or back, but they can arise almost anywhere. Other sites include the gums and palate, and internal organs such as the lungs, liver, spleen, pancreas, lymph nodes, adrenal glands, gastrointestinal tract, and testes. KS can be fatal, but its progress tends to be slower than that of opportunistic infections, which therefore are more immediately life-threatening.

In Western countries, HIV-associated KS is the most common malignancy in men with AIDS. It occurs about 20 times more frequently in homosexual and bisexual men than in hemophiliacs and male injection drug users with AIDS, and 50 to 100 times more often in men than in women. It does not occur in children, and whites are more frequently affected than blacks.

This distribution of the disease has led epidemiologists to believe that HIV-associated KS is caused by a sexually transmitted infectious agent other than HIV. As mentioned already, recent research linked a sexually transmitted human herpesvirus, KSHV, also known as HHV-8, in the development of KS. Although the association of this virus with KS is still somewhat controversial, evidence for its role continues to grow. Researchers also found KSHV associated with body cavity–based lymphomas in people with HIV disease (see below).

Treatment of HIV-associated KS depends on the status of the person's immune system and the stage and severity of HIV disease. If the immune system is relatively strong (i.e., CD4 lymphocyte counts of 250 or 300 cells per mm^3 or higher), and the individual is in otherwise good health, a period of "watchful waiting" may be appropriate. During this time, no treatment is administered and the disease is not likely to worsen. Individual lesions can be removed by cryotherapy (freezing), laser surgery, or radiation for the purpose of reducing local swelling, removing painful lesions, or for cosmetic reasons.

Systemic treatment involves combination antiretroviral therapy. In severe cases, treatment involves the use of chemotherapeutic drugs or interferon. Treatment may be delayed in people who are beginning antiretroviral therapy because improvements in immune status due to antiretroviral therapy can sometimes lead to the decrease and disappearance of KS lesions. The use of interferon-alpha is also effective in some patients with CD4 counts higher than 200 cells per mm^3.

■ Lymphomas

Lymphomas are malignancies that arise in T lymphocytes and B lymphocytes. Most HIV-related lymphomas tend to involve B lymphocytes and are known as "B-cell lymphomas." (Lymphomas that involve T lymphocytes also occur, but the incidence of T-cell lymphomas in people with HIV disease is no greater than it is in the general population, so T-cell lymphomas are not included as HIV-associated cancers.)

Non-Hodgkin's Lymphoma

NHL occurs in an estimated 4% to 10% of people with advanced HIV disease (AIDS). It is the second most common malignancy associated with HIV disease after KS, and it is the most common malignancy in injection drug abusers. The incidence of NHL is expected by some to increase as people with AIDS live longer, owing to more effective antiretroviral therapy and antimicrobial prophylaxis; others believe the NHL incidence will decrease because earlier and better control of HIV infection will sustain a relatively healthy immune system.

NHL more often occurs in people with a CD4 lymphocyte count below 50 cells per mm^3, although it can also occur in people with higher CD4 cell counts.

Symptoms of HIV-associated NHL include fever, night sweats, and weight loss of more than 10% of normal body weight. Lymphomas often begin in lymph nodes but may arise in or spread to a number of organs in the body. Occurrence of the disease outside the lymph nodes, which is very common in people with HIV disease, is referred to as extranodal disease or extranodal involvement. Sites of extranodal involvement can include the mouth and gums, brain and spinal cord, muscle, heart, adrenal glands, anus, and rectum. The variety of symptoms experienced by particular patients depends on the sites at which their lymphoma has occurred.

Treatment of HIV-associated NHL usually involves the use of multidrug chemotherapy. Treatment is complicated because the disease has usually spread to sites such as the bone marrow and CNS at the time of diagnosis. Also, because of the damage chemotherapy can cause to bone marrow cells (as described previously), individuals who already have a weakened immune system cannot tolerate the intensive chemotherapy regimens used to treat advanced NHL in non-HIV-infected patients. In people with HIV disease, such treatments might bring the lymphoma into remission but exacerbate a potentially fatal opportunistic infection. For this reason, regimens are being tested that use lower drug doses combined with hematopoietic growth factors that stimulate bone marrow cell function. Drugs that are less damaging to bone marrow cells are also being tested. The ultimate means of preventing NHL is to maintain immune function.

The cause of HIV-associated NHLs is unknown. They probably arise through several mechanisms that involve loss of immune function, chromosome or gene damage, and imbalanced cytokine production. EBV is associated with about half of all NHL cases (including those in non-HIV-infected people), but it is not thought to be the primary cause. EBV, however, is known to play an important role in a non-HIV-associated form of lymphoma that is endemic in parts of Africa, and it may also prove to be an important cause in AIDS patients.

Primary Central Nervous System Non-Hodgkin's Lymphoma

Primary CNS lymphoma is a form of NHL that rarely occurs in the general population, but it is seen in 4% to 6% of people with AIDS. Patients who develop primary CNS lymphoma almost invariably have a severely depressed immune system, with CD4 counts below 50 cells per mm^3. The disease usually occurs in the brain (rather than the spinal cord) and can cause a variety of symptoms during its progression, including headaches, confusion, lethargy, memory loss, partial paralysis, speech impairment, and personality changes.

Diagnosis of CNS lymphoma involves computed tomography (CT)

scans, which produce an X-ray–like image of the brain. But the characteristics of CNS lymphoma on CT scans are often difficult to distinguish from those produced by toxoplasmosis and other opportunistic infections that occur in the brain. Therefore, a brain biopsy may be needed for a definitive diagnosis. CNS lymphoma patients tend to fare worse than patients with systemic forms of lymphoma, with an average survival time of 2.5 months after diagnosis, even with therapy.

Treatment involves the use of steroids such as dexamethasone to reduce brain swelling and radiation therapy to shrink the tumor (although the use of steroids in AIDS patients can increase their susceptibility to disseminated fungal and bacterial infections). Experimental trials testing the use of chemotherapy are currently under way.

Body Cavity–Based Lymphoma

Body cavity–based lymphoma is a distinct class of HIV-related NHL that occurs in some patients with advanced HIV disease. Body cavity–based lymphoma develops as an accumulation of fluid, an effusion, that contains white blood cells. This effusion can occur in the spaces around the lungs, heart, or abdominal organs. There is no tumor mass as such. The cells involved are mature B cells that have become malignant. Cancerous cells from these tumors have shown signs of infection by both KSHV and EBV. This lymphoma can occur in patients who do not have KS.

Symptoms of body cavity–based lymphoma depend on the location of the effusion. Shortness of breath occurs if the effusion develops around the lungs; palpitations and compression of the heart accompany effusion around the heart; and swollen abdomen (ascites) occurs if the fluid accumulates in the abdominal cavity.

Hodgkin's Disease

There is growing evidence that Hodgkin's disease, a form of lymphoma, also occurs at a higher-than-usual incidence in people infected with HIV. Furthermore, the disease tends to follow a different course in individuals infected with HIV. The type of cell that gives rise to Hodgkin's disease remains unknown. Possibilities include B lymphocytes, T lymphocytes, and macrophages (these cells are described in Chapter 16). A diagnostic characteristic of Hodgkin's tumors is the presence of large, multinuclear cells known as "Reed-Sternberg cells."

In non-HIV-infected individuals, Hodgkin's disease usually first shows up as enlarged lymph nodes in one area of the body. The disease then progressively spreads to connecting groups of lymph nodes. This is sometimes accompanied by fever, night sweats, and weight loss. Eventually, tumor cells invade the liver and spleen.

In people infected with HIV, Hodgkin's disease is likely to be more advanced, more disseminated in the body, and more often accompanied by systemic symptoms (fever, night sweats, and weight loss) at the time of its diagnosis.

It also tends to be more resistant to treatment. The full-dose chemotherapy regimens used as standard therapy for Hodgkin's disease in the non-HIV-infected population usually cannot be used in people infected with HIV. As in the case of NHL, the immune and bone marrow deficiencies caused by HIV infection make the use of full-dose chemotherapy hazardous for HIV-positive people. Lower-dose chemotherapy regimens, some of which include hematopoietic growth factors, are being tested in clinical trials in people with HIV disease.

■ Cervical Cancer

Cervical cancer is a malignancy that arises in the epithelial tissue that covers and lines the cervix. Women with HIV disease are at a much higher risk of developing cervical cancer than are women in the general population (see also Chapter 11).

Cancer of the cervix progresses through several well-defined stages. It begins as an abnormal growth—a dysplasia—of the cervical epithelial cells. This precancerous condition is known as "cervical intraepithelial neoplasia," or CIN. The abnormal cells can be detected by a Papanicolaou test (also known as a "Pap test" or "Pap smear").

In non-HIV-infected women, untreated CIN spreads over a period of eight to ten years by the growth of abnormal cells throughout the thickness of the epithelial layer. However, it will not have yet broken through the lower boundary of the epithelium to invade neighboring tissue. This early stage of tumor development is known as "carcinoma in situ." With further progression, the tumor cells become malignant—they break through the thin membrane at the base of the epithelium and invade the wall of the uterus. At that point, the tumor becomes an invasive cervical cancer. Invasive cervical cancer is an AIDS-defining illness in women infected with HIV.

Cervical cancer is strongly linked to infection with human papillomavirus (HPV) types 16 and 18. These HPVs are sexually transmitted viruses (other types of HPV cause various kinds of common warts). When compared to women without HIV infection, women with HIV disease are more often infected with HPV and they are much more likely to develop CIN. Those with advanced HIV disease are more likely to develop CIN than are those with asymptomatic HIV disease. All of this suggests that HIV-caused immune suppression plays an important role in the rate of development of CIN, and probably in the rate of development of invasive cervical cancer itself. In addition, CIN in women infected with HIV is likely to be diagnosed at a more advanced stage, it is more likely to recur following treatment, and it is more likely to be associated with other carcinomas, including anal carcinoma (see "Cancer of the Anus").

Therefore, women with HIV infection should be monitored for CIN with a Pap test every six months. Some physicians also perform an initial colposcopy, the examination of the tissues of the vagina and cervix using a colposcope. A positive Pap test result should be confirmed by colposcopy and biopsy. Women with HIV disease should also be monitored for precancerous changes in the vulva, vagina, and anus.

Treatment of cervical cancer depends on the extent and stage of the disease at the time of diagnosis, and the woman's CD4 count. If the CD4 count is above 350 cells per mm^3, localized CIN can be treated by laser surgery, cryosurgery, or electrocautery; women with a lower CD4 count may require more aggressive therapy. This may include surgical removal of the opening of the cervix (a procedure known as "conization") or hysterectomy. Invasive cervical carcinoma is usually treated with radiation therapy, with or without surgery. Some regimens also use chemotherapy.

Although the prevalence of CIN is high in HIV-infected women, few have survived with advanced HIV disease long enough for CIN to progress to life-threatening invasive cervical cancer. This may change, however, as advances in antiretroviral treatment now allow HIV-positive people to live longer, even those with advanced disease. As was described for NHL, the incidence of CIN and cervical cancer may increase or decrease in the future.

■ Cancer of the Anus

Gay men practicing anal intercourse are at a relatively high risk of developing anal cancer. More than 95% of anal cancers are associated with HPV infection, primarily HPV 16 and 18, the same viruses responsible for cervical cancer. The immunosuppression caused by HIV infection may increase the risk of developing anal cancer still further. For this reason, HIV-positive gay men who practiced anal intercourse should receive routine inspection of the anal canal and the area around the anus (i.e., the perianal region) for signs of anal cancer or for precancerous changes known as "dysplasia." Some physicians now recommend a Pap-type test for gay men practicing anal intercourse, regardless of their HIV status. The test involves gently scraping superficial cells from the anal canal and examining them for dysplasia.

Anal cancer is treated using cryotherapy, electrocautery, surgery, radiation, or radiation plus chemotherapy, depending on the size and location of the tumor. Dysplasia, which is far more common, is treated with local therapies such as surgery, electrocautery, and occasionally cryotherapy or trichloroacetic acid for small lesions. Dysplasia of the perianal region may also be treated with direct application of the chemotherapeutic drug 5-fluorouracil.

Chapter 9

PREVENTION OF HIV INFECTION

Preventing HIV infection is of paramount importance at both individual and collective levels. In the absence of an effective vaccine against HIV, refraining from behaviors and practices that increase the risk of acquiring HIV (if one is HIV negative) and of transmitting it to someone else (if one is HIV positive) is the only means available now, and for several years to come, of slowing the HIV epidemic.

HIV is transmitted in three principal ways: through sexual activity; through contact with infected blood, primarily during injection drug use (IDU); and from HIV-infected pregnant women to their babies before or during birth, or during breast-feeding (see Chapter 3). In each case, there are ways to minimize the risk of transmission.

It is incumbent on everyone to reduce the rate of HIV transmission. This means everyone should know their HIV status and behave in an appropriate and responsible manner. Those who are HIV negative are responsible for protecting themselves from HIV. They should keep in mind not only their own health, but also the emotional and economic consequences that HIV disease would have for their loved ones. While anyone who is HIV positive is entitled to receive the best medical care available, that individual also has a moral obligation to do all that he or she can to avoid transmitting HIV to others. This means informing past and present lovers of one's HIV-positive status, and if in a relationship, working as a mutually caring couple to set jointly agreed upon standards of safe sexual behavior.

Acknowledging one's HIV status need not drive a couple apart. Rather, a shared emotional ordeal often increases the emotional involvement in a relationship. The value of a relationship and its emotional levels can acquire new depth.

Tom Coates, who is HIV positive and the executive director of the University of California San Francisco AIDS Research Institute, has said: "The very last thing I want to do is pass this virus along to anyone else." Certainly, the vast majority of people living with HIV share this feeling.

■ PREVENTING SEXUAL TRANSMISSION OF HIV

Sexual transmission is responsible for nearly two-thirds of AIDS cases in the United States, according to the Centers for Disease Control and Prevention's (CDC's) 1996 *HIV/AIDS Surveillance Report.*[1] Therefore, preventing the sexual transmission of HIV can do more than any other activity to slow the HIV epidemic.

Men having sex with men accounted for 40% of the new AIDS cases reported in the United States in 1996; men who have sex with men and also inject drugs made up an additional 4% of that year's new cases. Worldwide, however, heterosexual intercourse is the predominant mode of HIV transmission (see Table 3.1). In the United States, heterosexual intercourse accounted for 13% of new AIDS cases reported in 1996; this accounted for 6% of AIDS cases reported in men and for 40% of AIDS cases reported in women that year. HIV infection in women in turn leads to HIV-infected babies. Most heterosexual transmission occurs through vaginal intercourse, although a significant number of heterosexual couples in the United States also practice anal intercourse (see below). (For more on HIV transmission and the factors that increase its rate, see Chapter 3.)

■ General Recommendations for Preventing Sexual Transmission

The most effective means of protecting one's HIV-negative status is for two HIV-negative individuals to commit to mutually monogamous and faithful relationships in which neither person injects drugs. Any sexually active individual who is not in such a relationship should consistently practice safer sex. There is no way to guess whether an individual is HIV positive simply by looking at or talking with him or her. In fact, today, most HIV-infected individuals are unaware of their own infection because too many have neglected to be tested for HIV. Unfortunately, there is also no way to know when someone is lying about occasional infidelities and past use of injected drugs. It is therefore imperative for anyone, particularly someone with multiple sex partners, to use condoms during each act of intercourse (see "Using Condoms Correctly"). Condom use also helps prevent transmission of hepatitis and other sexually transmitted diseases (STDs).

Safer-sex practices include dry kissing (no case of HIV transmission has been traced to kissing, but the risk of transmission is increased during open-mouth or French kissing, particularly if one or both people have mouth sores or bleeding gums); kissing areas of the body other than the genitals and anus; caressing, hugging, and cuddling; rubbing body to body until climax; and masturbation, alone or mutually. For additional suggestions on safer-sex practices, contact the local AIDS service organization.

■ Condom Use

Studies have shown that the use of a condom during each act of intercourse is the most effective way to prevent HIV transmission during both anal and vaginal intercourse. A 1994 study by the European Study Group on Heterosexual Transmission, for example, examined the effectiveness of condoms in preventing HIV transmission in heterosexual discordant couples (couples in which one person was HIV infected and the other not).[2]

Among 124 couples who used condoms consistently, none of the HIV-negative partners became infected; of 121 couples who used condoms inconsistently, 12 uninfected partners (12%) became HIV infected. In that study, withdrawal prior to ejaculation was also associated with a lower risk of male-to-female transmission. Furthermore, the study found that the risk of infection was higher when the infected partner had advanced HIV disease, when genital sores were present, and when the couple practiced unprotected anal sex.

When used correctly during every act of intercourse, latex or polyurethane male condoms are the most effective means of preventing HIV transmission during vaginal and anal intercourse; on the other hand, lambskin or "natural membrane" condoms have pores that permit the passage of particles the size of HIV. Male condoms made of polyurethane plastic are also available. Laboratory tests have shown that particles the size of HIV cannot pass through this material. A study of the effectiveness of the polyurethane male condom in the prevention of pregnancy and STDs is under way. Polyurethane condoms can be made thinner than latex condoms, have no odor, are safe for use with oil-based lubricants, and, importantly, offer an alternative to people allergic to latex. The female condom, described later, also provides an effective barrier.

Condoms sold in the United States are regulated by the Food and Drug Administration (FDA) and are manufactured with stringent quality-control procedures. Condom failure rates in the United States are about 3%. Failure due to breakage is often due to improper storage or use. Condoms are weakened by age and by exposure to heat, sunlight, and oil-based lubricants. They can also be torn by teeth or fingernails. Cases of HIV transmission among couples using condoms are more often due to inconsistent or inappropriate use than to breakage or failure of the condom.

■ Women and HIV Prevention

The HIV epidemic is more than 15 years old, but women still have few means of HIV protection that are solely under their control. AIDS prevention programs have focused almost exclusively on the use of condoms by male partners. This requires the active cooperation of the male

■ Using Male Condoms Correctly

For maximum protection, all condoms must be used correctly and with each act of intercourse. Incorrect use can cause the condom to break or leak. Use a male condom correctly as follows:

- Use a new condom for each act of vaginal, anal, or oral intercourse.

- Put the condom on as soon as erection occurs and before the penis has any contact with the vagina, anus, or mouth.

- To put the condom on, hold the tip of the condom and unroll it onto the erect penis. To reduce the risk of breakage, leave space at the tip of the condom, ensuring that no air is trapped there.

- Adequate lubrication is important to prevent condom breakage. Use only water-based lubricants with latex condoms. Water-based lubricants include glycerin or lubricating jellies that are available at any pharmacy. Oil-based lubricants such as petroleum jelly, cold cream, hand lotion, baby oil, or substances such as cooking fats and oils can weaken latex condoms, although they have no effect on polyurethane condoms.

- Withdraw from the partner immediately after ejaculation, holding the condom firmly to the base of the penis to keep it from slipping off.

- Condoms lubricated with the spermicides nonoxynol 9 or octoxynol 9, both of which have been shown to kill HIV under research conditions, may provide additional protection should the condom rupture (although the anti-HIV effects of these spermicides remain controversial).

- Risk of HIV transmission is further reduced if the partner wearing the condom withdraws before climax. ■

partner or the ability of the woman to negotiate the conditions under which they will agree to engage in intercourse. If the man refuses to co-operate, the woman must choose between refusing to have sex with him—and possibly suffer dire repercussions—or participate in unprotected sex. This situation continues to have tragic consequences, particularly for women in coercive or abusive relationships, women who must trade sex for money or drugs, and women who have no education or say in sexual matters due to social circumstances.

Thus, there is an acute need for effective HIV prevention methods women can use without the consent and preferably even the knowledge of male partners. The need is all the more urgent because HIV is transmitted more effectively from male to female than from female to male during heterosexual intercourse. This is one reason why women are at higher risk than men of becoming HIV infected through heterosexual transmission of HIV in the United States, and why throughout the world, HIV-infected women outnumber men.

Two promising forms of protection for women are the female condom and chemical barriers—spermicides and microbicides that kill HIV.

Female Condom

The female condom is the most effective means of preventing vaginal HIV transmission presently available to women. It was approved by the FDA in 1993.

The female condom is a soft, loose-fitting plastic pouch about six inches long and two inches in diameter with a closed end that slips up into the vagina. When in place, the condom lines the entire length of the vagina. A soft, flexible ring at the closed end holds the condom in position in front of the cervix; a similar ring at the open end remains outside the body to protect the labia, or lips, of the vagina. During intercourse, the pouch catches and holds semen, thereby preventing pregnancy and transmission of HIV and other STDs. For information on use, see "Using the Female Condom."

As a contraceptive device, the female condom has a failure rate (measured in terms of slips, leaks, or tears) of 5% when used correctly during every act of intercourse; male condoms have a failure rate of 3% during similar "perfect" use. Under "typical-use" conditions, which means it might not have been used correctly or during every act of intercourse, the female condom has a failure rate of 21%, a rate expected to drop as people become more familiar with using it (the typical-use failure rate for the male condom is 12%). The effectiveness of the female condom in preventing HIV and STD transmission during typical use is under study.

■ Using the Female Condom

Directions for inserting the female condom are included with the product, along with a small container of additional lubricant. Recommendations and steps for proper use include the following:

- Use a new female condom for each act of intercourse.

- The female condom should not be used with a male condom.

- Spermicides can be used with the female condom. They can be applied to the vagina prior to insertion of the condom or to the inside of the condom if they are being used as a lubricant, or both.

- Before using the female condom the first time, practice inserting it two or three times in privacy to become accustomed to its application. (A new condom should then be used for sexual intercourse.)

- Inserting the female condom involves compressing the ring at the closed end of the condom and slipping it up into the vagina. When properly positioned, the condom is held in place by the pubic bone, as is a cervical cap. About one inch of the open end of the condom, which includes a second soft plastic ring, will remain outside the body to protect the lips—labia—of the vagina. It is important that the condom lies straight, not twisted, in the vagina.

- During intercourse, be sure that the outer ring is not pushed up into the vagina (if this begins to happen, stop and reposition the ring, add lubricant, or use a new condom) and that the penis is in the pouch and not under or alongside the condom and in contact with the vaginal wall.

- After intercourse, remove the condom by squeezing and twisting the outer ring to keep the semen inside. ■

A single female condom product is currently available over the counter under the brand name Reality (Female Health Company, Chicago, Illinois; toll-free phone number: 1-800-274-6601).

Chemical Barriers to HIV: Microbicides and Spermicides

A microbicide is a chemical that kills bacteria and viruses. A microbicide gel, cream, film, or suppository that could be applied to the vagina or rectum and kill HIV and other STD-causing pathogens during intercourse could protect a woman from HIV and be used without the knowledge or consent of her partner. Microbicides are not available yet, although they are under development. Ideally, two types of microbicides will emerge. One will kill sperm as well as HIV, and therefore will serve both as a contraceptive and as an anti-HIV agent. The second type will kill HIV but not sperm. Such a microbicide would protect women from HIV but also give them the option of becoming pregnant.

A spermicide is a chemical designed to kill sperm. In the United States, the spermicide nonoxynol 9 has been used for more than 40 years in contraceptive films, creams, foams, and gels and as a lubricant on condoms. Laboratory studies have shown that nonoxynol 9 also kills HIV on contact, suggesting it might also serve as an anti-HIV microbicide. Octoxynol 9, a chemical cousin of nonoxynol 9, shows similar spermicidal and anti-HIV activity. Both are detergent-like chemicals that disrupt the lipids in the cell membrane of sperm, killing them and thereby preventing conception. Similarly, they disrupt the lipids that compose the envelope of HIV, thereby destroying the virus.

Nonoxynol 9 is an effective contraceptive when used consistently and as directed. Whether nonoxynol 9 is equally effective in killing HIV in the environment of the vagina during intercourse remains unknown, and its effectiveness in preventing HIV transmission is controversial. Some studies have shown that topical use of nonoxynol 9 can reduce the risk of HIV transmission, but others suggest that its frequent use at high concentration can cause inflammation of the vagina and perhaps increase the risk of HIV transmission. Some studies have shown that topical use of nonoxynol 9 can reduce the risk of HIV transmission, while others suggest that it has no effect. These studies differed in such things as the form and concentration of nonoxynol 9 used and the length of time it was used. Thus, the effectiveness of nonoxynol 9 as a microbicide for HIV under typical day-to-day conditions remains unresolved. However, nonoxynol 9 has been recommended as one of several risk-reduction options in a ladder of options suggested for women by the Philadelphia Department of Health. (See "Safer-Sex Hierarchy for Women.")

Diaphragms and Cervical Caps

Controlled studies have not been done on the effectiveness of diaphragms and cervical caps as barriers to HIV or other STDs. Although some protection might be provided by these methods, they are certainly not recommended by themselves for protection against HIV infection.

Douching

Douching has been associated in some studies with an increase in risk of acquiring certain upper reproductive system infections. It is not known whether this is related to how the douching is done, or whether it is due to the douching itself. For example, douching could drive pathogens into the cervix and could remove natural protective lubricants and protective cells from the surface of the vagina. For these reasons, douching is not thought to be beneficial in preventing HIV transmission, and it may even increase the risk of HIV infection.

Female-to-Female Sexual Transmission

The risk of HIV transmission through female-to-female sexual contact is thought to be low, although the degree of risk remains unknown and possible cases of female-to-female HIV transmission have been reported in the medical literature. For these reasons, a barrier should be used during oral-genital contact (see "Oral Sex"). Sex toys such as dildos and vibrators should be sterilized between each use.

■ Oral Sex

No form of sexual activity between an infected and an uninfected person should be considered safe if it does not involve the use of a condom to prevent contact with semen or a barrier to prevent oral contact with vaginal fluid.

Oral stimulation of the penis (fellatio) is thought to have a lower risk of HIV transmission than vaginal or anal intercourse, but the degree of risk remains unknown. For this reason, a condom is recommended during fellatio. (Although the risk of transmission by oral sex is thought to be low, recent animal experiments suggest that it can happen. See Chapter 3.)

■ Safer-Sex Hierarchy for Women

The Philadelphia Department of Health recommends a ladder of options that women can use to reduce the risk of HIV transmission during vaginal intercourse. These options are ranked in order from most effective to least effective as follows[3]:

- Male or female condom

- Diaphragm or cervical cap with spermicide

- Spermicide alone

- Withdrawal (removal of penis from vagina prior to ejaculation) ■

Oral stimulation of the clitoris and vulva (cunnilingus) is also thought to have a lower risk of HIV transmission than vaginal or anal intercourse. Again, however, its degree of risk remains unknown. For this reason, a barrier such as a new condom cut along its length, should be used between the mouth and genitals (avoid using lubricated condoms and condoms with spermicide). Plastic food wrap is sometimes used as a barrier during cunnilingus. This material may not provide a completely safe barrier but it is preferable to no barrier at all.

■ Anal Intercourse

Anal intercourse is practiced not only by some gay men, but also by a significant proportion of heterosexual couples. Surveys of the general population indicate that 10% to 25% of women have engaged in anal intercourse. The proportion can reach 40% to 50% in some ethnic groups that use anal intercourse as a form of contraception and for protection of virginity (adolescents, too, can practice anal intercourse for the same reasons).

Anal intercourse is generally considered the behavior presenting the highest risk of HIV transmission, particularly for the recipient, because it is much more likely than vaginal intercourse to cause tissue damage and bleeding.

To prevent HIV transmission, condom use should be considered mandatory with each act of anal intercourse, but for those unwilling to use a condom, withdrawal—removal of the penis before climax—should be attempted. This practice may reduce the dose of virus to which the recipient partner is exposed.

Whereas withdrawal may reduce the risk of HIV transmission to some degree, it is not nearly as effective as condom use. This is so for the following reasons: Withdrawal may not occur soon enough; it does not protect against pre-ejaculatory fluid, which can be infectious, or against semen released early; it does not protect against skin abrasions or tears and so leads to possible blood-blood contact; and it does not protect against transmission of other STDs, which may be cofactors for the transmission of HIV.

A few clinics treating men who have sex with men have done informal studies testing the use of the female condom during anal intercourse. When used this way, the inner ring of the condom is removed and the device inserted with the penis.

■ Other Sexual Practices

It appears that a part of human nature is to use sexual activity for purposes other than reproduction, not only for pleasure and play but also to act out desires of dominance and aggression. In this respect, humans are no different from other primates. Uniquely, however, humans sometimes also use sexual acting out to express contempt and hate. Short of outright criminal assault, as in rape, humans have developed some odd consensual behaviors—as in sadomasochism and its variations—that despite being consensual, often cause physical damage to the body. Many of these behaviors invariably cause bleeding, or expose fragile and vulnerable body parts to foreign objects or to the blood or excrement of others, all of which exposes an individual to numerous disease-causing microbes. HIV is only one such dangerous infectious agent among many.

Therefore, it is important to the health of young people and to their understanding of the rationale for, and the adoption of, the practice of safer sex that they grow up in a society that gives them a sober grasp of what may be considered harmless play and what is unacceptable physical trauma or intolerable danger to the biological integrity of the body.

In addition to inculcating respect for oneself and others, the educational process must achieve habits of good personal hygiene and provide a solid grounding in the reality of infectious diseases, especially STDs. Only then can the young grow up equipped with the knowledge they need to set sensible limits to their sexual behavior.

■ Unsafe Sex among Young Gay Men, 1996

During well over a decade of self-initiated and largely self-financed educational and support efforts, the gay community has achieved exemplary success in promoting safer-sex practices among its members. In the San Francisco gay community, for example, HIV transmission rates dropped from more than 10% per year in the early 1980s to 1.4% in 1990. The prevention practices that were promoted have included the consistent and correct use of condoms, a reduction in the number of sexual partners and in the frequency of anal intercourse, the avoidance of mind-altering drugs, and, in particular, the avoidance of nonsterile needles and syringes for drug injection. By 1993, however, the rate of HIV infection among young gay men aged 18 to 29 in San Francisco had risen to an estimated 2.6% per year. A 1995 study[4] of gay men aged 18 to 24 in New York found that 9% of the men were infected with HIV and the transmission rate was 2%. These figures are too close for comfort to those of the 1980s: According to one 1991 study,[5] a 20-year-old gay man today has about a 50% chance of becoming infected by HIV during his lifetime.

These increases in the rate of infection are believed to occur largely because young gay men tend to ignore safer-sex practices. Many have admitted to engaging in anal intercourse and nearly half of them do not use condoms or use them inconsistently. The need for prevention programs targeting young gay men remains urgent. Like other adolescents, they do not see the ravage of AIDS among their contemporaries because of the long incubation period between the time of HIV infection and the onset of AIDS. They often consider AIDS a disease of older gay men only. For gay adolescents, however, the level of risk represented by each new unprotected sexual encounter is very high because the prevalence of HIV infection is much higher in the gay population than it is in the heterosexual population.

Young gay men represent one example of the continuing need for educational programs stressing the importance of safer-sex practices that are directed toward those at highest risk for HIV transmission, as well as to the general public. Prevention efforts are needed to specifically target African Americans, Hispanics, and immigrants. Among them are many men who have sex with men but who do not regard themselves as homosexuals. They are not members of the gay community, and they remain out of reach of its AIDS-related educational and service organizations.

Also largely out of reach of gay educational organizations are gay men in smaller cities. According to a 1992 survey,[6] the incidence of HIV infection was 9% among gay men of all ages in 16 small cities. Nearly a third of them admitted having engaged in unprotected anal intercourse an average of eight times during the two months preceding the survey.

IDUs everywhere have the highest prevalence of HIV infection. They are at the dual risk of acquiring HIV through the sharing of injection equipment (see Chapter 3) and through sexual contact within their circle of drug users. People who trade sex for drugs or money are also more likely to engage in high-risk behaviors. So are "closeted" gay men because opportunities to have male-to-male sex are infrequent for them. When the opportunity does occur, they may fear losing it by raising the topic of safer sex.

Also at high risk are people with STDs. The presence of sores or ulcerations caused by many STDs increases the risk of acquiring or transmitting HIV during a single sexual encounter by 10 to 100 times. Immediate treatment of STDs and refraining from having sexual contacts until the infection is eliminated are essential for preventing the sexual transmission of HIV. Even STDs such as gonorrhea, chlamydia, and trichomoniasis that do not produce sores will also increase risk (see Chapter 3).

The association between treatment of STDs and prevention of HIV transmission was demonstrated unequivocally in a 1995 study done in six Tanzanian villages in Africa.[7] This study showed that improvement in the treatment and management of STDs reduced the incidence of HIV infection by 42% over two years.

■ Emerging Prevention Issues for People Who Are HIV Positive

Several questions about HIV prevention are emerging for people who are responding to treatment with combination antiretroviral therapies. They live longer, have a better quality of life, and may want to be sexually active.

Is It Safe to Have Unprotected Sex with Someone Else Who Is Also HIV Positive?

No. Some HIV-positive people feel it is okay to have unprotected sex with another HIV-positive individual. There is a risk, however, that HIV strains in one partner or the other may have developed drug resistance, and that the resistant strain will be transmitted during sexual activity. Therefore, even when both partners are HIV positive it is important to practice safer sex.

Is Unprotected Sex Safe When Viral Load Is Nondetectable?

No. A nondetectable viral load does not mean HIV is not present in the blood, semen, or vaginal secretions. Viral load is a relative measure of the amount of HIV in blood plasma. A nondetectable viral load does not mean that no virions are present; it means merely that the level of free virus in the plasma is too low to be detected by the test used. Even HIV-positive individuals with a nondetectable viral load should practice only safer sex.

Will Protease Inhibitors Taken as a "Morning-After Pill" Protect against HIV Infection?

No. While there are anecdotal reports of individuals who, after engaging in unprotected sex, take protease inhibitors or other drugs as a morning-after pill, there is no evidence that this use of an antiretroviral drug, particularly on a one-time basis, can protect against infection. Quite the contrary, there is ample evidence that unless antiviral drugs are taken in appropriate combinations, and following a strict, medically prescribed regimen over the long term, possibly irreversible drug resistance may develop. Even worse, resistance to one protease inhibitor could confer resistance to all of them (see Chapter 5).

■ BLOOD TRANSMISSION

HIV is transmitted very efficiently through blood-to-blood contact. In the early days of the HIV epidemic, before the virus was discovered and named and a test was developed to detect it, blood transmission occurred through the use of HIV-contaminated blood for blood transfusions, through the administration of HIV-contaminated clotting factors to hemophiliacs, and through the sharing of needles and syringes by IDUs (who remain a major source of transmission today; see Chapter 3).

Since early 1985, the screening of all blood donations with the HIV antibody test (the ELISA test) and the discarding of any blood that yields a positive result have effectively prevented the transmission of HIV through blood transfusions and blood products (see below).

Furthermore, in 1985, manufacturers also began using heat to destroy viruses, including HIV, during the preparation of clotting factors for the treatment of hemophiliacs. Clotting factors are no longer a source of HIV infection, and hemophiliacs born after 1985 have been in no danger of contracting HIV through treatment with clotting factors.

■ Other Preventable Risks

Operators of tattooing shops or people (including teenagers) who pierce their ears or other body parts and who share these needles without sterilizing them between each use also run a risk of HIV infection. The risk is less, however, than when people share needles and syringes for injection because syringes transfer a larger sample of blood. However, all of these individuals, as well as beauticians, should disinfect any instruments or tools used to cut through skin (including cuticle scissors, in the case of beauticians) between uses.

■ Injection Drug Use

The sharing of needles and syringes by drug users for the injection of heroin, cocaine, methamphetamine, and other drugs is responsible for 25% of AIDS cases reported in 1996, making it the second leading means of HIV transmission, after sexual transmission, in the United States. The practice also transmits hepatitis B virus, hepatitis C virus, and other blood-borne microbes. In addition, the practice of needle sharing by IDUs has contributed significantly to the spread of HIV in the heterosexual population. Once infected with HIV because of needle sharing, IDUs, who are for the most part heterosexuals, can then transmit the virus to their sex partners. When their female partners (in some 30% of cases they are not themselves drug users) become pregnant, often without suspecting that they are HIV infected, they may transmit HIV to their newborns.

Transmission of HIV among IDUs occurs primarily through the sharing of injection equipment (also known as "works," "gimmicks," and "sets"). This happens because an IDU will draw blood into a syringe to be sure the needle has penetrated a vein. In addition, after injecting the drug, he or she will repeatedly refill the syringe with blood to flush out any remaining drug. However, some blood will remain in the needle and the sides of the syringe. If the user is infected with HIV, and that same needle and syringe are passed on to someone else, HIV from the infected individual will be transmitted to the next user. This is, in fact, a very efficient method of transmitting HIV (see Chapter 3).

Reducing the Risk of HIV Transmission through Contaminated Needles

Discontinuing the use of illicit drugs is, of course, the safest option. But when that is not achievable in the short term, there are several things that can be done to reduce the risk of transmitting HIV and other blood-borne infections through contaminated drug-injection equipment. These include the following, in decreasing levels of effectiveness:

- Never share works, that is, needles and syringes, filters (cottons), spoons (cookers), or glasses. Always use new sterile needles and syringes obtained through a needle-exchange program (see below) or purchased over the counter in states where this is legal.

- If sterile works are not available, clean the equipment with full-strength bleach. See "Cleaning Injection Drug Works to Reduce the Risk of HIV Transmission."

■ If full-strength bleach is not available, rinse the blood from the needle and syringe with clean water, then flush at least three times with detergent or soap; or flush three times with household disinfectant, or high-proof whiskey, rum, or vodka (do not use beer or wine because the alcohol content is too low and would not destroy the virus). Note that this is less safe than using bleach, and using bleach is less safe than using new sterile needles and syringes.

■ Cleaning Injection Drug Works to Reduce the Risk of HIV Transmission

The Centers for Disease Control and Prevention recommends that needles and syringes never be shared. When obtaining sterile injection equipment is impossible and needles and syringes are to be shared, the following procedure can reduce the risk of HIV transmission.[8]

■ Immediately after use and again just before reuse, wash out the needle and syringe by filling them several times with clean water. (This reduces the amount of blood residue remaining in the syringe. Blood, especially clotted blood, reduces the effectiveness of bleach when disinfecting needles and syringes.)

■ Next, completely fill the needle and syringe with *full-strength* liquid household bleach at least three times. Leave the syringe full of bleach at least 30 seconds each time—the longer the better.

■ Then rinse the needle and syringe by filling them several times with clean water. *Do not reuse water from the initial prebleach washing because it may be contaminated.*

■ Each time the needle and syringe are filled with prebleach wash water, bleach, and rinse water, fill the syringe completely to the top.

■ Shake and tap the syringe to remove any air bubbles when using the prebleach wash water, bleach, and rinse water.

Removing the plunger from the syringe and treating it separately as above disinfects areas, such as behind the plunger, that are not reached by solutions in the syringe. ■

- Be wary of "new" works bought on the street. Used equipment and needles are often rebagged and sold on the street as new. Before use, always sterilize needles bought on the street with bleach as described in "Cleaning Injection Drug Works to Reduce the Risk of HIV Transmission."

- Use new, ideally sterile water and works to prepare drugs, and disinfect the skin at the injection site with an alcohol swab to reduce the risk of local bacterial infection.

- Safely dispose of used needles and syringes. Return them to a local needle-exchange program, if one is available; never discard them in public places or where children may find them.

Syringe-Exchange Programs

The practice of needle sharing by IDUs is largely attributable to a shortage of sterile needles and syringes due to state prescription and drug paraphernalia laws that restrict syringe sales and possession. (For the purpose of this discussion, the term "syringe" refers to both needles and syringes.) Many states have prescription laws that prohibit the sale, distribution, and possession of syringes without a valid medical prescription. Furthermore, most prescription laws also require that the syringe be used in the treatment of a bona fide medical condition such as diabetes. Drug paraphernalia laws exist in nearly all states and prohibit the sale, distribution, possession, manufacture, or advertisement of any item that can be used to introduce illicit drugs into the body.

A number of states, however, have allowed pilot syringe-exchange programs to exist as a way of reducing HIV transmission among IDUs. Syringe-exchange programs provide sterile needles and syringes in exchange for used, potentially HIV-contaminated ones, and they safely dispose of contaminated syringes. Such programs have been used with success in Australia, Canada, the Netherlands, and the United Kingdom. The first syringe-exchange program in the United States began in Tacoma, Washington, in 1988. That same year, Congress made it illegal to use federal funds to support needle-exchange programs. The law was passed out of concern that such programs would encourage injection drug use; it also contained a proviso saying that the ban could be lifted if evidence showed that syringe exchange reduces HIV transmission and does not increase drug abuse. Since then, there have been a series of federal prohibitions in different pieces of legislation prohibiting the use of federal funds for exchange programs.

The status of syringe-exchange programs is classified by the Chemical Dependency Institute of the New York City Beth Israel Medical Center, which periodically surveys them, as legal, illegal but tolerated, and illegal/underground. Legal syringe-exchange programs exist in states that have no laws requiring a prescription for obtaining syringes, or states that have exemptions to such laws to allow operation of syringe-exchange programs. Illegal-but-tolerated syringe-exchange programs are those that operate in states with prescription laws, but allow syringe-exchange programs to operate with the support or approval of local officials. Illegal syringe-exchange programs are those that operate without formal support from local officials in states with prescription laws. In 1997, researchers at Beth Israel Medical Center's Chemical Dependency Institute surveyed 87 syringe-exchange programs in 71 cities in 28 states and one territory and found that 53% were legal programs, 23% were illegal but tolerated, and 24% were illegal/underground programs. In 1996, syringe-exchange programs exchanged 14 million syringes.

In addition to providing new sterile injection equipment and collecting and safely disposing of contaminated equipment, many syringe-exchange programs also provide alcohol swabs, condoms, counseling and social services such as HIV safer-sex counseling and referral to HIV testing, tuberculin skin testing, and addiction treatment programs.

Syringe-exchange programs thus far probably have been too limited in number and outreach capacity to have a significant impact on the rate of the spread of HIV nationally, but a number of studies indicated that they are effective locally in reducing HIV transmission. A recently published study showed such effectiveness directly by using a saliva test to measure seroconversion rates of exchange participants and comparing them to those of nonparticipants.[9] The rate of HIV transmission was reduced by 60% within three years among the participants in five experimental syringe-exchange programs in New York City.

A recent report by the National Academy of Sciences/Institute of Medicine[10] reviewed 17 studies that addressed the question of whether syringe-exchange programs lead to increased drug use. Eleven of the studies examined drug use at the individual level. These were primarily comparisons of the participants' self-reported frequency of drug injection before and after they had used a syringe-exchange program. Among these 17 studies, 5 reported decreases in drug injection frequency, 5 reported no change, and only 1 reported an increase. The remaining 6 studies examined drug use at the community level. They used objective indicators such as drug-related emergency-room visits (which were studied nationwide) or the mean age of the local population of IDUs, which would decrease if there were new recruits injecting drugs. None of these studies showed either a rise in drug-related emergency-room visits or a lowering in age of the drug-using population after the implementation of syringe-exchange programs.

According to the *New England Journal of Medicine,* a National Institutes of Health Consensus Development conference on Interventions to Prevent HIV Risk Behaviors held in February 1997 recommended that syringe-exchange programs be "implemented at once."[11] Nevertheless, the ban on federal funding of needle-exchange programs remains in effect, as do most state paraphernalia and prescription laws.

To learn if a particular city has a needle-exchange program, contact the local AIDS service organization or call the North American Syringe Exchange Network at 1-206-272-4857.

■ Safety of the Blood Supply

HIV testing of the blood supply began in 1985 (see Chapter 3). This, added to the self-exclusion of people at high risk of infection with HIV from donating blood, has made the transmission of HIV through blood transfusion an extremely rare event. In 1996, the risk of transmission of HIV through a blood transfusion in the United States was estimated to be 1 unit in 700,000 (0.00014%).

However, the transmission rate of HIV infection by contaminated blood and blood products is estimated to be responsible for about 3% to 5% of cases worldwide and for 3% of cases in most developed countries other than the United States. This percentage is steadily dropping in most developed countries because of donor testing that was implemented starting in 1985.

Prevention of accidental transmission of HIV infection through transplanted organs or tissues started improving in 1993, when the U.S. Public Health Service (USPHS) released guidelines for screening and testing of organ and tissue donors.

■ Prevention following Percutaneous Exposure of Health-Care Workers

Health-care and laboratory workers can become infected with HIV if they accidentally stick themselves with a sharp object that is HIV contaminated, such as a needle, scalpel, or broken glass. HIV can also infect through an open wound—even a tiny one—that comes in contact with HIV-infected blood. Exposure to infectious agents through any break in the skin is referred to as "percutaneous exposure."

The average risk for acquiring HIV infection through percutaneous exposure has been studied and is believed to be about 0.3% per exposure (see Chapter 3).

Some types of percutaneous exposure, however, are presumed to carry a higher risk than others. The high-risk exposures identified by the Centers for Disease Control and Prevention (CDC) include the following:

- A deep injury

- The presence of visible blood on the object that caused the injury

- An injury caused by a device that had been placed in an infected person's vein or artery, such as a needle used to draw a blood sample

- An injury caused by a device used for an infected patient who died as a result of AIDS within 60 days of the injury, and who therefore was presumed to have a high viral load of HIV

For these highest-risk exposures only, the CDC advises that a three-drug antiretroviral therapy be administered promptly and be continued for several weeks to reduce the risk of infection. The regimen should be implemented by an individual in consultation with someone experienced in antiretroviral therapy and HIV transmission. Such preventive treatment is known as "postexposure prophylaxis."

The effectiveness of antiretroviral drugs for postexposure prophylaxis is still unknown. The CDC recommendation is based on limited data, derived from the effectiveness of AZT in reducing transmission from HIV-infected mothers to their newborns, and from animal experiments.

These recommendations were *not* developed to address other forms of HIV exposures, such as sexual exposure.

Health-care or laboratory workers who receive postexposure prophylaxis are encouraged to enroll in an anonymous registry to provide the CDC with the data needed to determine the effectiveness of the treatment.

■ Universal Precautions

Precautions for health-care workers working with people who have symptoms of AIDS were first proposed by the USPHS in 1982. In 1987, and in recognition that AIDS is caused by HIV and that this virus can infect for years without causing disease symptoms, the USPHS recommended that all health-care personnel regard all patients as potentially infected with HIV, hepatitis B virus, and other blood-borne pathogens. The safeguards recommended are known in the medical world as "universal precautions." In brief, universal precautions require the following:

- That health-care workers wear appropriate barrier items such as gloves, gowns, aprons, and eye wear to protect their skin and mucous membranes when exposure to blood or other bodily fluids of patients is expected

- That their hands and skin be washed immediately and thoroughly following accidental contact with other people's blood or bodily fluids

- That precautions be taken to prevent injuries caused by needles, scalpels, and other sharp instruments

- That the need for mouth-to-mouth resuscitation be minimized

- That health-care workers with open sores refrain from direct patient care and from handling patient-care equipment until the condition heals

- That pregnant women strictly adhere to these precautions to minimize risk of HIV transmission to them and to their infants

Universal precautions do *not* apply to the following bodily fluids unless they contain visible blood:

■ Nasal secretions, sputum, sweat, tears, vomitus, urine, and feces. (Note that these fluids can transmit other pathogens and that proper infection-control procedures should always be followed.)

■ Saliva. It is not necessary to wear gloves when feeding a person infected with HIV or when removing saliva from the skin. Dentists, however, should apply universal precautions and practice thorough infection control because dental procedures routinely involve saliva that contains blood.

■ Breast milk. Although breast milk can transmit HIV, it has not been implicated in transmitting HIV to health-care personnel and universal precautions are not required in the care of lactating mothers.

In the absence of an anti-HIV vaccine, adhering to the prevention measures described in this chapter will be the only means available to significantly slow the spread of HIV. But several approaches to prevention—other than through a vaccine—can and must be improved. Women are in serious need of alternatives to the male condom. In particular, they need a means to protect themselves that can be used without the knowledge and consent of male partners. The ongoing research to develop microbicides for just this purpose must be given highest priority.

The continuing ban on federal funding for syringe-exchange programs must be lifted. There is now strong evidence that syringe-exchange programs *do* decrease the rate of HIV transmission among drug users and *do not* increase IDU. In addition, exchange programs remove from circulation contaminated needles and syringes that would otherwise be discarded in neighborhood parking lots, parks, and playgrounds. Syringe-exchange programs work because they embody—not approval of drug use—but empathetic concern. They foster dialogue between program staff and usually fearful and diffident "clients." As part of a comprehensive prevention program targeting the drug-using population, they are demonstrably effective as a source of referrals to medical, social, and drug-addiction treatment services. It is essential, however, that drug treatment programs be made available promptly on demand.

Educational efforts targeting ethnic groups, young gay men, and others who remain at high risk need considerable expansion.

Finally, prevention of HIV infection can occur only through a real awareness of why prevention is necessary and how it is accomplished. This education must begin early. By adolescence, all children should have a solid understanding of the nature of drug abuse and of infectious diseases, particularly STDs, and of how to avoid them. It is easy to blame teenagers for taking risks and feeling immortal, but adults often do not give them the information they need to grow up any wiser.

ENDNOTES

1. Centers for Disease Control and Prevention. *HIV/AIDS Surveillance Report* 1996;8(2):10.

2. De Vincenzi I, et al. A longitudinal study of human immunodeficiency virus transmission by heterosexual partners. *New England Journal of Medicine* 1994;331:341–346.

3. Personal communication. Erica Gollub, Director, AIDS Epidemiology, Philadelphia Department of Public Health, Philadelphia, Pennsylvania.

4. Dean L, Meyer I. HIV prevalence and sexual behavior in a cohort of New York City gay men (aged 18–24). *Journal of Acquired Immune Deficiency Syndromes and Human Retrovirology* 1995;8:208–211.

5. Hoover D, et al. Estimating the 1978–1990 and future spread of human immunodeficiency virus type 1 in subgroups of homosexual men. *American Journal of Epidemiology* 1991;134:1190–1199.

6. Kelly JA, et al. Acquired immunodeficiency syndrome/human immunodeficiency virus risk behavior among gay men in small cities: findings of a 16-city national sample. *Archives of Internal Medicine* 1992;152:2293–297.

7. Grosskurth H, et al. Impact of improved treatment of sexually transmitted diseases on HIV infection in rural Tanzania: randomised controlled trial. *Lancet* 1995;346:530–536.

8. Centers for Disease Control and Prevention. *HIV/AIDS Prevention Bulletin* April 19, 1993.

9. Des Jarlais DC, et al. HIV incidence among injection drug users in New York City syringe-exchange programmes. *Lancet* 1996;348:987–991.

10. Normand J, Vlahov D, Moses LE, eds. *Preventing HIV Transmission: The Roles of Sterile Needles and Bleach.* Washington, DC: National Academy Press, 1995.

11. Editor's Note. *New England Journal of Medicine* 1997;336:1034–1035.

Chapter 10

VACCINES AGAINST HIV INFECTION

The methods of prevention discussed in the previous chapter are very effective in protecting individuals from either acquiring or transmitting HIV infection. When applied properly, consistently, and widely, in a population at risk for HIV, they will slow the spread of the HIV epidemic within that population. But the worldwide HIV epidemic—the HIV pandemic—will ultimately be controlled only by immunization against HIV using a protective, cheap, simple, and widely available vaccine.

Vaccines prepare the immune system—the body's means of controlling infection—to respond quickly and effectively against a virus or other microbe before it has a chance to cause disease. A person whose immune system can fight off a pathogen before it can cause disease is said to be immune to that particular pathogen. Some of the vaccine strategies described in this chapter may also be useful for people already infected with HIV. Such vaccines are known as "therapeutic vaccines."

The widespread use of vaccines in the United States has dramatically reduced the incidence of several viral diseases, including measles, mumps, and poliomyelitis. As yet, no effective vaccine exists to prevent

HIV infection, and few candidate vaccine preparations have even been tested in human subjects. Many features of HIV make it difficult to develop a vaccine against it. Before reviewing why this is so, it is useful to become familiar with what vaccines are and how they work.

■ VACCINES IN GENERAL AND HOW THEY WORK

Most viral vaccines fall into one of three categories:

- Attenuated live-virus vaccines contain a live virus that has been weakened—attenuated—such that it no longer causes disease in the vast majority of recipients. This is usually the most effective type of vaccine because it provides long-lasting immunity, but it has a higher level of risk in that it can lead to disease in rare instances (the oral [Sabin] poliomyelitis vaccine, for example, leads to polio in about one in a million people who receive it). Examples include vaccines for measles, mumps, and rubella.

- Inactivated vaccines contain a disease-causing microbe that has been killed by exposure to heat or chemicals. Examples include the first (Salk) poliovaccine and influenza vaccines.

- Subunit vaccines contain only viral components, those necessary to raise an immune response against the virus. Examples include the hepatitus B vaccine and some types of influenza vaccines.

To be effective, a vaccine must stimulate a strong immune response; that is, it must be "immunogenic." Within the body, the components of a vaccine are perceived as foreign substances, or antigens. The antigens trigger an immune reaction, usually the production of antibodies and the appearance of long-lived memory cells. Memory cells enable the immune system to recognize and respond quickly to the virus in the future. Often, booster doses of a vaccine must be given months or years after the initial dose to extend the life of the memory cells and the effectiveness of the vaccine. In this way, a vaccine can protect against an infectious agent for decades.

■ Steps in Developing a Vaccine

In the face of any infectious disease, vaccine development begins with the observation that some infected people recover from their infection and are protected thereafter from developing the same disease again. Microbiologists then isolate and identify the microbe responsible for the infection. Next, they must determine which proteins belonging to the microbe are most important for stimulating the protective immune response.

Other scientists, meanwhile, study the immune response itself to determine its nature. They want to know, for example, whether antibody-mediated immunity or cell-mediated immunity is more important in conferring protection against the microbe. This information is known as the "correlates of immunity" (or correlates of protection). Identifying the correlates of immunity may require several years of research.

Knowledge about the microbe's antigens and its correlates of immunity is then used to develop candidate vaccines. These in turn are tested in laboratory animals, a phase of vaccine development known as "preclinical testing." Preclinical testing is essential for demonstrating the safety and degree of protection offered by a candidate vaccine before the vaccine is tested in humans.

Not just any species of laboratory animal will work for preclinical vaccine testing. It must be an animal that when infected by the microbe develops a disease that is similar to the disease in humans (and, in the case of HIV, it must do so within a practical period of time). Furthermore, the animal should develop an immune response to the microbe that is similar to the immune response in humans; that is, the correlates of immunity should be the same both in the animal and in humans.

During preclinical testing, researchers give the candidate vaccine to animals and study the strength and durability of the resulting immune response. They wait weeks, months, or even years and then expose "vaccinated" and unvaccinated animals to a live form of the microbe to measure the candidate vaccine's success in protecting the animal against the specific disease. Scientists refer to this step as "challenging" the animals.

If animal testing shows that a candidate vaccine is safe and effective, a vaccine developer (in the United States it is usually a pharmaceutical company) applies to the Food and Drug Administration (FDA) for approval to begin testing in humans. The pharmaceutical company must also develop a safe, efficient, and cost-effective method for manufacturing the candidate vaccine in large quantity. If FDA approval is given, phase I testing can begin in humans. Phase I and II studies are typically carried out at medical-research centers.

Phase I studies focus primarily on the safety of the candidate vaccine. It is given at gradually increasing doses to a small number—usually fewer than 100—of carefully selected healthy volunteers. During the study, researchers watch for any undesirable side effects and for the strength and type of immune response elicited. If the outcome of a phase I study is promising, the sponsor seeks FDA approval to begin a phase II study.

Phase II studies can involve up to several hundred selected volunteers from a population that is at risk for the disease. Again, safety is of primary concern, but particular attention is now paid to the nature and strength of the immune response. Researchers also work to determine the best dose, route, and schedule by which the candidate vaccine should be administered.

When these are known, phase III tests are done using thousands or tens of thousands of volunteers who are people at high risk for the infection. These studies continue to investigate safety, dose, route, and schedule of administration, but the goal now is to determine efficacy, that is, the degree of protection the candidate vaccine gives against disease. Phase III studies are also likely to reveal unexpected side effects that almost inevitably occur in a small number of people among the many thousands vaccinated in large phase III trials. If a vaccine can be shown to be both safe and highly protective, the developer will apply for a license from the FDA for the right to market the new vaccine for general use.

In December 1992, the National Institutes of Health (NIH) AIDS Vaccine Evaluation Group initiated the first phase II trial of a candidate vaccine against HIV. To date, several candidate vaccines against HIV have reached that stage of development, but only one, a gp120 vaccine, has gone on to phase III testing. (The trial is being conducted in the United States and Thailand.)

Because of the urgency and importance of developing an HIV vaccine, six AIDS Vaccine Evaluation Units have been set up by the NIH at different medical-research centers in the United States for the expeditious testing of candidate AIDS vaccines.

■ FEATURES OF HIV AND HIV DISEASE THAT MAKE VACCINE DEVELOPMENT DIFFICULT

HIV is very different from all other viruses against which vaccines have been developed, and HIV infection is different in many important ways from other viral infections (in fact, no single vaccine exists today against any of the three known human retroviruses). These differences include the following:

- Precise correlates of immunity remain insufficiently known for HIV, although cell-mediated immunity is thought to be more important than antibody-mediated immunity for controlling HIV infection. In contrast, existing vaccines primarily stimulate antibody-mediated immunity (i.e., the production of antibodies) and only to a lesser degree, cell-mediated immunity.

- Compared to most other viral infections, HIV infection establishes itself quickly in the body. This happens because the primary targets of the virus—helper T lymphocytes and monocytes/macrophages (i.e., cells with CD4 molecules on them)—are present wherever HIV enters the body. A successful HIV vaccine might have to prepare the immune system to respond exceptionally quickly to the virus.

- HIV mutates frequently (see Chapter 18). This means that while all HIV particles have the same basic structure, their various proteins can differ slightly from one virus particle to the next. While the immune responses generated by a vaccine would recognize the proteins of the HIV strain(s) used to make the vaccine, they may not recognize genetic variants of HIV. (The influenza virus also has a high mutation rate—though it is lower than that of HIV—which is why people must get a different flu shot every year.)

- There are multiple subtypes of HIV worldwide (see Chapter 18). It is unlikely that a single vaccine will protect against all of them. Thus, several vaccines will probably be needed, each protecting against a few subtypes or perhaps even only one of them.

■ Other than the rare, protected, impractical, and costly chimpanzee, no animal has yet been found to develop an AIDS-like immune deficiency when given HIV (HIV-infected chimpanzees, like humans, can take ten years to develop AIDS). The best animal model currently available is the macaque infected with the simian immunodeficiency virus (SIV), resulting in an AIDS-like disease. SIV is closely related to HIV, but it is nevertheless a different virus. So while vaccine experiments with SIV are useful, they cannot predict the safety or effectiveness of a vaccine designed for use against HIV in humans.

In addition to all the difficulties just listed, ethical, legal, and economic hurdles have dampened the pharmaceutical industry's interest in developing an HIV vaccine. For example, for ethical reasons, volunteers participating in the testing of anti-HIV candidate vaccines must be thoroughly counseled about how to achieve and maintain low-risk behavior. They are also warned not to expect protection from the vaccine they are helping to test. Such counseling complicates the planning and analysis of a study's results.

Furthermore, people who volunteer to help test a candidate HIV vaccine will thereafter test positive for antibodies to HIV even though they are not HIV infected. Because their serostatus can lead to discrimination in employment, housing, and insurance, as well as to other kinds of social stigmatization, protections must be devised for them. For example, participants of phase I and phase II trials have been given photo identification cards stating that they have participated in an HIV vaccine trial. Researchers can also provide vaccine-trial participants with letters to give to sexual partners, employers, and insurance companies that explain the reason for their positive serostatus. Last, while vaccine-trial participants may test positive for HIV antibodies by an ELISA test, a confirmatory Western blot test (see Chapter 2) will reveal the presence of antibodies only to the antigen or antigens used in the vaccine (e.g., a gp120 vaccine will elicit antibodies to the gp120 protein; other proteins characteristic of HIV infection such as gp41 or p24 will be missing). In such cases, viral genome tests such as reverse transcriptase–polymerase chain reaction (RT-PCR) or branched-chain DNA amplification (bDNA), both of which measure the amount of HIV particles in the blood (see Chapter 2), can also verify that participants in vaccine trials are not HIV infected.

Then, too, companies fear the threat of liability if an HIV vaccine should fail to protect certain individuals or should incompletely protect a proportion of a vaccinated population.

■ THE NEED FOR AN HIV VACCINE

The need for an HIV vaccine is most acute in developing countries, where 90% of all new HIV infections are occurring. And the epidemic is expanding rapidly in many of those countries. In Bombay, India, the prevalence of HIV infection in sex workers went from 1% to 51% between 1987 and 1993; among people arriving in sexually transmitted disease (STD) clinics, the rate of HIV infection jumped from 2% to 3% to 36% between 1989 and 1994, and by 1994, 2.5% of pregnant women visiting prenatal clinics in Bombay were HIV positive. The prevalence of HIV infection among blood donors in Phenom Penh, Cambodia, rose from 0.1% in 1991 to about 10% in 1995. By early 1997, 40% of pregnant women in Zambia were HIV infected. Current estimates indicate that more than 300 million people would require vaccination today. For worldwide use, an anti-HIV vaccine should have the following qualities:

- It should be inexpensive and easy to administer.

- It should be easy to transport and store; for example, it should not require refrigeration.

- It should induce long-lasting immunity with a single immunization and require few, if any, booster doses.

- It should be compatible with other vaccines.

- It should provide protection against many strains of HIV.

■ EVIDENCE THAT AN HIV VACCINE CAN BE DEVELOPED

Despite the numerous difficulties, there is also evidence that an HIV vaccine can be successfully developed:

- Early in HIV infection, during the acute infection phase and despite the presence of a very high viral load, the immune system mounts a response sufficiently effective to virtually eliminate HIV from the blood within weeks. In general, progression of the infection thereafter occurs slowly—an average of 10 years passes before clinical symptoms develop. It is now known that during this long period, the immune system fights the disease by rapidly replacing immune-system cells lost to HIV (see Chapter 4).

- About 2% of HIV-infected individuals have survived for 10 to 15 years with no signs of disease or impaired immunity. They are known as long-term nonprogressors. Although some of these individuals have genetically determined resistance to HIV (see Chapter 4), others show merely high levels of antibody and cell-mediated immunity against HIV.

- There is evidence that infection by HIV-2 confers some degree of immune protection against HIV-1 disease.

- Researchers have produced two types of vaccines that in one case protected macaques against strains of SIV, and in the other, to a certain degree, protected chimpanzees against HIV. The protection conferred by these vaccines, however, was against only the strains of virus used in the preparation of the vaccine. (See "Vaccine Strategies Undergoing Laboratory Study.")

■ CANDIDATE VACCINES THAT HAVE UNDERGONE CLINICAL TESTING

About 20 candidate anti-HIV vaccines have undergone phase I testing in uninfected humans, and a number of these have gone into phase II testing. During phase II testing, many of these candidate vaccines elicited the production of antibodies, as mentioned already, but at levels below that seen in natural HIV infection. Since antibody levels seen in natural infection are insufficient to prevent HIV disease, it was felt that the lower levels elicited to date by candidate vaccines would be ineffective. The following approaches have been used in the preparation of these candidate vaccines.

■ Subunit Vaccines Based on HIV Envelope Proteins

Candidate vaccines based on the gp120 envelope protein have been among the most widely tested. Two of them have gone through phase I and phase II testing, but in June 1994 the NIH decided not to proceed with phase III testing. The vaccines were faulted for their inability to produce neutralizing antibodies and to elicit cell-mediated immune responses.

■ Synthetic Peptide Vaccines

Synthetic peptide candidate vaccines consist of short chains of amino acids—peptides—that are assembled by machines. The structure of the synthetic peptides mimics that of small fragments of certain HIV proteins. These fragments are believed to be those to which neutralizing antibodies bind. The so-called V3 loop, for example, is a fragment of the HIV gp120 envelope protein that is important to that protein's function (gp120 enables HIV to attach to CD4 cells; see Chapter 18). At least two candidate synthetic peptide vaccines mimicking portions of the V3 loop that are common to several strains of HIV have undergone early testing in humans. However, this type of vaccine has elicited only weak antibody responses and has not stimulated cell-mediated immunity.

■ Recombinant Subunit Vaccines

Recombinant subunit vaccines use viral proteins produced using recombinant DNA technology. In this case, recombinant DNA technology involves transplanting the genes for certain HIV proteins into bacteria or other microorganisms, or mammalian cells. The host cells then churn out large quantities of the "recombinant" HIV protein. This method of production is a safer and more cost-effective way to obtain large quantities of HIV protein than the alternative, which requires growing large amounts of infectious HIV particles.

Recombinant gp160 proteins and p24 proteins (rgp160 and rp24) have been tested in early clinical trials. Their apparent drawback resided in a component of the recombinant product that was subtly different from that of the natural HIV proteins. As a result, the antibodies elicited by the recombinant proteins did not effectively neutralize strains of HIV that are commonly transmitted.

■ Live Recombinant Vector Vaccines

These candidate vaccines use a non-disease-causing virus—an avirulent virus—other than HIV in which certain genes from HIV have been inserted through recombinant DNA technology. The avirulent virus serves merely as a vehicle, or vector, that carries the HIV genes, along with its own, into body cells. There, the avirulent virus replicates harmlessly but produces both its own proteins and those encoded by the HIV genes. In theory, all the viral proteins should elicit an immune response, including a response against HIV proteins.

Several live recombinant vector HIV vaccines are currently undergoing development and early testing. They include vaccinia and canarypox viruses as vectors for the HIV gene coding for gp160, the protein that forms the knobs on the envelope of HIV.

■ VACCINE STRATEGIES UNDERGOING LABORATORY STUDY

■ Attenuated Live-HIV Vaccines

Attenuated live-virus vaccines use a weakened—attenuated—form of the virus. The virus actually replicates within cells of the host, but without causing disease (or by causing very minor symptoms). In this way, attenuated live-virus vaccines imitate a natural infection and activate both cell-mediated and antibody-mediated arms of the immune system. As a result, these vaccines are very effective—attenuated live-virus vaccines are used to protect children against measles, mumps, rubella, and polio and were successful in eradicating smallpox.

The feasibility of an attenuated live-HIV vaccine has been tested using SIV in macaques. The SIV virions used in the vaccine had been attenuated by removing the *nef* gene from the virus. The *nef* gene was believed to be required for SIV (and HIV) to be infectious. When the SIV lacking *nef* was tested in macaque monkeys, it was found to protect adult macaques from later challenge with SIV given naturally, but it did not protect infant macaques.

Attenuated live-virus vaccines carry an important risk, however. Attenuated viruses can sometimes mutate back to a virulent form. In the case of SIV and HIV, for example, they might acquire a *nef* gene from a preexisting but latent infection with another retrovirus. Therefore, an attenuated live-virus vaccine that uses HIV itself has been considered too dangerous for testing in humans, but research using SIV in animal models continues.

■ DNA Vaccines

This entirely novel type of vaccine imitates the activity of an attenuated live-virus vaccine, but with much less risk. DNA vaccines are made up of rings of harmless bacterial DNA that also include one or two viral genes. The viral genes are spliced into the rings of bacterial DNA using recombinant DNA techniques. When the vaccine is injected into muscle, the DNA rings are taken up by body cells. If all goes well, the cells begin producing the viral proteins, which then elicit immune responses that will protect against the virus.

Furthermore, because the cells that have taken up the DNA produce viral proteins, the proteins would be displayed on the cell surface, which activates the cell-mediated immune response (see Chapter 16). Thus, they can elicit both cell-mediated and antibody-mediated immune responses, as do attenuated live-virus vaccines. (As mentioned already, other types of vaccines predominately activate the antibody immune response.)

DNA vaccines have a number of advantages over other types of vaccines. They may be safer for individuals with a compromised immune system, they are easier to prepare, and they do not require refrigeration. For these reasons, DNA vaccines could potentially be produced in large quantities and distributed worldwide at reasonable cost.

Candidate DNA vaccines have been tested in animals, including chimpanzees, and a phase II trial of a DNA vaccine designed to test whether it stimulates cytotoxic T-cell activity in people who are already infected with HIV has shown promising results.

The chimpanzee study[1] involved four animals, three of which were given a vaccine containing the *env, rev,* and *gag/pol* genes from HIV. The animals were given eight injections of the vaccine over the course of a year. All three animals developed antibody responses; two of the animals developed cell-mediated immune responses.

At week 60, two of the vaccinated chimpanzees and the one unvaccinated animal were challenged with a high dose of HIV; the third vaccinated chimpanzee was used as a control. Virus was detectable by RT-PCR testing in one of the vaccinated animals six weeks after challenge, and in the other vaccinated animal after eight weeks. The virus levels were low, however (below 500 virus particles per ml). The control animal, on the other hand, had 10,000 virus particles per milliliter of serum at both six and eight weeks. Forty-eight weeks later, both vaccinated animals had nondetectable virus levels.

This candidate vaccine is now undergoing clinical trial testing in humans.

■ Pseudovirions

Research on attenuated live-virus HIV candidate vaccines has led to the finding that the *gag* gene of HIV could on its own direct the assembly of virus-like particles. These particles—known as "pseudovirions," or false viruses—have much of the outer structure of a normal HIV particle but do not contain genetic material. Pseudovirions, therefore, cannot replicate, but they do display many important HIV antigens, and they are in preclinical testing for use in a candidate anti-HIV vaccine.

■ HAZARDS TO AN ANTI-HIV VACCINE

No vaccine is completely safe for everyone. In addition, there are several potential hazards unique to anti-HIV vaccines. For example, several proteins produced by HIV are very similar to proteins produced naturally by human cells. An immune response to these viral proteins might result in an immune response against normal cell proteins. This could result in an autoimmune disease, perhaps one leading to the destruction of CD4 cells. This in turn would further impair the immune system and its ability to mount an effective immune response to the vaccine itself and, later, to HIV.

There is also evidence from laboratory studies that antibodies that bind to HIV but that do not neutralize the virus might actually aid HIV infection. Such antibodies could facilitate the infection of macrophages, which ingest virus-antibody complexes. There is no evidence, however, that HIV disease has been accelerated in persons who enrolled in trials of gp160 candidate vaccines.

■ PHASE III VACCINE TRIALS REQUIRE LARGE POPULATIONS AT HIGH RISK

Phase III trials of any candidate vaccine will require a large population of people who are at high risk of HIV infection. A large population is needed to minimize the duration of phase III HIV vaccine trials. For this reason, trials of many candidate vaccines will have to be done in developing countries that have a high prevalence of HIV infection. Many countries in Africa and Asia, for example, welcome the opportunity to participate in vaccine studies, particularly because these nations cannot provide the antiretroviral drug therapies available in developed countries. They also lack the resources and personnel to develop, organize, and conduct vaccine trials on their own, or to purchase the equipment needed to conduct the studies (e.g., microscopes, refrigerators, freezers, centrifuges, laboratory glassware, and autoclaves for sterilizing equipment); in fact, health-care budgets in many developing countries are so small that physicians are forced to reuse disposable syringes.

Such trials raise a number of ethical problems in their design and follow-up. Thus, the trials will be planned and overseen by knowledgeable medical ethicists as well as clinical researchers, along with public-health officials in the host countries.

■ CONCLUSIONS

An anti-HIV vaccine remains a long way off. An additional and substantial basic-research effort is needed to overcome difficulties resulting from both the unusual biology of HIV and the nature of HIV disease. The news here is not entirely discouraging, however. Evidence from immunological, epidemiological, and animal studies suggests that an anti-HIV vaccine is a realistic possibility, and entirely new approaches to immunization such as that offered by "DNA vaccination" provide additional hope.

The problems that can be anticipated in vaccine development are not limited to the laboratory. There are also logistical, organizational, economic, political, and ethical challenges to overcome. Phase III trials for an anti-HIV vaccine will have to be largely conducted in developing countries, where the prevalence of HIV infection is high. They should be carried out with very large numbers of volunteers (in order to shorten the duration of the trials). Such trials will be primarily under the direction of researchers from developed countries. The planning and implementation of such field trials will require effective cooperation at the international level among scientists, physicians, governments, pharmaceutical companies, and population groups at high risk.

These issues, both scientific and organizational, have been the object of recent intense analysis and evaluation. Both the Office of AIDS Research at the NIH and AmFAR have created targeted research-grant programs to address major unanswered questions, principally regarding the correlates of immunity to HIV. The International AIDS Vaccine Initiative (IAVI), undertaken by the Rockefeller Foundation, seeks to organize a consortium of government and private agencies, including pharmaceutical companies, to move forward with the planning of vaccine trials in various countries with international financial support and local approval.

If true control of the HIV epidemic is to be achieved, development of an anti-HIV vaccine is an absolute must. The mode of HIV transmission—predominately sexual—and the nature of HIV disease—specifically, that it is caused by a retrovirus and that symptomatic disease takes years to develop—predictably make HIV an infectious agent whose spread will not be controllable in any significant way other than through universal immunization.

■ INFORMATION ON HIV VACCINE TRIALS

For information about protective vaccine trials for HIV infection, see the *AmFAR AIDS/HIV Treatment Directory* or call the AIDS Clinical Trials Information Service or check its web site (these sources are all listed in Appendix 1).

ENDNOTE

1. Boyer JD, et al. Protection of chimpanzees from high-dose heterologous HIV-1 challenge by DNA vaccination. *Nature Medicine* 1997;3(May): 526–532.

Chapter 11

WOMEN AND HIV DISEASE

HIV/AIDS in women has long been a neglected aspect of the HIV epidemic. Until recently, little scientific attention has been paid to many fundamental questions about HIV disease in women. Scientists still do not know exactly how HIV is transmitted from men to women, and many questions remain about the course of HIV disease in women. Women desperately need methods to prevent heterosexual HIV transmission that are under their own control. And while a number of microbicides (preparations applied to the vagina that would kill HIV and other pathogens) are under development, at best it will be several years before any become licensed and widely available.

HIV infection in women often represents a threat to two or more people: a mother and her progeny. HIV transmission from mother to child (perinatal transmission) is now responsible for virtually all new cases of HIV infection in children. Research on the prevention of perinatal transmission has been extraordinarily successful, and the risk of perinatal HIV transmission can now be greatly reduced (see Chapter 12).

However, the incidence of HIV infection continues to grow among women, and the rate at which it is growing is now higher than that among men. From the beginning of the epidemic through December

1996, 85,500 cases of AIDS had been reported in women in the United States, making up 15% of all adult AIDS cases. Whereas women accounted for 7% of AIDS cases in 1985, they made up nearly 20% of the cases reported in 1996.

During 1996 alone, 13,820 new AIDS cases were reported in women. Thirty-four percent of these infections were acquired through the woman's own injection drug use, but 40% were acquired through sexual contact with an HIV-infected man. The remainder included cases due to HIV acquired from contaminated blood, blood components, or tissues (2%); cases due to HIV infection resulting from treatment for a coagulation disorder (less than 1%)[1]; and cases for which risk factors were still undetermined at the end of the reporting period (24%). The "undetermined" category included cases that were still under investigation, cases in women unwilling to disclose their route of exposure or unaware of a clear-cut exposure, and cases that were incompletely investigated because of death or because the women were lost to follow-up or had declined to be interviewed.

In 1995, heterosexual transmission overtook injection drug use as the leading cause of HIV infection in women. (Injection drug use accounted for 43% and 40% of AIDS cases in women in 1994 and 1995, respectively, while heterosexual transmission accounted for 40% and 42% over the same period. These figures were obtained after investigation of the risk factors for the "undetermined" category; similarly, the number of 1996 AIDS cases in the heterosexual and injection-drug-use categories will likely increase from the end-of-year figure cited previously for 1996.) It is important to note that all these figures pertain to cases of "full-blown" AIDS—that is, to HIV infections acquired an average of ten years earlier. Today, HIV infection has increased among women in the United States, and in developing countries it is even more prevalent in women than in men.

In the United States, HIV infection is more likely to occur among women of color, particularly African-American and Hispanic women. In 1993, the Centers for Disease Control and Prevention (CDC) found that HIV disease had become the fourth leading cause of death among women 25 to 44 years old, but by then it was already the leading cause of death among African-American women and the third leading cause of death among Hispanic women in the same age group. By 1996, CDC figures showed that there were 3.5 cases of AIDS per 100,000 white women. That rate was 17 times higher among African-American women (61.7 per 100,000) and six times higher for Hispanic women (22.7 per 100,000). Also, in 1996, white women accounted for 21% of all AIDS cases in women, while African-American women accounted for 59% and Hispanic women accounted for 19% of cases (Asian, Pacific Islander, American Indian, and Alaskan native women made up less than 1% of 1996 AIDS cases in women).

■ WOMEN ARE AT HIGHER RISK THAN MEN OF ACQUIRING HIV INFECTION

Both biological and psychosocial factors place women at higher risk than men of acquiring HIV infection. In terms of biology, when an HIV-infected male ejaculates during intercourse, the several milliliters of semen he releases are rich in both free virus and virus-infected lymphocytes and macrophages. This semen is brought into contact with a broad surface of mucosal tissue in the vagina and on the cervix. These tissues contain high numbers of CD4 lymphocytes, which can become infected by HIV from the semen.

When an HIV-infected woman has intercourse with an uninfected man, the primary source of transmission from her to him is free virus and virus-infected cells present in the vaginal and cervical secretions. These secretions have contact mainly with the skin of the penis. If the skin is intact, the virus cannot penetrate it. HIV-infected vaginal secretions have little access to the mucosal tissue lining the male's urethral canal, making transmission of the virus a less likely event.

But sexual intercourse is rarely a single event between two members of a sexually active couple. Each instance of unprotected sexual intercourse with an infected female statistically increases the risk that an uninfected male will acquire HIV.[2] Thus, in the long run, the rate of female-to-male HIV transmission becomes similar to the rate of male-to-female transmission. This explains why the prevalence of HIV infection is similar in both men and women in the developing world today.

A number of psychosocial factors also increase a woman's vulnerability to HIV infection:

- Women have little or no control over the means to practice low-risk sexual behavior: There is nothing they can do to protect themselves without the knowledge and consent of their male sexual partner.

- Because of their inferior social standing in relation to men, virtually worldwide, women are generally unable to negotiate the frequency and nature of sexual interactions. Sometimes they are not even able to choose who their partner will be. Worldwide, untold numbers of women are prevented from learning about, and certainly from insisting on, the use of condoms and behaviors recommended for practicing safer sex. Throughout the world, 90% of all HIV-infected women have acquired their infection through heterosexual contact.

- Other important sources of HIV infection for women living in developing countries include transfusions with untested or poorly tested blood; nonsterile medical equipment used during childbirth; and reused, unsterilized needles and syringes used to inject medications.

- Lesbian and bisexual women are also at risk for HIV/AIDS. Transmission of HIV during homosexual sex between women is uncommon (although it has been reported) and remains fairly unresearched (see also Chapter 3). However, lesbians may engage in the same high-risk behaviors as heterosexual women (e.g., injection drug use with shared needles), and because they often socialize with gay and bisexual men, they are at higher risk than heterosexual women when they have unprotected sex with men.

■ PREVENTION OF HIV TRANSMISSION IN WOMEN

All sexually active women, including pregnant women, should consider themselves at risk for HIV infection. Granted, the level of risk for a woman who is not an injection drug user varies greatly, depending on her sexual practices. For a woman who has no sexual relations, the risk is virtually nil; for a woman in a stable monogamous relationship, the risk is small, although it depends on her partner's degree of faithfulness; for a woman who engages in casual sex with multiple partners, the risk can be very high. Here, the level of risk rises with the prevalence of HIV infection in her social circles and geographic area, as the HIV status of a potential new sex partner can rarely be known in advance. In certain areas or communities of the United States, the prevalence of HIV can be very high—20% to 50%—so that even a single act of unprotected sex with a new partner (let alone a relationship involving repeated intercourse) poses a significant risk for acquiring HIV infection.

The danger and uncertainty for both women—and men—spring from the fact that HIV disease follows an insidious course. In most adults, HIV infection does not manifest itself through any overt or characteristic symptoms for an average of ten years after infection. Therefore, the appearance of a potential sex partner, or his claims of good health, cannot be interpreted to signify the absence of HIV infection. Even a prospective partner who has been tested for HIV cannot claim to be free of infection unless that man has been recently tested twice, over the course of several weeks (completely abstaining from risky sexual behavior and drug use in the interval) and was given negative results on both blood tests.

The safest course for a woman who wants to be sexually active is to enter into a monogamous, committed, and mutually faithful relationship, and that before entering such a relationship, both she and her partner undergo HIV testing twice, as mentioned already. Only after both partners test negative for HIV, and after complete trust of faithfulness has been established between them, can they forego safer-sex practices and engage in unprotected sex with each other and *only* with each other. Under all other circumstances, sexually active women should always practice safer sex: Use a male latex or polyurethane condom, or a female condom, during every act of vaginal or rectal intercourse. During oral-penile sex, use a male condom; during oral-vaginal sex, use a latex or polyurethane barrier such as a condom split lengthwise to form a sheet (see also Chapter 9).

The single alternative to the male condom that is now available to women is the female condom (see Chapter 9). As mentioned earlier, research is also under way to develop chemical barriers—microbicides—that can be applied to the vagina to kill HIV (see Chapter 9).

■ HOW DOES HIV ENTER A WOMAN'S BODY DURING SEXUAL INTERCOURSE?

Actually, scientists still cannot answer this question completely. Researchers are trying to determine, for example, whether it is virus-infected cells such as HIV-infected T lymphocytes and macrophages (which are abundant in semen) or the relatively small amount of free virus particles also present in it that are more important for transmitting the infection. Researchers are also trying to learn which regions of the female reproductive tract are most susceptible to HIV infection. Indeed, answers to both questions are important to the development of microbicides for female-controlled prevention of infection.

Vaginal epithelial cells lack CD4 receptor molecules so that free virus particles are not believed capable of binding to them and infecting them. (There is laboratory evidence, however, that HIV-infected lymphocytes can attach to epithelial cells and transfer HIV to those cells through fusion of the cell membranes; the role of cell-to-cell transfer in HIV infection is unknown.) Many researchers believe that the most significant form of HIV transmission occurs when HIV-infected T lymphocytes and monocytes/macrophages in the semen attach to and penetrate the vaginal and cervical epithelia. These HIV-infected immune cells lead to the infection of CD4 lymphocytes belonging to the female. In addition, lymphocytes and macrophages are found in abundance in the tissue just below the female epithelium, thereby providing a large population of target cells for initial infection. This would explain why inflammation, sores, or other kinds of lesions in the vagina or cervical epithelium—lesions that not only offer gaping entry points to the virus but also attract the female's immune cells that bear CD4 molecules—increase the risk of HIV transmission. It is well established that women with sexually transmitted diseases are at increased risk of HIV infection. Therefore, women should have any sexually transmitted infection treated promptly.

■ COURSE OF HIV INFECTION IN WOMEN

One of the few studies looking at the course of HIV disease in women was published in 1994[3] and involved 768 women and 3,779 men. It found that women had a 38% greater risk of developing bacterial pneumonia. Women also had a 33% greater risk of death during the study's 15-month follow-up period, even though the rates of disease progression did not differ significantly between men and women in the study. Why women had poorer survival than men did during this study remained unknown, but the investigators speculated that it might be due to social factors such as limited access to health care and lower socioeconomic status including homelessness, domestic violence, and lack of social support.

■ PSYCHOSOCIAL FACTORS AND THE COURSE OF HIV DISEASE IN WOMEN

Indeed, psychosocial factors play a significant role also in the course of HIV disease in women:

- Women are often diagnosed later in their disease than are men, largely because HIV infection is still regarded by many—sometimes including women themselves—as a disease of men or gay men. This delays the start of antiretroviral therapies and the use of prophylaxis for opportunistic infections in women. Older women are usually diagnosed and treated even later because they and their doctors have still lower expectations of HIV infection; their way of life typically presents none of the risk factors associated with HIV infection.

- Women have less access than men to routine and state-of-the-art HIV/AIDS care. They are often less mobile than men and more likely to face language and cultural barriers, all of which reduce access to health care and interfere with a woman's ability to comply with demanding treatment regimens.

- There are few support groups organized for women with HIV disease. Older women in particular have few resources to turn to for support.

- Women often neglect their own health care to take of others. As a result, many learn of their HIV-positive status only after giving birth to a child who later develops AIDS. As primary caregivers, such women may devote themselves to the care of their HIV-infected child (and perhaps also their HIV-infected husband and/or other children) and place their own health-care needs last.

- Fewer than 10% of all participants in HIV-related clinical trials are women. Being fewer in numbers than men in the early years of the epidemic, having less control over their mobility, and facing more language and cultural barriers, women with HIV/AIDS have always been underrepresented in clinical trials, which are often portals to expert care and promising new drugs. To this day, the number of women enrolled in clinical trials is too low to allow statistical calculations that might reveal whether the response of women to a treatment is different from the response of men.

■ BIOLOGICALLY UNIQUE ASPECTS OF HIV DISEASE IN WOMEN

The HIV-related conditions that occur uniquely in women involve infections or malignancies of the female reproductive tract. Most of these gynecological problems also occur in HIV-negative women. Since few studies have compared the incidence of these conditions in women with and without HIV disease, a debate continues over whether they truly occur more frequently in women who are HIV infected. It is well agreed, however, that these diseases are more aggressive in women infected with HIV. They include certain vaginal infections, pelvic inflammatory disease (PID), and precancerous cellular changes of the cervix (cervical intraepithelial neoplasia, or CIN). CIN progresses more rapidly to invasive cervical cancer in women infected with HIV (for this reason, the CDC has included invasive cervical cancer as an AIDS-defining illness; see Chapter 8).

■ Vaginal Infections

Vaginal infections suspected of being associated with HIV infection include the following:

- Genital ulcers of unknown origin occur in women with HIV disease, as they do in other severely immune-suppressed men and women. The appearance of these ulcers seems to be rare, and they have not been associated with abnormal cell growth (i.e., neoplasia) or with any known viral or bacterial infection. Instead, they are often categorized by physicians as acute or chronic inflammation. They can be confused with ulcerations caused by herpes simplex infection that do not respond to treatment. HIV-related genital ulcers sometimes respond to antiretroviral therapy.

■ Vaginal candidiasis, or yeast infection of the vagina, is thought by some investigators to have a higher incidence in HIV-positive women, but research findings are mixed. The HIV Epidemiology Research Study (HERS) found vaginal candidiasis occurring in 22 (8%) of 273 HIV-negative women and in 38 (10%) of 382 HIV-positive women, a difference that was not statistically significant.[4] Preliminary results of the Women's Interagency HIV Study (WIHS), however, showed the incidence of vaginal candidiasis in HIV-positive women to be twice that of HIV-negative women.[5] In addition, vaginal candidiasis tends to be more prolonged and difficult to treat in women infected with HIV. As in men, oral and esophageal candidiasis are common problems in women with HIV disease. (For descriptions of these conditions, see Chapter 7.)

■ Bacterial vaginosis (a bacterial infection of the vagina) and trichomoniasis (a protozoal infection that causes inflammation of the vagina) may also occur more frequently in HIV-positive women. Some evidence suggests that sexually transmitted infections, including gonorrhea and chlamydia, are more common in HIV-positive women, but it is not clear yet whether this is a result of HIV infection or of high-risk behaviors that are also responsible for acquiring HIV infection itself.

■ Pelvic Inflammatory Disease

PID, also known as salpingitis, is an inflammation of the fallopian tubes. PID can be caused by a variety of bacterial or viral infections. Other sites of infection include the ovaries, uterus, and cervix. PID most often occurs in sexually active women younger than 25 years and is usually caused by an infection acquired during intercourse, childbirth, or abortion. Women who use intrauterine devices (IUDs) have an increased risk for PID. Symptoms include severe lower abdominal pain and fever.

Many physicians believe that PID occurs with higher frequency in HIV-positive women, although some studies refute this. On the other hand, there is evidence suggesting that PID becomes a recurring or chronic problem as the immune system weakens during progression of HIV disease.

■ Human Papillomavirus Infection and Cervical Cancer

Women who are HIV positive are at high risk of infection by human papillomavirus (HPV). There are many types of HPV, some of which are harmless and produce no sign of infection, while others are responsible for warts on hands, feet, and the anogenital area. Preliminary data from a WIHS study indicate a tenfold increase in the incidence of genital warts in HIV-positive women.[6]

Other types of HPV are associated with CIN and cervical cancer. CIN is an abnormal proliferation or growth of the epithelial cells that line the cervix. Left untreated, CIN can progress to cervical cancer. Like PID, CIN is associated with early sexual activity and multiple sex partners. It is detected by Pap tests. The incidence of CIN is higher in HIV-positive women. When it does occur in these women, CIN must be closely monitored with a Pap test every six months. In any woman, if CIN does not resolve on its own (which can occur in HIV-negative women), it must be treated to prevent progression to cervical cancer (see Chapter 8).

■ Menstrual Disorders

Women who are HIV positive often report changes in their menstrual cycle. Few scientific data exist, however, to know whether these changes occur in HIV-positive women with greater frequency than they do in HIV-negative women.

■ MEDICAL MANAGEMENT OF WOMEN WITH HIV DISEASE

As noted in the first chapter, perhaps the most important step for any person living with HIV is to obtain care from a physician experienced in treating HIV disease. In addition, for women infected with HIV, medical care is likely to be better if all their care needs—including gynecological and family-planning needs—can be met by the same physician or within the same clinic.

Women who are HIV positive should receive a complete gynecological exam, including a Pap test, during their initial medical visit (see Chapter 1). A second Pap test should be done six months later. If both tests reveal no sign of CIN, women with asymptomatic HIV disease can later be given annual Pap tests. However, HIV-positive women should receive subsequent Pap tests every six months if they have symptomatic HIV disease or if they show evidence of HPV infection, as suggested by the presence of CIN through a positive Pap test result or the finding of genital warts.

The initial medical evaluation of HIV-positive women should also include the following:

■ A complete menstrual, sexual, obstetrical, and gynecological history

■ Breast and pelvic exams

■ Screening for vaginitis, urinary tract infection, syphilis, gonorrhea, and chlamydia

■ Prophylaxis and Anti-HIV Therapy

Nonpregnant HIV-positive women should receive prophylaxis for *Pneumocystis carinii* pneumonia (PCP) and for *Mycobacterium avium* complex (MAC) (see Chapter 7) on the same basis as men. However, certain prophylactic drugs must be prescribed with caution during pregnancy because of risks to the fetus.

Women should also be offered antiretroviral therapy using the same standards of care that are used for men (see Chapter 5); they must also have the same opportunities as men to participate in clinical trials (see Chapter 6).

■ Wasting in Women with AIDS

Weight loss and wasting are common complications of HIV disease. Wasting is a life-threatening condition that results in the loss not only of fat tissue, but also of muscle (i.e., "lean body mass"). Use of the male sex hormone testosterone is widely accepted for the treatment of HIV-associated wasting syndrome in men and women, but it is not yet approved by the Food and Drug Administration. Its possible role in the treatment of wasting in women is even less well established than in men. In addition, it has a number of side effects in women such as suppression of menstruation, hair loss, and growth of facial hair.

Megestrol acetate (Megace) is an appetite stimulant also used in the treatment of HIV-associated wasting. Megestrol acetate is a progestin, a chemical related to progesterone, a hormone produced by the ovaries. When taken by women, megestrol acetate produces significant irregular vaginal bleeding. An AIDS Clinical Trials Group study (ACTG 313) is examining the use of megestrol acetate alone and in combination with testosterone for the treatment of wasting in HIV-positive men and women. (For more information on wasting, see Chapter 4 and Chapter 13.)

■ Menopause and Hormone Replacement Therapy

Women who are HIV positive can receive hormone replacement therapy for managing the symptoms of natural or premature menopause. Symptoms of menopause can be overlooked in HIV-positive women, or they can be attributed to the symptoms of HIV infection. Menopausal symptoms can include hot flashes, sweating, cystitis, atrophic vaginitis, urethritis, vaginal dryness and itching, and discomfort during urination or intercourse.

■ Pregnancy and HIV Infection

Some concerns have been raised about whether pregnancy hastens the course of HIV disease. While the evidence is still incomplete, pregnancy seems to have no significant effect on the rate of progression or course of HIV disease or on the health of the mother. Moreover, antiretroviral treatment is not known to have a harmful effect on pregnancy or on "embryonic and fetal development (nonetheless, some women may elect to delay or interrupt antiretroviral therapy until the end of the first trimester; for more explanation, see Chapter 5). Antiretroviral drugs do not seem to increase the complications of pregnancy, or to affect its outcome; that is, they have not been shown to affect the incidence of miscarriages, ectopic pregnancies, stillbirths, or the birth of preterm or low-birth-weight babies.

Over the next few years, data from several major studies now under way should help clarify many of the gynecological, behavioral, psychological, social, and cultural aspects of HIV disease in women. These studies include the following:

- The HIV Epidemiology and Research Study (HERS), conducted jointly by National Institute of Allergy and Infectious Diseases (NIAID) and the CDC, involves 800 HIV-positive women and 400 HIV-negative women.

- The Women's Interagency HIV Study (WIHS) is conducted by the NIAID. WIHS is following 2,080 HIV-infected women and 575 HIV-negative women.

- The New York City Cervical Disease Study is evaluating HIV-related gynecological manifestations of HIV disease.

- The Women and Infants Transmission Study (WITS) is evaluating pregnancy-related questions about HIV infection and its transmission during pregnancy. It was a study sponsored by WITS, the famous ACTG 076 trial, that first revealed in 1995 that treatment with AZT during pregnancy and delivery can greatly reduce the incidence of perinatal transmission of HIV (see Chapter 12).

The story of women in the HIV/AIDS epidemic well illustrates the additional price in ill health there is to pay by those who are members of a group, no matter how large, that still has subservient status in human society. While laws have been passed to protect women from such things as sexual harassment and job discrimination, women often still hold a subordinate standing in their personal relations with men. Yet, women remain the chief caregivers within the family, often shoulder the primary responsibility for raising children, and are often the anchors of families. When they die, many times they leave children behind who are uprooted, sad, disoriented, and lonely. What will become of them? In New York City alone, there could be as many as 100,000 AIDS orphans by the year 2000. This, too, is part of the growing cost to society of the HIV/AIDS epidemic as it continues its spread among women.

■ RESOURCES FOR WOMEN WITH HIV

See Appendix 1 for a listing of organizations that provide hotlines and information for women about HIV disease.

ENDNOTES

1. Note that the cases of HIV infection contracted from contaminated blood, blood components, or tissues and those resulting from treatment for a coagulation disorder were reported as AIDS in 1996, but the HIV infection that caused them occurred much earlier, at a time when blood, blood products, and tissues for transplantation were not as yet tested for HIV.

2. This should not be interpreted to mean that it is safe for an uninfected male to have unprotected sex even once with an infected female because the risk of transmission is lower than the risk for male-to-female transmission. Risk is assessed statistically, which means it is useful for predicting the likelihood of an event in a population. Risk numbers cannot be used to predict the outcome of a single event—in this case, whether transmission of HIV will occur during a single episode of sexual intercourse. Risk numbers are helpful for predicting how often HIV will be transmitted when 100, 1,000, or 10,000 couples have one episode of intercourse. Note, too, that there are many factors (e.g., the presence of sores from sexually transmitted diseases) that increase the risk of HIV transmission during intercourse. See Chapter 3.

3. Melnick SL, et al. Survival and disease progression according to gender of patients with HIV infection. *Journal of the American Medical Association* 1994;272:1915–1921.

4. Cu-Uvin S, et al. Prevalence of genital tract infection in HIV seropositive women. *Program and Abstracts of the HIV Infection in Women Confer-*

ence: Setting a New Agenda. February 1995; abstract FC1-178. Richmond, VA: Philadelphia Sciences Group, 1995.

5. Greenblatt RM, et al. Lower genital tract infections among HIV infected women and high risk seronegatives: the Women's Interagency HIV Study. *International Conference on AIDS.* 1996;11(2):126 (abstract no. We.C.3402).

6. *Ibid.*

■ *Chapter 12*

CHILDREN AND HIV DISEASE

AIDS was first described in children in 1982, a year after the syndrome was first identified in adults. By 1992, HIV disease was the seventh leading cause of death in children one to four years old in the United States. Today, early diagnosis and antiretroviral treatment and the use of prophylactic drugs for protection against opportunistic infections have enabled some HIV-infected children to live into their teens.

In many ways HIV disease in children resembles HIV disease in adults. In many other ways pediatric HIV disease is very different. Important differences include the following:

- The course of the disease is more uncertain in children. Some children born with HIV progress to advanced disease in three years, while others live into their teens with few signs of illness.

- The immune system is still developing and maturing in infants and children. In addition, infants possess a higher number of CD4 lymphocytes than adults, and the number of their lymphocytes changes at rates different from that of adults during disease progression. All this adds to the complexity of determining the timing and course of antiretroviral therapy.

- The amount of virus in the blood of infants (i.e., their viral load) during acute HIV infection is higher than it is in adults. In addition, the levels of free virus in the blood of HIV-infected infants decline more slowly than do those of adults, often taking three to four years to reach a baseline level (i.e., to reach a "set point").

- Advances in antiretroviral therapy for children lag behind those made for adults. This happens in part because new treatments for pediatric HIV disease must be tested through clinical trials conducted in children to show that the treatments are safe and that the dose is correct for children in various age groups (see also Chapter 6). Because the number of HIV-infected children is much smaller than the number of infected adults, it takes longer to enroll the number of children needed to complete a pediatric trial. For this reason, it is important that as many HIV-infected children as possible receive treatment through clinical trials. In addition, pharmaceutical companies appear less interested in pediatric clinical trials because children represent a much smaller commercial market for new drugs.

- Many children develop lymphocytic infiltrating pneumonitis, a chronic lung disease uncommon in adults (see below).

- HIV-related cancers, which occur frequently in adults, are much less common in children. Kaposi's sarcoma, a common cancer in adults, is extremely rare in children.

HIV infection in children is also complicated by a number of unique social and psychological problems:

- More than 98% of HIV infections in children result from mother-to-child—perinatal, or vertical—transmission. For nearly every HIV-infected child, there is an infected mother and often an infected father or sibling.

- Often, the HIV-infected child's caregiver is a single mother who struggles to care for her HIV-infected child while infected herself.

- HIV-infected children often come from homes already troubled in many ways.

- By the year 2000, an estimated 80,000 to 125,000 children will have lost their mothers to HIV/AIDS in this country alone.

■ DIAGNOSIS OF HIV INFECTION IN INFANTS AND CHILDREN

■ Treatment of HIV-Infected Pregnant Women Reduces the Rate of Perinatal Transmission

The source of HIV infection in children has changed considerably since the beginning of the HIV epidemic in 1981. In the first years of the epidemic, some children contracted HIV through transfusions of then-untested contaminated blood; others, born with hemophilia, contracted it through contaminated clotting factors. The testing of blood for anti-bodies to HIV, which began in the United States in 1985, and the use of heat-treated or genetically engineered clotting factors have virtually elim-inated these sources of infection. Surviving children who had developed AIDS after receiving contaminated blood transfusions or clotting factors before 1985 made up about only 8% of all pediatric AIDS cases at the end of 1996.

Today, nearly every new case of HIV infection among children in the United States and worldwide occurs through perinatal transmission, that is, during pregnancy, delivery, or breast-feeding. Studies have shown that HIV is transmitted from pregnant untreated HIV-infected mothers to about 25% of their newborns on average. In the early 1990s, some 7,000 HIV-infected women gave birth each year in the United States to more than 2,000 HIV-infected infants.

Today, the rate of mother-to-infant transmission is being dramat-ically reduced in this country with the use of AZT in pregnant HIV-infected women prior to and during delivery, and in their infants for six weeks after birth. This remarkable finding was made through the AIDS Clinical Trials Group (ACTG) 076 study, which showed that the rate of mother-to-child transmission could be cut by two-thirds—down to 8%—by this treatment.[1]

(As is typical of clinical research, the 076 study was preceded by animal studies—preclinical research—that first demonstrated the effectiveness of the strategy. Animal experiments first showed that anti-retroviral drugs would prevent perinatal transmission of a leukemia-causing retrovirus in mice. This led to studies in monkeys, which showed that antiretroviral treatment reduced the transmission of the simian immunodeficiency virus [SIV] from macaque mothers to their new-borns. Success in these studies led to the ACTG 076 study. For more in-formation on how new treatments are developed, see Chapter 6.)

Research that followed the 076 study showed that a high level of free virus in the mother's blood—a high viral load—at the time of delivery appeared to increase the risk of perinatal transmission. AZT given be-ginning in the second trimester may have helped reduce the risk of mother-to-child HIV transmission by reducing the mother's viral load before delivery (although there can be exceptions to this; mothers with a low viral load may transmit HIV, or mothers with a high viral load may not).

Clinical trials are now under way to determine if the use of a combi-nation of antiretroviral drugs in HIV-infected pregnant women will re-duce perinatal transmission still further. Arthur Ammann, M.D., of the American Foundation for AIDS Research (AmFAR), has predicted that the use of combination antiretroviral therapy would reduce the rate of perinatal transmission to less than 2% of births to HIV-positive women, or fewer than 100 new cases per year in the United States. With AZT alone, it is estimated that fewer than 500 newly infected infants are now born in the United States each year.

The findings of the 076 study were a true breakthrough. They showed for the first time that a treatment for HIV disease could reduce HIV transmission, and they raised the hope that this route of transmission might one day be eliminated entirely. The results prompted the U.S. Pub-lic Health Service, in July 1995, to offer guidelines for a national program that would universally provide HIV counseling to all pregnant women and offer voluntary testing to any pregnant women who desired it.

The results of the ACTG 076 study, however, also generated calls by politicians and others for mandatory HIV testing of all pregnant women or of all newborns. They argued that not identifying HIV infection in pregnant women denied protection to unborn children. This would delay, for example, the use of prophylaxis against deadly *Pneumocystis carinii* pneumonia (PCP), which can occur in HIV-infected infants as early as three months after birth.

Those who objected to the mandatory testing of pregnant women and newborns argued that this would deter many pregnant women from seeking prenatal care. Or, they said, women who had been tested but who did not wish to learn their HIV status would not return for further prenatal care. They also pointed out that many women at high risk for HIV already have a profound distrust of the health-care system, a distrust that stems from personal or communal negative experiences, language barriers, low educational level, and cultural differences. Women who are illegal immigrants fear imprisonment; women who use illegal drugs fear that their children will be sent to foster homes, and they fear imprisonment for themselves. At the same time, all women tend to be receptive to preventive health-care advice such as HIV counseling and to preventive measures such as testing and treatment when appropriate during pregnancy to protect the health of their unborn child. Counseling and voluntary testing, said the opponents of mandatory testing, are a more effective way to ensure that pregnant women receive perinatal care and that they receive the education needed to accept AZT treatment for the protection of their babies.

In 1996, the federal government initiated an attempt to require states to provide universal HIV counseling and voluntary testing to pregnant women. The original plan gave states two years to reduce the rate of perinatal transmission by 50% of its 1993 level. Those states that did not reach this target would have to implement mandatory HIV testing of either all pregnant women or all newborns, and they would lose federal funding for certain AIDS-related programs if they did not comply. However, the funding necessary for a universal counseling and voluntary testing program for pregnant women was never appropriated by Congress, and the requirement for the states to establish such a program was never enforced.

Instead, the government seems to have taken a wait-and-see approach. There is a sense that most state health departments and physicians will routinely provide counseling and testing without a federal mandate. In addition, federal funding has been provided to improve the monitoring of perinatal cases of HIV infection by states. In 1998, the Secretary of Health and Human Services was to review the success that states achieved in reducing the rate of perinatal HIV transmission, either through voluntary or through mandatory programs. The secretary was then to determine whether a federally mandated national program is necessary.

A number of states have taken steps to implement universal counseling and voluntary testing programs for pregnant women. Some of these programs were mandated through legislation, but many states have encouraged counseling and voluntary testing through advisories and public campaigns aimed at physicians and the public. In 1996, New York State took steps to implement what is tantamount to a program of mandatory testing of newborns. Since 1988, New York State had tested all newborns for antibody to HIV as a way of monitoring the prevalence of HIV infection in women. This testing program, done only to monitor the pattern of HIV spread in the population, was "blinded." Blood samples taken from newborns were identified only by a number; the infants were not identified and the parents were not, and could not be, contacted when their infant tested HIV positive. State legislation in 1996 changed that. It now requires the identification of all HIV-positive newborns and the automatic notification of their parents.

■ Screening of Infants

All children born to HIV-infected mothers will test HIV positive at birth by the standard HIV antibody test (which is why the testing of newborns can be used to follow the epidemic of HIV infection in their mothers). But about three-fourths of these children will not be infected with HIV. Non-HIV-infected newborns can nevertheless test positive because certain antibodies produced by their mothers—including antibodies against HIV—pass into the fetus's blood during pregnancy. Traces of these maternal antibodies remain in the child's blood for up to 18 months. Only after the age of 18 months does the HIV antibody test reliably reveal whether a child is HIV infected or not, that is, whether he or she produces his or her own antibody in response to HIV infection.

This creates an important dilemma: HIV-infected infants should be started on antiretroviral treatment early and are at high risk of developing PCP as early as three months after birth. Thus, unless the truly HIV-infected infants can be identified within the first few weeks of life, all infants born to infected mothers will be given PCP prophylaxis to prevent this life-threatening infection in only the 25% of them who are truly HIV infected.

To reduce this problem, the Centers for Disease Control and Prevention (CDC) recommends first identifying pregnant women who are HIV infected—perhaps through universal counseling and by encouraging voluntary testing, as described—and then screening their newborns using new tests that identify the presence of the virus itself in blood, rather than antibodies to it. These new tests can accurately identify 90% of truly HIV-infected infants within the first month or two of life. Such tests include viral culture, polymerase chain reaction (PCR), and branched-chain DNA (bDNA) testing (see Chapter 2). HIV-infected pregnant women should ask their physician about the availability of these tests for their baby in the area where they live. Newborns of HIV-infected mothers should also be screened for other infections such as syphilis and hepatitis B.

■ ROLE OF CD4 LYMPHOCYTE COUNTS IN HIV-INFECTED CHILDREN

In adults, CD4 lymphocyte counts help assess the health of the immune system and help determine when to begin preventive treatments for opportunistic infections. CD4 counts in children are used in a similar way, but children have a much higher number of CD4 lymphocytes at birth than do adults (Table 12.1). These numbers decrease as children age and as the immune system matures. This means that the CD4 lymphocyte counts used as standard measures in adults to mark disease progression cannot be applied in the same way to children, which adds to the difficulty in determining when to begin preventive treatments and antiretroviral therapy in HIV-infected children.

Table 12.1 ■ *CD4 Lymphocyte Count and Level of Immune Suppression at Different Ages*

Age	CD4 Lymphocyte Count (per mm³)	
	Moderate Immune Suppression	Severe Immune Suppression
1–11 months	750–1,499	<750
1–5 years	500–999	<500
6–12 years	200–499	<200
Adults	200–499	<200

CD4 counts are typically determined at the ages of 1 month and 3 months in infants born to HIV-infected mothers. HIV-infected infants should have additional CD4 counts at the ages of 6, 9, and 12 months. These counts are important for assessing the health of these infants' immune systems, for determining their response to treatment, for monitoring progression of HIV infection, and for determining the need for PCP preventive treatments beyond the age of 1 year.

Note, however, that measurements of viral load will probably soon replace CD4 lymphocyte counts as a more accurate marker upon which to make decisions regarding the use of anti-HIV therapy (see "Antiretroviral Therapy in Infants and Children").

■ DISEASE PROGRESSION IN CHILDREN

HIV disease in children seems to follow two distinct patterns. About 10% to 15% of infected untreated infants experience an early onset, with rapidly progressing HIV infection. They develop severe immune suppression, opportunistic infections, and encephalopathy during their first few months of life. Most of these children die from advanced disease by age 5.

The remaining 85% to 90% of children are long-term slow progressors. They develop immune deficiency gradually over a period that can last ten years. The course of their disease is similar to that of adults (although the AIDS-defining illnesses are different), and they often survive into their teens. About half of these surviving children experience moderate or serious illness; the other half continue to survive without experiencing serious illness.

A French study published in 1996 followed 267 infected infants to see if those who developed rapidly progressing disease exhibited characteristics that set them apart from infants with slower progression.[2] They found that infants with early-onset, rapidly progressing disease tended to be born with swollen lymph nodes and an enlarged liver or spleen, or both. Another important indicator was a low proportion of CD4 lymphocytes. If CD4 lymphocytes made up less than 30% of the child's total lymphocyte count, the child had a threefold higher risk of early and severe disease. Other observations suggest that rapid progression is also re-lated to high viral loads during acute infection.

The reason for the two patterns of HIV disease is not known. Scien-tists suspect that time of infection may be a determining factor: Children who are infected in the womb might develop severe disease early, while children infected during birth or breast-feeding might have the slower form of disease.

■ Can Some Babies Eliminate HIV from Their Body?

There have been occasional reports in the medical literature about HIV-infected infants who later appeared to have eliminated the virus from their body. The reports were met with skepticism, however, because de-finitive evidence that the infants had actually been truly infected was lacking.

■ CARE OF THE HIV-INFECTED NEWBORN

Most HIV-infected infants are asymptomatic at birth, although those born to women who use drugs may be jittery and irritable. In the United States and other developed countries, breast-feeding by an HIV-infected mother is discouraged because it can transmit the virus. (Breast-feeding by HIV-infected, poverty-stricken mothers is encouraged in developing countries, however, because the risk of death from malnutrition or diarrhea-associated diseases in these infants is much higher if they are not breast-fed.)

All HIV-positive babies should be followed routinely by physicians and nurses who are familiar with the signs and symptoms of HIV disease. Parents should watch for signs of fever, breathing problems, poor weight gain, feeding difficulties, severe vomiting, and diarrhea, and report them immediately to the child's physician. If they sense that the child, even if well, is not developing physically or intellectually as he or she should, they should express their concern to the physician.

The medical management of the HIV-infected child involves prophy-laxis for PCP (see below) and antiretroviral therapy if symptoms of HIV disease or deterioration of the immune system become apparent. It is essential that the child's caregivers be educated about HIV disease. It is also essential that the child be provided with nutritional support (including supplementations when appropriate), adequate housing, and clothing; that the child and caregiver be given emotional support, including relief support for the caregiver; and that visiting-nurse and home-health aide services be provided. Lastly, the mother should call her state HIV/AIDS hotline for information on the entitlement programs for which she and her child may qualify.

■ CHILDHOOD IMMUNIZATION

Immunization for childhood diseases is one of the most effective and least expensive means of preventing some of the viral and bacterial infections that occur in HIV-infected children. HIV-infected infants and children should receive the same immunizations according to the same schedule as non-HIV-infected children, although in some cases the nature of the vaccine preparation used may be different. Recommendations for these vaccinations are provided and periodically reviewed and revised by the Committee on Infectious Disease of the American Academy of Pediatrics and by the Advisory Committee on Immunization Practices of the U.S. Public Health Service.

Immunizations should include hepatitis B vaccine; diphtheria-pertussis-tetanus (DPT) vaccine; enhanced inactivated poliovirus vaccine (EIPV), used in place of the live attenuated oral vaccine usually given to children in the general population; *Hemophilus influenzae* type b vaccine; measles-mumps-rubella (MMR) vaccine; and polyvalent pneumococcal vaccine.

The effectiveness of immunizations depends on the health of the child's immune system at the time the vaccinations are given; the effectiveness of a vaccination decreases as the child's HIV disease progresses and the immune system weakens.

■ CLASSIFICATION OF HIV DISEASE IN CHILDREN

The CDC currently uses four categories of increasing disease severity for classifying children with HIV disease. The category in which a child is placed depends on the degree of immune suppression and the kinds of complications and infections the child has developed. A brief description of each category follows.

- Asymptomatic (CDC Category 'N'): children who show no signs or symptoms attributable to HIV infection, or who show only one of the conditions for category 'A.'

- Mildly symptomatic (CDC Category 'A'): children with two or more symptoms such as swollen lymph nodes (lymphadenopathy), enlarged liver or spleen, dermatitis, or recurrent or persistent respiratory tract infections, sinus infections, or middle-ear infections (otitis media).

- Moderately symptomatic (CDC Category 'B'): children who develop conditions considered to be of intermediate severity. These include oral candidiasis that persists for more than two months, bacterial meningitis, pneumonia, recurrent or chronic diarrhea, and lymphoid interstitial pneumonitis (LIP).

- Severely symptomatic (CDC Category 'C'): children who have opportunistic infections, cancers, or other conditions characteristic of advanced disease. These include serious bacterial infections such as septicemia or pneumonia (two or more in a two-year period), PCP, bone or joint infections, abscesses of an internal organ or body cavity, dementia (encephalopathy), cryptococcal disease, cryptosporidiosis, esophageal or pulmonary candidiasis, tuberculosis (TB), or lymphoma.

■ OPPORTUNISTIC INFECTIONS IN INFANTS AND CHILDREN

HIV-infected children are subject to most of the opportunistic infections that can occur in adults. Some that are particularly notable in HIV-infected children are described here. See Chapter 7 for separate listings on bacillary angiomatosis, candidiasis, coccidioidomycosis, cryptococcosis, cryptosporidiosis, cytomegalovirus (CMV) infection, diarrhea, herpes simplex infection, histoplasmosis, microsporidiosis, *Mycobacterium avium* complex (MAC), oral hairy leukoplakia, PCP, shingles (varicella-zoster virus [VZV]), toxoplasmosis, and TB.

■ Bacterial Infections

After PCP, recurrent severe bacterial infections are the second most common AIDS-defining illness in American children with HIV disease. Bacterial infections are caused by the same bacteria that cause illnesses in non-HIV-infected children. They include bacteria responsible for middle-ear infections, or otitis media; sinusitis; gastrointestinal illness (e.g., *Salmonella*); lower respiratory tract infections, including pneumonia; and meningitis.

Urinary or indwelling venous chest catheters—tubes placed in the chest wall for injection of intravenous drugs or withdrawal of blood samples for testing—can be a significant source of bacterial infection in children. Proper catheter care is important in reducing this source of infection. The child's physician should be promptly notified of any problem involving a catheter.

■ Candidiasis and Other Fungal Infections

Candidiasis is caused by the yeast-like fungus *Candida albicans*, a microbe found commonly on human skin and mucous membranes. Candidiasis also occurs in non-HIV-infected infants and children. (Candidiasis is also a common opportunistic infection in adults with HIV disease; see Chapter 7.) Infants acquire *Candida* organisms during birth and during breast-feeding. The most common sites of infection in infants are the mucous membranes of the mouth, throat, and esophagus. Candidiasis can occur in the diaper area, where it sometimes requires prolonged therapy, and in the mucous membrane at the base of the fingernails, although this condition, known as "*Candida* onychomycosis," is very rare.

Oral Candidiasis (Thrush)

Oral candidiasis occurs in 15% to 40% of HIV-infected children. Signs of infection include creamy white plaques on the tongue, gums, throat, cheek linings, or roof of the mouth. Erythematous candidiasis appears as roughened red patches on the tongue or lining of the mouth. It can be severe enough to make eating difficult. Candidiasis can also cause angular cheilitis, which produces cracks and fissures in the corners of the mouth.

Left untreated, oral candidiasis can extend into the throat and infect the epiglottis. This can cause hoarseness and interfere with breathing, and it requires immediate medical attention.

Oral candidiasis can sometimes be confused with oral hairy leukoplakia, a viral infection that often occurs on the sides and surface of the tongue in immune-suppressed adults but is rare in children (see also Chapter 7).

Esophageal Candidiasis

Candidiasis of the esophagus is a diagnostic indicator for HIV disease. It occurs often in adults, but the frequency in children is unknown. Esophageal candidiasis can occur with or without concurrent oral candidiasis. Esophageal candidiasis sometimes produces no symptoms; other times, it causes difficulty and pain on swallowing.

Other Fungal Infections

Ringworm and athlete's foot infections can occur in HIV-positive children, and they can be extensive and severe. The major fungal infections that often occur in adults with HIV disease—cryptococcosis, histoplasmosis, and coccidioidomycosis—are rare in HIV-infected children.

■ Herpesvirus Infections

Herpesviruses include CMV, VZV (which is responsible for both chickenpox and shingles), herpes simplex virus types 1 and 2, and Epstein-Barr virus (EBV). Herpesviruses are common sources of infection in both adults and children with HIV disease. For further information, see the sections on CMV disease, herpes simplex infection, and shingles in Chapter 7. In addition, infection by human herpesvirus (HHV) type 6 or 7 is a common cause of high fever in children. HHV-8, a human herpesvirus associated with Kaposi's sarcoma, is not usually found in children in the United States, and this may explain why children infected with HIV rarely develop Kaposi's sarcoma.

An HIV-infected child who has no previous history of chickenpox and who is exposed to someone with either chickenpox or shingles should receive an injection of gamma globulin promptly (i.e., within a day or two of exposure) to prevent the infection or reduce its severity.

■ Measles Virus

The measles virus is one of the most contagious viruses known. Measles infection can cause serious complications in non-HIV-infected children, but it can be very dangerous and even fatal in HIV-infected children, especially in those with advanced HIV disease. Symptoms of infection include rash, fever, conjunctivitis, cough, runny nose, watery eyes, and sometimes croup and pneumonia.

The measles virus spreads rapidly indoors by droplets produced when a person with active measles coughs and sneezes. It is important that HIV-infected children be immunized against measles. In addition, if exposure to measles occurs, the child should receive an injection of gamma globulin promptly, within days of the exposure. Gamma globulin is a mixture of antibodies that includes antibodies against measles. An injection of gamma globulin supplements the child's immune response to the measles virus and helps prevent or lessen the severity of a measles infection.

■ *Mycobacterium avium* Complex

As children live longer with HIV disease, MAC is seen with increasing frequency. It is an indicator of markedly advanced disease and requires treatment with multiple drugs. (For more information on MAC, see Chapter 7.)

■ *Pneumocystis carinii* Pneumonia

PCP is the most common opportunistic infection in children with HIV disease. The disease produces in them an acute, diffuse, life-threatening pneumonia that results from inflammation and destruction of lung tissue. (For more information on PCP, see Chapter 7.)

Symptoms include shallow rapid breathing, cough, shortness of breath, and fever. (In HIV-infected children, similar symptoms can be caused by CMV infection and a variety of bacterial and viral infections.) LIP also causes a type of pneumonia, but LIP has a subtle onset, progresses slowly, and usually occurs in older children (see below).

In both adults and children, PCP was a leading cause of death in people with HIV disease before prophylactic drugs were available to prevent it. In perinatally infected infants who do not receive PCP prophylaxis, PCP can suddenly occur as early as three months after birth. It is fatal if left untreated.

Unlike adults, children may not indefinitely require PCP prophylaxis. If a baby's CD4 lymphocyte count is back to normal at 12 months, PCP prophylaxis can be discontinued until and unless disease progression makes resumption imperative. In some children, this may be when they are in their teens.

Prevention

U.S. Public Health Service guidelines recommend the following for PCP prophylaxis in infants and children:

- Any child born to an HIV-infected mother should begin PCP prophylaxis at the age of four to six weeks regardless of his or her CD4 cell count. However, it should never begin earlier than four weeks after birth because younger infants cannot tolerate the sulfa drugs used for PCP prophylaxis. There is also a danger of harmful drug interactions between these drugs and AZT in newborns being treated with AZT to reduce their risk of perinatal HIV infection.

- All truly HIV-infected infants should continue PCP prophylaxis until the age of 12 months, and so should those born to HIV-infected mothers but whose true HIV status is still unknown.

- Children older than 12 months should have regular CD4 lymphocyte counts to determine their need for continuing PCP prophylaxis.

- HIV-infected children who have had an episode of PCP should receive PCP prophylaxis indefinitely to prevent recurrence, regardless of their CD4 lymphocyte count or stage of disease.

- The recommended chemoprophylactic drug for PCP is trimethoprim-sulfamethoxazole (TMP-SMX). Children who cannot tolerate TMP-SMX can be given dapsone, aerosolized pentamidine, or intravenous pentamidine. A new experimental drug, atovaquone, is also available through the pediatric clinical trials network or when prescribed by AIDS-care specialists. Information can be obtained by calling the AIDS Clinical Trial Information Service toll-free at 1-800-874-2572.

- Regimens for PCP prophylaxis must be strictly followed for success.

■ Tuberculosis

All infants born to HIV-infected mothers should have a tuberculin skin test (the PPD test, see Chapter 7) at the age of 9 to 12 months as is recommended for all infants in the course of routine care.

TB is an uncommon illness in HIV-infected infants and children in the United States, but even in this country it can occur in children living with an adult who has active TB. Those at highest risk are children who live in crowded, poor conditions or in shelters for the homeless. Once exposed, they can develop a rapidly progressive form of TB. If TB exposure is suspected, the child must be tested. If the child tests positive, he or she should be treated promptly. Treatment is similar to that for adults (see Chapter 7).

■ OTHER IMPORTANT CONDITIONS IN CHILDREN WITH HIV DISEASE

■ Diarrhea

Diarrhea is not in itself a disease, but it is a common symptom of many opportunistic infections. The majority of people with HIV disease experience diarrhea at some time in the course of the disease. The condition can be caused by HIV itself, as well as by a variety of viral, bacterial, or protozoan infections. Acute diarrhea can also have noninfectious causes. Fever may or may not be present. Prolonged diarrhea requires medical attention; its effective treatment begins by identifying the underlying cause. Left untreated, diarrhea can result in dehydration and a loss of important salts (i.e., electrolytes). It may also interfere with absorption of nutrients, and thereby contribute to malnutrition.

■ Lymphoid Interstitial Pneumonitis

LIP produces a chronic, diffuse pneumonia. Onset of the disease occurs silently, with no symptoms, and this form of pneumonia progresses slowly. LIP occurs almost exclusively in HIV-infected children, and it can be the first sign of symptomatic disease. LIP can be diagnosed in children as young as two months, but it characteristically occurs in children older than one year (PCP also produces a diffuse pneumonia and can have symptoms resembling LIP, although PCP is a more aggressive disease and typically occurs in infants less than one year old).

LIP is caused by a gradual accumulation of lymphoid cells and other white blood cells in the tissues of the lung. This infiltration of the lung tissue interferes with the movement of oxygen from the air spaces of the lung—the alveoli—into red blood cells in the small blood vessels of the lung. Progression of LIP is marked by the continuing accumulation of infiltrating cells and a gradual decrease in the amount of oxygen entering the blood. Sometimes, the medium-sized airways in the lung lose elasticity and become stiff and dilated.

The rate of LIP's progression is variable. Some children experience very little change for long periods; others experience slowly progressive, chronic disease with occasional lung infections and occasional difficulty breathing.

In children with LIP, the level of oxygen in the blood is low, a condition known as "hypoxia." Therefore, the tissues of their body never receive the full amount of oxygen that they need. Chronic, progressive hypoxia causes children with LIP to become quickly winded from exercise. They must rest frequently when walking or playing. The lack of oxygen can give a blue cast to their lips and fingernail beds.

Other symptoms include a broadening of the ends of the fingers and toes, a condition known as "clubbing." Clubbing is also seen in children with other chronic respiratory diseases like cystic fibrosis and chronic severe asthma. Children with LIP can also experience slow growth and delayed development, a condition known as "failure to thrive."

There is no cure for LIP. Management of the disease involves use of antiretroviral therapy to slow progression of the underlying HIV infection, medications and treatments that improve the child's ability to breathe, and, according to some experts, corticosteroids to reduce the infiltration of lymphocytes into the lung.

Supportive care is important to reduce the risk of respiratory infections, and should include immunization for influenza (and if the child is not as yet vaccinated against them, pneumococcus, and *Hemophilus influenzae* type b); a nutritious diet; and monitoring for LIP progression. A child with advanced LIP may require oxygen treatments and bronchodilator therapy, which can be given at home.

The cause of LIP is unknown. Some specialists theorize that it is an abnormal immune response to antigens inhaled into the lungs or circulating in the blood. Others think it could be caused by infection of the lung tissue by EBV, which is often found in LIP tissue samples, or by coinfection of the lung with EBV and HIV.

■ HIV Encephalopathy

Progressive HIV encephalopathy occurs in about 10% of children with HIV disease. The condition is similar to AIDS dementia complex in adults, and is usually associated with a poor prognosis.

In young children, HIV dementia is accompanied by atrophy of the brain and a concomitant reduction in the size of the head, and a deficit in developmental milestones such as an ability to sit, stand, or walk. Older children may experience a deterioration of intellectual ability (e.g., difficulty with memory, writing, or arithmetic), weakness, spasticity, and difficulty walking.

Encephalopathy probably results from direct infection of the central nervous system with HIV, which is often found in brain tissue and cerebrospinal fluid of affected children.

Treatment with antiretroviral therapy sometimes produces temporary improvements in brain growth, mental ability, and developmental milestones. As the disease progresses, families often need the assistance of nurses or home health-care aids to manage the activities of daily living such as feeding, bed care, and pain control.

■ Malignancies in Children with HIV Disease

The progressive immune deficiency of HIV-infected people increases their risk of developing cancer (see Chapter 8). Kaposi's sarcoma rarely occurs in children with HIV disease, and the incidence of lymphomas and sarcomas that do occur is much lower than it is in adults. Soft-tissue sarcoma is a type of cancer that is seen somewhat more often in HIV-positive children than in HIV-negative children. These malignancies arise in connective tissue and muscle, often in unusual locations such as the spleen, liver, and lung. Leiomyosarcoma, a tumor of smooth muscle, is an otherwise rare malignancy increasingly seen in children with HIV disease.

■ ANTIRETROVIRAL THERAPY IN INFANTS AND CHILDREN

It is imperative that all HIV-infected pregnant women be offered antiretroviral therapy, which can reduce the risk of HIV transmission from HIV-infected mothers to their infants and thereby prevent HIV infection in children. Infants who are born HIV infected in spite of this preventive treatment are given antiretroviral drugs to slow the onset of HIV disease. If the therapy is successful, disease progression is halted or slowed, which results in a drop in viral load, increased CD4 counts, and even weight gain and improved mental function.

Important questions to be addressed with HIV-infected children include when to begin antiretroviral treatment, what drugs should be used, when to switch from one treatment to another, and when to stop treatment. Clearly, children with falling CD4 counts and high viral loads require immediate treatment, regardless of clinical symptoms (taking into account the normal age-related differences in CD4 lymphocyte counts of children compared to adults).

Clinical trials in both adults and children have dramatically shown that the use of several antiretroviral drugs simultaneously, starting early after diagnosis, is the most effective way to manage HIV infection.

The use of two or more antiretroviral drugs is known as "combination therapy" or multidrug therapy, while the use of a single drug is known as "monotherapy." Many physicians favor treating children with a combination of two antiretroviral drugs, often AZT (zidovudine) and ddI (didanosine), or AZT and 3TC (lamivudine). Others prefer other drug combinations, and a variety of new combinations will become available as more drugs receive approval for use in children.

The rapidly evolving standard of care is leading to early intervention with drug combinations and to the determination of both CD4 counts and viral load to assess response to treatment.

Because few antiretroviral drugs have been studied in children, combination therapy is difficult to apply in children. Clinical trials testing the various drug combinations in HIV-infected children are under way, but their results are not yet available. In addition, drugs are often not available in doses or formulations designed for children. These problems confront the pediatric HIV specialists wanting to treat children with protease inhibitors and other new or experimental drugs. Since even drugs not "approved for use in children" could be effective in controlling their disease progression, physicians must use their best medical judgment in treating HIV-infected children, and derive guidance from clinical trials done in adults.

The importance of entering as many children as possible in clinical trials cannot be overstated. For information on clinical trials for children with HIV disease, telephone the AIDS Clinical Trials Information Service toll free at 1-800-874-2572, or the Pediatrics Branch of the National Cancer Institute at 1-301-402-0696. Children who cannot gain access to clinical trials must be aggressively treated by an expert physician on an individual basis.

In the near future, treatment decisions in children will be increasingly based on changes in viral load, as they are now in adults. Viral load will be used to determine when to begin anti-HIV therapy, whether the therapy is effective, and when to change therapy in response to drug resistance.

■ TELLING A CHILD ABOUT HIS OR HER HIV INFECTION

One of the most difficult decisions facing the parent of an HIV-infected child is deciding when and how to tell the child about his or her condition. Parents may understandably dread this obligation. They may want to avoid the pain and guilt of telling the child how he or she became infected, and of answering the child's questions about whether his or her disease will lead to an early death. The parents may also fear telling their own friends, coworkers, and even family members, and worry that their child will be unable to keep the information confidential, and that the child and the family will be ostracized.

All are legitimate fears and concerns. But secrecy also carries a price. It cuts the parents off from the support they could otherwise receive from close friends and family. The child's doctors, nurses, social workers, and perhaps teachers also become enmeshed in the web of secrecy. They cannot discuss the child's situation without the parents' consent. This prevents them from openly discussing important issues of which the child should be aware, particularly by the time he or she reaches the age of nine or ten.

"This kind of secrecy has a tremendous psychological impact," says Warren Andiman, associate professor of pediatrics and epidemiology at the Yale University School of Medicine. "The child sort of knows what's going on, but can't say the word; the mother sort of hints at it, but can't say the word; and if there are other people in the family who are sick, the child kind of picks up on it, but can't say the word, so no one can talk about it. It makes a difficult situation much worse."

Often, however, the child overhears the medical talk and grasps the meaning of the caregiver's serious tones, sees stories about HIV on television, and figures out what's wrong on his or her own. How do children respond when they do finally find out? "They usually handle it pretty well," says Andiman, "because then we can extend the emotional and psychological support that are traditionally provided for other catastrophic illnesses. We can sit down with the family and work through how they're going to deal with it."

Andiman recommends that when an HIV-infected child reaches

school age, the parents begin discussing their situation between themselves and with their doctor to determine at what age and under what circumstances they would like the child to be told of his or her infection. It is also sometimes helpful for parents to rehearse their answers to some of the more common questions that children will ask. Some parents prefer to tell the child themselves in a peaceful situation at home; others prefer to receive help from the child's social worker or physician.

■ WHEN A CHILD ENTERS THE FINAL STAGE OF HIV DISEASE

When their child reaches late-stage HIV disease and becomes terminally ill, the parents or guardian should seek advice from the child's physician regarding decisions such as whether to authorize the use of a ventilator and other life-extending treatments. A child in late-stage HIV disease requires constant, vigilant care. It is often helpful for the caregivers to seek respite care, which provides someone who can stay with the child to give them time to seek medical care for themselves, to attend to their other children or to other responsibilities, or just to get much-needed rest. Caregivers can learn about respite programs in their community by telephoning a local hospice or by talking with social workers at community hospitals and larger pediatric AIDS programs.

Many communities also have children's hospice programs. Hospice programs provide medical care—including pain control—spiritual and psychological support, and bereavement counseling to the family (see Chapter 13). The traditional admission criterion for adult hospice programs is a life expectancy of six months or less. The child with AIDS often has a life expectancy longer than six months and may endure life-threatening illnesses several times. For this reason, admission to a children's hospice program varies and is often made on a case-by-case basis.

For information on children's hospice programs, call Children's Hospice International toll-free at 1-800-2-4-CHILD or the National Pediatric HIV Resource Center at 1-800-362-0071.

■ ADOLESCENTS WHO ARE NEWLY INFECTED WITH HIV

According to recent CDC statistics, one of every four new HIV infections to occur in 1996 was in someone under the age of 20. Adolescents who become infected by HIV confront a set of problems and challenges different from both those of younger children and those of adults. By 1997, a total of 2,754 adolescents had developed AIDS in the United States, making up only 0.5% of the total number of people with AIDS.[3] But those small numbers present only a small part of the picture. Also by 1997, a total of 21,097 cases of AIDS had been reported in young adults ages 20 to 24.[4] Because there is an average ten-year time lag between the time of HIV infection and the development of AIDS, most young adults diagnosed with AIDS became infected during adolescence.

Surveys conducted among high school students (grades 9 through 12) by the CDC report that about three-fourths of high school students have had sexual intercourse by grade 12. About one-fifth have had more than four sexual partners, and fewer than half report using latex condoms consistently. Many report using alcohol or drugs when they have sex, which impairs judgment and increases the risk of unsafe sex.

Ironically, the CDC reports that most teenagers understand how HIV is transmitted. The adolescents' strong sense of immortality and invincibility—"it can't happen to me"—is the major obstacle that family-, school-, and community-based education programs need to overcome.

Because of this general attitude and the time lag between the time of infection and the development of symptoms, reports of AIDS diagnosis in adolescents are rare. When HIV testing reveals HIV infection, adolescents often respond with denial, guilt, and fear. They often resent the resulting new dependence on parents and the medical community. It is important that HIV-infected adolescents have the chance to openly discuss their infection and their future. Individual and family counseling can help improve family communication, resolve feelings of guilt, and provide reassurance.

Adolescents with HIV infection should be encouraged to enroll in appropriate clinical trials, and they usually qualify for adult studies. Consent from parents or guardians may be required for those younger than 18, however. All clinical trials require that potential participants understand the risk and benefits of the trial before enrolling and provide informed consent before joining the trial (see Chapter 6). Usually, both the adolescent and his or her parent or guardian must provide their consent, although state laws can vary. The consent of the child may be waived if he or she is not capable of providing informed consent because of age, maturity, or psychological condition.

■ CONCLUSIONS

The number of infants and children with HIV/AIDS has always represented a relatively small part of the epidemic, but a particularly heart-wrenching part. Fortunately, it is also a part of the epidemic that early on came under at least partial control.

First, in 1985, blood testing for HIV led to the prevention of HIV transmission through blood transfusions, which was the cause of the earliest HIV infections in children. Soon after, elimination of HIV from clotting factors spared children born with hemophilia.

In 1994, the remarkable results of the clinical trial ACTG 076 almost immediately reduced the rate of mother-to-child HIV transmission. Within two years, the number of babies born each year with HIV infection dropped from an estimated 2,000 to fewer than 500—and the number is still decreasing. In fact, some major metropolitan areas have not reported a newly infected infant for more than one year. This nation owes a large measure of gratitude for this outstanding achievement to farsighted scientists, dedicated physicians, and the many courageous women who volunteered for this seminal study.

But all is not well yet. The treatment regimen used in the ACTG 076 trial is not practical for, or affordable by, millions of women who desperately need it—particularly those living in the developing countries hardest hit by the HIV epidemic. Unfortunately, an art we have not yet mastered is how to make medical progress achieved in wealthy and technologically advanced societies beneficial to the world's poorer nations. New approaches are needed for prevention of perinatal transmission in these countries. The lives of millions of children across the world could be saved through further clinical research and determined international cooperation between governments and pharmaceutical companies.

And there is another population of children among whom HIV infection is not abating but growing: adolescents. Because the human immune system is fully mature by age 13, adolescents with HIV/AIDS can be medically treated as adults. But adolescents are still children, and one out of four new HIV infections now occurs among them. However, the very real psychosocial and developmental factors that account for much of the higher-risk behaviors of adolescents should not provide an excuse for their widespread ignorance of pertinent biological and medical facts. It is the responsibility of adults, parents, and other authority figures, in addition to school teachers, to create an environment of trust and honesty in which such information can be imparted in a frank and timely way. This is an area where many adults must do much better, and soon, to stem the spread of HIV among youth.

ENDNOTES

1. Connor HM, et al. Reduction of maternal-infant transmission of human immunodeficiency virus type 1 with zidovudine treatment. *New England Journal of Medicine* 1994; 331:1173–1180.

2. Mayaux M-J, et al. Neonatal characteristics in rapidly progressive perinatally acquired HIV-1 disease. *Journal of the American Medical Association* 1996;275:606–610.

3. Centers for Disease Control and Prevention. *HIV/AIDS Surveillance Report* 1996;8(2):14.

4. *Ibid.*

■ *Chapter 13*

LIVING WITH HIV DISEASE

As mentioned in Chapter 1, the single most important step in living with HIV disease is to seek care from a physician experienced in treating it. However, there are a number of steps an individual can take to help maintain a high quality of life when living with HIV infection. They include gaining knowledge about HIV disease so that the individual can make informed decisions about medical care, staying as healthy as possible, and preparing for future contingencies.

■ GAINING KNOWLEDGE ABOUT HIV DISEASE AND ITS TREATMENT

It is extremely helpful for someone who is HIV positive to learn all he or she can about HIV disease and its treatment. However, the amount of information a person with a potentially serious illness wants varies greatly from person to person. Some people actively seek information and want to learn as much as possible about their disease and they may want—and may demand—to play an active role in determining the course of their treatment. Others prefer neither to discuss their illness nor to read about it and choose to leave treatment decisions to their physician. Both are ways of coping with the disease. But the people who are knowledgeable about it and its treatment, who ask questions of their physician, and who are familiar with treatment options and clinical trials are more likely to receive better care and to successfully follow their treatment regimen.

A highly useful resource for learning about experimental anti-HIV treatments and therapies for opportunistic infections is the *AIDS/HIV Treatment Directory* published by AmFAR. It is available directly from AmFAR and from the National AIDS Clearinghouse. Addresses and telephone numbers for both are listed in Appendix 1, as are other sources of information. In addition, appendix 1 includes information about how to read medical-research papers. It is intended to help people who are unfamiliar with the medical literature but who would like to read original scientific papers describing experiments and their results or the state of the art in an area of basic or clinical research.

The World Wide Web (WWW) is still another valuable source of information on HIV disease (AmFAR's *HIV/AIDS Treatment Directory,* for example, is on the Web; see Appendix 1 for its location). Medical information on the Web should be approached with caution, however, because anyone with the right computer and software can set up a Web site and present information there. Be aware also that the WWW is used by people trying to sell all kinds of products, including medical treatments. A selection of authoritative HIV-related Web sites is also listed in Appendix 1.

In the end, however, information is helpful only if it is put to wise use. "The key to success in living with HIV and AIDS is putting information into practice," said Allen Gifford, M.D., assistant professor of medicine, University of California San Diego, and coauthor of *Living Well with HIV and AIDS.* "This means setting goals and collaborating with health-care professionals in making treatment plans."

■ STAYING HEALTHY

Staying healthy involves getting sufficient exercise and rest, following a nutritious diet, storing and preparing food safely, avoiding sources of infection, coping with the stress caused by HIV disease, and recognizing certain general or nonspecific changes in one's health that might indicate changes, for better or worse, in disease progression.

■ Diet and Nutrition

Good nutrition and maintaining body weight by consuming sufficient healthy calories are of vital importance to the person who is HIV positive, even if asymptomatic.

Some of the most important recommendations in each of these areas are provided below, although this list is not exhaustive. People who are HIV positive should consult with a registered dietitian to help evaluate their eating patterns and establish a healthy diet that will meet their circumstances. To talk with a registered dietitian about HIV/AIDS nutrition, or for referral to a registered dietitian, call the American Dietetic Association's (ADA) consumer nutrition hotline at 1-800-366-1655. One can also request a copy of the ADA's booklet, *Living Well with HIV and AIDS: A Guide to Healthy Eating* (this publication is unrelated to the book mentioned on the previous page).

Changes in diet and eating routines should be made one step at a time. For example, a person who commonly eats on the run could begin by eating more regularly. When eating more regularly becomes routine, begin substituting more nutritious foods for those that are less nutritious. This may involve eating vegetables with every dinner or substituting fruits for cookies or chips when snacking. Recommendations for maintaining weight and establishing a healthy diet include the following:

- Keep a weekly record of body weight. Weight should be measured in the morning after urinating and before eating. Weight loss that occurs over a week or two should be reported to the doctor.

- Eat regularly every day. Depending on one's lifestyle, that may mean three healthy meals and two or three snacks per day, or it may mean four or five small meals over the course of a day. Meals should include a variety of foods to provide adequate amounts of protein, carbohydrates, fats, vitamins, and minerals. Drink plenty of fluids.

- Eat foods that are high in calories and protein. Calories should come from foods high in carbohydrates such as breads, cereals, potatoes, noodles, and rice. Protein can come from meats, poultry, fish, eggs, milk, cheese, and dried beans.

- Vegetarians can obtain protein from beans, tofu, soybean milk, breads, and grains. Eggs and dairy products are also excellent sources of protein.

- Eat at least four servings of vegetables and three servings of fruit daily for vitamins, minerals, and fiber.

- Foods that are high in fat and sugar are good for increasing caloric intake, but use them sparingly. High-fat foods include margarine, mayonnaise, sour cream, and some salad dressings; sweet foods include honey, jelly, jam, syrup, and sugar.

- Snack on foods that are high in nutrients such as fruits, vegetables, and peanut butter; eat candy, cookies, and potato chips in moderation as these items are high in calories and low in nutrients (i.e., food components necessary for the body's normal function).

- Vitamin and mineral supplements in moderation can be helpful, but avoid taking large doses of vitamins or minerals without the guidance of a doctor or dietitian. Large doses of some supplements can be toxic, are associated with diarrhea, and can suppress, rather than help, the immune system.

- The timing of some medications with respect to meals is also important. Some HIV medications must be taken on an empty stomach, while others are taken on a full stomach. Still others work best when taken with certain types of foods. Talk with the physician and with the pharmacist who dispenses the medications about their timing, and plan meals accordingly.

- The dietary needs of a person with AIDS, as well as the texture and quantity of food that can be eaten and the frequency of eating, will vary with the condition of the individual.

Drinking Water

Drinking water can be a source of exposure to microbes responsible for cryptosporidiosis and other infectious diseases in people with HIV disease. The risk of exposure to *Cryptosporidium parvum,* which causes cryptosporidiosis, from ordinary municipal tap water is uncertain. Certainly, some municipal water systems experience *Cryptosporidium* outbreaks from time to time. In these situations, tap water can be boiled to make it safe, or filtered or bottled water can be used for drinking and for making ice cubes. Care must be exercised in the type of bottled water or filter system chosen. (For more information on water, see "Cryptosporidiosis" in Chapter 7.) Untreated water is also a source of *Cryptosporidium,* and people with HIV disease should avoid drinking water directly from lakes or rivers, and accidentally swallowing water while swimming in lakes, rivers, or public swimming pools.

Combating Weight Loss and Wasting

Involuntary weight loss is a common symptom of HIV disease. It can also be the first sign of wasting, or cachexia. Wasting is defined as involuntary weight loss associated with diarrhea of more than two stools a day for more than 30 days. Wasting is dangerous because it involves the loss of lean body mass as well as the loss of body fat. Lean body mass refers to the nonfat tissue mass of the body, particularly muscle tissue. The cause of HIV-associated wasting syndrome remains a matter of debate. Malnutrition, malabsorption, and altered metabolism may play a role. However, rapid weight loss during HIV disease is usually associated with an opportunistic infection of the intestines, while slower weight loss can be due to HIV itself.

Metabolic disorders can also contribute to wasting. These can be caused by gastrointestinal disorders or the presence of certain cytokines in the blood (particularly tumor necrosis factor-alpha [TNF] and the interleukins, IL-1 and IL-6, which are associated with inflammation). Metabolic disorders are also caused by an HIV-associated drop in production of testosterone by the testes.

It is also common for someone with HIV disease to lose interest in eating, which can accelerate weight loss and wasting. Losing interest in eating can occur because of a loss of appetite (anorexia), mouth sores that make eating painful, depression, nausea, and fatigue. Loss of appetite can also occur as a side effect of medication.

Because wasting can be a life-threatening condition, even gradual weight loss in a person with HIV disease should be discussed with his or her doctor. Treatment of weight loss begins by identifying and treating any underlying cause, plus aggressive nutrition therapy. Nutrition therapy often involves consuming more foods or drinks that are high in nutrients and calories and low in fat (to avoid feeling full) and eating smaller-but-more-frequent meals. Nutritional supplements are also used. Bouts of weight loss can be reversed, but the amount of weight gained is often less than the amount of weight lost.

Loss of appetite due to mouth sores or pain from swallowing can be caused by candidiasis, herpes infection, other infections, or by Kaposi's sarcoma. Sores can also alter the taste of food. When mouth sores are present, foods that are served cold or at room temperature are easier to eat, as are foods that have a soft, smooth texture. Examples include eggs, yogurt, pudding, and tuna salad. Avoid foods that are salty, spicy, crunchy, or dry.

The appetite stimulants dronabinol and megestrol acetate (Megace) have been approved by the Food and Drug Administration (FDA) for the treatment of HIV-associated wasting or unexplained weight loss. Other therapies are currently being tested in clinical trials. These include human growth hormone, testosterone, and thalidomide (which has anti-TNF activity). See the *AIDS/HIV Treatment Directory* published by AmFAR for information on clinical trials of new treatments for wasting.

Weight loss can also be caused by diarrhea. Left untreated, diarrhea can result in dehydration, the loss of important salts (electrolytes), and malnutrition, and so can contribute to wasting. The most common cause of diarrhea in people with HIV disease is an underlying opportunistic infection, although it can also be caused by some drugs, pancreatitis, and lactose intolerance. Whatever the cause, it must be identified and treated. Diarrhea also results from the deterioration of the lining of the small intestines by HIV, a condition known as "villous atrophy."

Management of diarrhea involves identifying and treating any underlying cause and giving supportive care. General antidiarrheic drugs will sometimes ease symptoms. Supportive care includes providing plenty of electrolyte-containing liquids for rehydration and foods that provide a source of soluble fiber, which promotes the formation of a solid stool. These foods include bananas, rice, applesauce, and noodles. Nutritional supplements taken by mouth and used under the direction of a doctor or dietitian can also help. Avoid foods that are high in insoluble fiber. These include cereals, granola, seeds, and raw vegetables and most fruits.

■ Food Safety

Many bacteria and fungi are found naturally in and on food. These microbes multiply more rapidly on food that is improperly stored, handled, or prepared, thereby causing spoilage. These microbes also pose a risk of illness or infection for people who are HIV positive, making it important that foods for these individuals be stored and handled properly. Recommendations by the American Dietetic Association for the safe handling of food include the following:

- Purchase and use packaged foods before the expiration date listed on the label, and make every effort to consume foods prior to their expiration date.

- Choose fresh fruits and vegetables with unbroken skins.

- Shop for cold and frozen foods last, and ask that they be packaged in the same bag. Keep a cooler in the car to store cold and frozen foods if the trip home is longer than 30 minutes.

- Cold foods should be stored immediately in a refrigerator that is 40°F or lower; frozen foods should be stored at 0°F or lower. Measure temperatures with a refrigerator thermometer.

- Thaw frozen foods in a microwave or the refrigerator. Place leftover foods containing meat, eggs, or milk products in the refrigerator or freezer immediately after eating.

- Wash hands thoroughly with soap before preparing food. After handling raw foods, wash hands again with soap before handling cooked food.

- Bacteria can grow on cutting boards and in cracked or chipped china or crockery. Wash these items in a dishwasher or in soapy water hotter than 140°F. Sanitize cutting boards after working with raw meats, fish, and poultry in a mixture of 1 tablespoon of bleach to a quart of water. Clean countertops with a similar solution.

- Avoid raw red meat; poultry; or fish, including raw oysters, carpaccio, sashimi, and sushi; raw or runny eggs; and homemade food and drinks that might contain raw eggs (e.g., Caesar salad dressing, some frostings, homemade eggnog). Raw or undercooked red meat can cause serious infection; pork, lamb, and venison in particular are sources of toxoplasmosis. Raw seafood carries a risk of hepatitis, while raw eggs can be a source of salmonella.

- Cook all meats to 165°F or higher; cook poultry to 180°F. Use a meat thermometer to ensure that a safe cooking temperature was reached.

- Wash fresh fruits and vegetables thoroughly. Peel the skin if it might hide soil particles.

- Avoid fruits, vegetables, and cheeses that show signs of mold.

- Drink only pasteurized dairy products; eat only pasteurized cheese.

When Eating Out

- Be sure eating utensils, beverage glasses, and place settings are clean. Return dirty utensils, or cold and undercooked food.

- Avoid salad bars. The vegetables and fruits being served may not have been cleaned or stored properly. Meats may be undercooked.

■ Avoid Exposure to Contagious Diseases

People with AIDS should avoid contact with people who have contagious illnesses until their symptoms have cleared. This includes illnesses such as colds, flu (influenza), and gastroenteritis. If contact is unavoidable, the person with these conditions should wear a surgical mask and wash hands before touching the person with HIV disease.

It is recommended that both the person infected with HIV and his or her caregiver be immunized against the flu (influenza) every year. Other recommendations for avoiding infection that are particularly important for a person with advanced HIV disease include the following:

- A person with HIV/AIDS should avoid being in the same room with someone with chickenpox until all the chickenpox blisters have crusted over. Also, someone who never had chickenpox can be infectious if he or she was recently exposed to a person with chickenpox. A person with HIV/AIDS should notify his or her physician of any exposure to chickenpox and ask for possible treatment.

■ Shingles is caused by the same virus that is responsible for chickenpox (see Chapter 7), and exposure to someone with shingles can lead to chickenpox in anyone who has not previously had chickenpox. For this reason, a person with HIV/AIDS should also avoid contact with anyone who has shingles.

■ A person with HIV/AIDS should avoid contact with anyone having skin infections such as boils or cold sores (the latter, also known as fever blisters, are caused by the herpes simplex virus). A caregiver who has skin sores or rash should cover the diseased skin and wear gloves during contact with a person with advanced HIV disease.

Pets can also be a source of infection for the person with HIV/AIDS. It is not necessary for someone with HIV disease to give up a pet, but pets must be handled with caution:

■ A person with HIV disease should wash his or her hands after handling a pet.

■ Cats in particular can be a source of a number of infections, including bacillary angiomatosis, cryptosporidiosis, and toxoplasmosis (see Chapter 7).

■ Empty litter boxes daily; to avoid producing litter dust, do not sift the litter.

■ Sick pets should be checked immediately by a veterinarian. A person with advanced HIV disease should not handle a sick pet or its litter.

■ Stress, Anxiety, and Psychological Complications

Individuals who are HIV positive can be confronted with a variety of psychological and emotional stresses. Stress and anxiety can be associated with learning of one's HIV seropositive status and deciding who to tell about it (see Chapter 1). Other sources of stress include the uncertainties that surround HIV disease, fear of abandonment, loss of control, loss of employment, coping with the health-care system, and the expense of drugs and health care. Anxiety can also be associated with preparing a will.

Ironically, recent advances in highly active antiretroviral therapy (HAART), which have resulted in better survival at all stages of HIV disease and often remarkable beneficial effects in individual patients, can contribute to stress for people with HIV/AIDS. Deciding on an optimal combination therapy, expecting its effects, and, if all goes well, even psychologically adjusting to being fit for work again and being able to contemplate a longer life expectancy require new adjustments and can be causes of new stress and anxiety. This is particularly so at a time when so little is known regarding the long-term duration of the therapeutic effects of the new treatments or their possible long-term side effects.

Managing stress is important in people with HIV infection because stress itself can weaken the immune system, as well as greatly impair a person's quality of life. People cope with the stress of HIV infection in a variety of ways. Unhealthy ways include denial (which can take the form of habitually missing medical appointments, not getting follow-up tests done, or not taking medications) and drug or alcohol abuse.

Healthy ways of managing the stress of HIV disease include participating in an HIV support group and talking with a counselor or psychologist. Spirituality, meditation, positive thinking, and staying busy through work, reading, and hobbies can also help in managing stress.

People who develop clinical depression are usually successfully treated with the help of counseling and antidepressant medications. Depression can also occur as a side effect of certain drugs, including sedatives, seizure medications, blood-pressure medications, and many others. Treating these patients may involve decreasing the drug's dose, discontinuing the drug, or changing drugs.

■ Indicators of Possible HIV Disease Progression

Staying healthy with HIV infection also involves being alert to symptoms that might signal the presence of an opportunistic infection. Early detection of an opportunistic infection permits early and aggressive treatment. Thus, it is essential that a person living with HIV disease promptly notify his or her doctor of any new symptoms or health-related experiences. Common symptoms of disease progression include the following:

- Unexplained fever

- Swollen "glands" (refers to swollen lymph nodes, or lymphadenopathy, particularly in the neck or groin)

- Night sweats

- Unusual bleeding or bruising

- Unexplained cough

- Severe headache or diarrhea

- Sudden or unexplained weight loss

■ THE ADVENT OF SYMPTOMATIC HIV DISEASE

Certain opportunistic infections eventually occur in most people with HIV disease (see Chapter 4). The appearance of one of these diseases signals the transition from asymptomatic to symptomatic HIV disease. Examples of early HIV-associated opportunistic infections include oral candidiasis and oral hairy leukoplakia.

The appearance of one of these early "indicator diseases" can produce a psychological crisis for some people infected with HIV. The condition itself may present with only mild symptoms, and it may be readily treated, but it reminds the individual of the reality of his or her HIV disease and of its progression, which may lead to anxiety or depression. Individuals facing these problems can derive solace from talking about their fears and concerns with someone who has experienced the same anxieties. Such individuals can be found in HIV support groups, or through peer counseling or buddy programs organized by local AIDS service organizations. Other sources of help include the person's physician or social worker.

■ COMPLEMENTARY AND ALTERNATIVE TREATMENTS

Many individuals with HIV infection believe that complementary and alternative treatments—treatments other than those recognized by medical science—such as certain vitamin preparations, food or mineral supplements, special diets, Chinese herbs, and plant extracts will help control their HIV infection. They believe that these can strengthen their immune system, protect their immune cells from HIV, and slow the progression of their disease. Alternative treatments also give many patients a sense of control over their illness and for that reason, they can make these patients feel better. Therefore, complementary or alternative treatments can be helpful.

The effectiveness of these treatments has often not been tested through clinical trials or other methods of Western science (see Chapter 6), and their usefulness is largely open to question or doubted by most physicians. Occasionally, an alternative treatment can even be toxic or harmful at certain doses. Usually, though, it will not interfere with the drugs that are prescribed by physicians for antiretroviral therapy or the prevention or treatment of opportunistic infections.

It is imperative, however, that anyone who is considering trying an alternative or unproven treatment first investigate it carefully. Beware of claims that a treatment is a "cure" or will have miraculous effects. Unfortunately, there presently is no cure for HIV disease, and both the safety and the effectiveness of any treatment have to be properly studied through clinical trials (see Chapter 6). If a treatment has been properly tested for safety and efficacy in HIV disease, the results of such testing should have been published in a peer-reviewed medical journal or presented at a significant medical conference. It is also helpful to seek information on the treatment from reputable buyers' clubs (for information on buyers' clubs, see Chapter 5) and from organizations such as the Treatment Action Group in New York and Project Inform in California (see Appendix 1).

A person taking any alternative treatment should also *always* tell his or her doctor about the treatment. This way the doctor can determine whether the compound in question poses any risk of toxicity or of drug interactions with the prescription medicines the person is taking.

Project Inform includes the following points in its recommendations for evaluating new or alternative treatments for HIV disease:

■ Extraordinarily high prices for an alternative or experimental treatment may be evidence that the treatment is a fraud. Beware of charlatans who are out to make a buck, even by selling a potentially harmful treatment.

■ Interview the person who is promoting the treatment. How much does he or she know about HIV and AIDS? What is their training? How do they explain the cause of AIDS?

■ How has the treatment been evaluated? What is the justification for using this particular treatment for AIDS? If the treatment has not been objectively evaluated (tested through a clinical trial and the results published in a peer-reviewed journal or presented at a recognized medical conference), proceed with caution.

■ Is the person promoting the treatment interested in specific information about your condition or are you treated as a faceless customer? Do they answer your questions patiently in understandable language, or do they talk down to you? Are their explanations about the treatment either overly simplistic or overly complex?

■ Do they seem eager to foster a sense of distrust between you and your current health-care providers? Are they attempting to separate you from your current support network?

■ If you have a funny feeling about someone pitching a treatment, listen to your instincts and do not act impulsively.

■ PREPARING FOR THE FUTURE: ADVANCE DIRECTIVES

An important aspect of maintaining control of one's medical care is planning ahead for the kind of medical treatment that would be preferred in the event that one becomes incapacitated or unable to make one's own decisions. This is done through advance directives. Advance directives are legal documents that instruct physicians and other health-care professionals about the use of resuscitation, life support, and other types of medical care a person might receive to maintain life if that person is unable to make the decision for himself or herself. Advance directives include durable power of attorney for health care (DPAHC), living wills, and do-not-resuscitate (DNR) orders.

■ Durable Power of Attorney for Health Care

A DPAHC is the most important type of advance directive. It is a legal document that authorizes another person to make health-care decisions for someone who is unable to make those decisions for himself or herself. A DPAHC has no effect until the individual is unable to provide informed consent. If a person is incapacitated and incapable of making an informed decision about medical treatment and has not signed a DPAHC, state law determines who makes decisions on the patient's behalf. This is usually the closest relative by marriage or blood.

States generally do not recognize domestic partners or lovers as relatives, no matter how close or long the relationship. If someone has been named under a DPAHC, he or she has sole authority over health-care decisions for the patient, regardless of the wishes of relatives.[1] It is usually not necessary to visit a lawyer to get a DPAHC. Many state medical associations now distribute DPAHC forms, and they are often available at hospitals.

The individual's physician should help him or her to be clear and specific when completing a DPAHC. It should include, for example, whether and when nutrition and hydration are to be withheld or withdrawn; not doing so leaves a very painful decision solely in the hand of the holder of the DPAHC.

■ Living Will

Some states have "natural death" laws that give adults the right to direct their physician in writing to withhold or withdraw life-sustaining procedures if the patient is permanently unconscious or in a terminal condition. These are often called "living wills." Life-support measures include cardiopulmonary resuscitation (CPR), use of electric shock to start the heart (defibrillation), use of a respirator or ventilator, and the use or withholding of artificial feeding and hydration.

Complications arise if a patient has both a living will and a DPAHC and they say different things. Some states specifically say that the power of attorney prevails over the directive; other states, unfortunately, do not address the possible conflict.

■ Do-Not-Resuscitate Order

A DNR order means that if a person's breathing or heart stops, the doctors and nurses will not use machines and other methods to restart them or keep the person alive. A DNR order is more common with individuals who have experienced long-term disease and are in the late stages of their illness. The admitting doctor should discuss the possibility of a DNR order with the patient upon admission to the hospital. In order to be effective, the patient's physician must sign the order and enter it into the patient's chart; the patient need not sign it.

Decisions about advance directives must be made carefully. Help and advice can be sought from doctors, nurses, social workers, clergy, and family and friends. Also, specific rights and conditions for advance directives vary from state to state. Without an advance directive, a family member will make decisions about the life support of a patient who is unconscious or unable to legally make such decisions. The order of priority as to who is responsible for these decisions differs from state to state. (For example, the patient's guardian might be the first person a hospital would seek. If there is no guardian, the responsibility might then go, in this order, to the spouse in a legally recognized marriage, the adult children, the parents, and adult siblings.)

■ HOSPICE CARE

Hospice care is an important option in the continuum of care for a person with advanced HIV disease. Hospice programs are designed to provide the best possible quality of life for people who have exhausted specific treatment possibilities and are at the end stage of life. Care is focused on both the patient and the family. Hospice programs seek to relieve physical, psychological, social, and spiritual suffering, a goal that is accomplished through aggressive pain and symptom control. Any treatment needed to control the pain and symptoms of HIV disease can be used in a hospice setting. These can include most kinds of antiretroviral therapy for HIV disease as well as prophylactic and suppressive therapies for opportunistic infections.

Hospices are staffed by a multidiscipinary team that includes specially trained physicians, nurses, social workers, counselors, clergy, physical and occupational therapists, and volunteers. In many cases, the patient's original physician also remains involved in his or her patient's care. All hospice patients are treated with nonjudgmental and compassionate respect.

Typically, hospice programs are available to individuals who are thought to have six months or less to live, as determined by both the patient's physician and the hospice physician. At all times, however, hospice care affirms life, but it does nothing to either prolong it or shorten it. Hospices also provide the medications, supplies, equipment, and services needed by the patient. Hospice services are available 24 hours a day, seven days a week. Care is administered in the home whenever possible, but it is also provided to people with HIV disease in settings that include hospitals, free-standing hospice centers, and AIDS residential facilities.

Hospice care also promotes reconciliation. Whenever possible, hospice facilitates the interaction of families, friends, and loved ones with the patient. This makes a hospice unlike any other component of the health-care system. At the same time, accomplishing this goal to the extent possible requires that a bond of trust exist between the patient, the family, and the hospice staff. With a bond of trust established, hospice staff can help the patient and family come together to heal possible past rifts and resolve differences that often still linger at the end of life.

This can be especially important for gay men and others with HIV disease who often have two families: a family of origin and a family of choice. Conflict may exist between these two families, but hospice staff can facilitate a dialogue that often enables the two families to pull together to help the patient reach the end of his or her life as peacefully and comfortably as possible. Hospice also later provides bereavement counseling.

Many people with HIV disease, however, postpone entry into a hospice program until the last few weeks of life. This may occur in part because people with HIV disease are in their 20s, 30s, and 40s, which is younger than most people who have a terminal illness. Therefore, they may be unwilling to acknowledge the end of life. Many people with HIV disease also become engaged in protest and political activism, and may view entering a hospice program as giving in to the disease. To be sure, a hospice can still help people who are in their final weeks or days of life, but less time will be available to build a bond of trust between patient, hospice staff, and others and to foster reconciliation.

To find the nearest hospice or to obtain additional information about hospices, call the toll-free National Hospice Organization help line at 1-800-658-8898.

■ INFORMATION FOR CAREGIVERS

Caring for a person with HIV disease is an act of love—a physically and emotionally demanding act of love. Caregivers for someone with HIV disease can often feel overwhelmed and find themselves in danger of burnout and depression, unless they take steps to ease their stress. This is particularly true of caregivers who are also struggling to hold down full-time jobs (see "Care for the Caregiver").

Caregivers who are themselves HIV positive are in particular danger because they may see themselves in the position of the person for whom they are caring. They can develop fears of their own future illness, and many may also be grieving or mourning the loss of other friends or family members to HIV disease.

Counseling or HIV support groups can help cope with such fears.

Other anxieties, such as fear of infection, can be addressed through practical information about caring for someone with HIV disease. It is essential for a caregiver to know, for example, that HIV is not transmitted by touching, hugging, ordinary kissing, or other forms of casual contact (see "How HIV Is Not Transmitted," Chapter 3). People with AIDS do not require separate dishes or eating utensils, and their dishes and eating utensils can be washed as dishes ordinarily are, with detergent and hot water. No special precautions are needed when washing the clothes and bedding of someone with AIDS; use cold or hot water as indicated by ordinary washing instructions. Clothing can also be dry-cleaned or hand washed.

However, because HIV is found in the blood from an infected person, it is not a good idea to share razors or toothbrushes with someone who has AIDS because these implements sometimes draw blood and therefore present a small risk of HIV transmission.

Blood and body fluids that contain visible blood, such as a bloody stool, are possible sources of infection. (Only a small number of health-care workers have become infected through contact with infected blood, and these infections usually occurred when a worker was accidentally stuck with a needle or when infectious blood was splashed on skin having cuts or open sores.) The risk of infection through contact with the blood of a person with HIV disease is low, but caretakers can reduce that risk further by wearing gloves whenever they expect to have contact with blood or items soiled by blood, semen, or vaginal fluids. For example, gloves should be worn by a caregiver when cleaning sheets, clothing, and other articles soiled with urine, feces, or vomit. This also protects them from disease-causing microbes other than HIV.

Liquid waste should be disposed of in the toilet. Avoid splashing. Wound dressings, paper towels, sanitary pads and tampons, and other items soiled with blood, semen, or vaginal fluid should be disposed of in a plastic bag which is then securely sealed. The doctor's office or the health department can advise about proper disposal of such bags.

Many people with AIDS are infected by cytomegalovirus (CMV), which is found in saliva and urine. For this reason, and to maintain good hygiene in general, the caregiver should always wash hands well after contact with saliva and urine. This is particularly important for pregnant women, who can transmit CMV to their unborn baby.

Caregivers should wear disposable latex hospital gloves when providing nursing care. The gloves are to be discarded after each use. Caregivers can wear household rubber gloves for household chores that involve contact with infectious blood. The gloves can be cleaned, disinfected, and reused; gloves that are cracked or peeling or have holes should be discarded. A convenient disinfecting solution is made by combining a tablespoon of household bleach per quart of water. Make it fresh each time it is needed. This solution can also be used to disinfect such things as sponges and mops and to disinfect bloodied floors, showers, tubs, and sinks.

■ Handling Used Needles and Syringes Safely

The use of needles and syringes may be necessary if the person with AIDS is a diabetic, is a hemophiliac, or is taking certain treatments at home. The Centers for Disease Control and Prevention recommends the following measures for the safe handling of needles and syringes:

- Handle needles and syringes carefully. Pick them up by the barrel of the syringe and carefully dispose of them into a puncture-proof container with a plastic top, such as a large coffee can.

- NEVER try to replace caps on needles, remove needles from their syringes, or bend or break needles.

- Keep the needle-disposal container in a room where the needles and syringes are used, but safe from children and visitors.

- Dispose of the needle-disposal container before it is full. Ask the doctor or nurse about how to dispose of the container safely.

- If you stick yourself with a used needle, wash the injury thoroughly with soap and water. Then contact your doctor for further evaluation and perhaps treatment.

■ Caregivers and AIDS Dementia Complex

AIDS dementia complex is a common complication of advanced HIV disease (see Chapter 4). The severity varies greatly in different patients. Symptoms can include agitation, loss of memory, reduced ability to concentrate, personality changes, mood changes, impaired judgment, loss of balance, unsteady gait, leg weakness, and frequent falls. Advanced AIDS dementia complex can result in profound memory loss—patients can even lose awareness of their disease—disorientation, inability to think, loss of speech, and abnormal reflexes. Antiretroviral therapy can sometimes slow, and occasionally reverse, progression of AIDS dementia complex.

The home of a person with AIDS dementia complex should be arranged to minimize the risk of injury and maximize freedom of movement. This can be done with the help of a home-safety assessment, which can be conducted by a social worker or home-health nurse. In general, keep living areas brightly lit and walkways clear and free of electrical wires and unstable furniture to reduce the risk of falls. Calendars and clocks should be prominently displayed to help keep the person oriented as to the date and time. Sharp objects, chemicals, poisons, power tools, and other dangerous objects should be safely stored, and knobs should be removed from the stove to prevent accidental injury and fire.

Talking with a person who has severe AIDS dementia complex can be difficult. Ask the doctor, social worker, or home-health nurse for guidance. Lisa Capaldini, M.D., assistant clinical professor of medicine at the University of California, San Francisco, makes the following recommendations to help caregivers communicate with someone who has severe AIDS dementia complex:

- Speak in a low-pitched, even tone.

- Ask simple yes or no questions.

- Respond to questions with answers that are short and to the point.

- Because long-term memory is often less affected, reminiscing about early experiences might be soothing to the individual. Immediate memory, on the other hand, is likely to be severely impaired, so trying to recall recent events could be frustrating.

■ Care for the Caregiver

Caring for a person with HIV disease can be frustrating, as well as physically and emotionally exhausting. It can be painful to watch someone become sicker despite one's best efforts. To help cope with these difficulties and perhaps their own fears, frustrations, and anger, caregivers also need a support system. This is especially true of caregivers who are themselves HIV positive.

A caregiver's support system can include a professional counselor, understanding and compassionate clergy, and a caregivers support group.

Contact your physician or local AIDS service organization for information or a referral. It is also important to have someone who can at times
stay with the person with AIDS to give the main caretaker time to rest
and meet other obligations. Such help may be available through respite
care programs. Information on local respite programs can be obtained
from the individual's social worker or primary physician, or from the
local AIDS service organization or hospice program.

■ NEW THERAPIES ALLOW MANY PEOPLE WITH HIV/AIDS TO LIVE LONGER AND BETTER LIVES

Until recently, preparing for the end of life was all most people with HIV
infection could look forward to. This is now changing. In 1996, deaths
among people with AIDS declined substantially for the first time ever. Between January and September of that year, the number of Americans
who died from AIDS dropped by 19% compared to the same period in
1995. The decline reflects improvements in medical care, better use of
prophylaxis and treatments for opportunistic infections, and the start in
the use of combination therapies. The trend in improved survival is expected to continue, as the period covered by the 1996 figures does not reflect the current early and widespread use of combination therapies that
include a protease inhibitor, which have greatly improved treatment effectiveness.

Today, many people with HIV/AIDS who had been planning for the
end of life find themselves seeking help to learn how to continue with life.
Many attend seminars and workshops organized to help them deal with
renewed health, finding jobs, and confronting issues of HIV in the workplace.

To be sure, this is good news for people with HIV/AIDS, but questions
and problems remain with potent combinations of antiretroviral drugs
(HAART). These drug regimens are rigorous and demanding, and full
compliance with their requirements is a challenge for anyone. At the
same time, complete compliance with the new treatment regimens is essential to prevent the emergence of HIV strains that are resistant to multiple drugs (see Chapter 5). Indeed, the development of HAART-resistant

strains is certainly possible. There is also uncertainty regarding the duration of the benefits these treatments offer and whether the resulting increases in CD4 counts represent a sufficient strengthening of the immune system to significantly ward off opportunistic infections and malignancies. Considerably more basic and clinical research remains to be done to answer these questions. Of particular importance is research in the area of immune reconstitution, believed to be a necessary future complement to antiretroviral therapy in order to truly reverse immune deficiency.

Currently, the most effective way to live in a world with HIV is to avail oneself of HIV testing and the benefits of early detection of HIV infection, as well as early and aggressive anti-HIV treatment provided by a physician experienced in HIV disease.

A true cure remains elusive. But further research holds the promise that HIV disease will become medically manageable, a chronic but not terminal illness, and that full-blown AIDS will one day be entirely preventable. This will probably happen first in people in whom HIV is detected early, before it can be achieved in people at later stages of HIV disease.

ENDNOTE

1. Most states give parents, children, spouses, health-care providers, and certain public-health officials the right to challenge the durable power of attorney for health care (DPAHC) in court. However, most states also allow the patient to eliminate the right to challenge by specifically saying so in the DPAHC.

The Medical Science of HIV/AIDS

Chapter 14

THE CELL

Just as buildings are made of bricks, the body is made of cells. On close examination, though, an individual cell bears a strong resemblance to a peach. Like a peach, a cell has three main regions:

- A thin outer skin, the cell membrane

- A pulp under the skin, the cell cytoplasm

- A sphere at the center, the cell nucleus

The cell membrane, cytoplasm, and nucleus, respectively, serve as doorway, hearth, and home to HIV. An understanding of the role played by each of these regions of the cell helps gain an understanding of how HIV replicates (described in Chapter 18).

■ THE CELL MEMBRANE AND CELL-SURFACE PROTEINS

The delicate membrane that surrounds the cell consists mainly of a double layer of lipid, or fat, molecules. This double layer is also known as the "lipid bilayer." Each lipid molecule resembles an old-fashioned clothespin, with a round head at one end and two prongs at the other. The molecules making up the two layers sit with their round heads facing out, and their double prongs pointing in (Figure 14.1).

FProtruding from the lipid bilayer and extending through its surface are various kinds of large protein molecules. These are also an integral part of the cell membrane. Some might be envisioned as large smooth rocks poking up from a surface of pebbles. Others coil or wind up and down through the lipid layers and protrude from it like lengths of garden hose

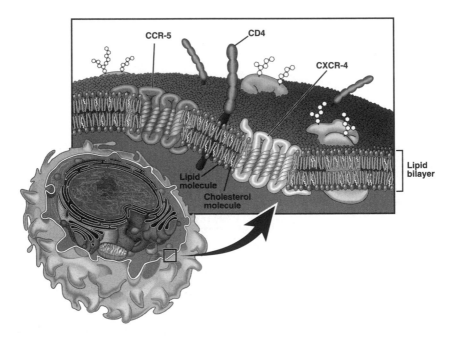

Fig. 14.1 ■ *The cell membrane of a helper T cell or macrophage. The cell membrane consists of two layers of lipid molecules—the lipid bilayer—and various types of protein molecules. The lipid bilayer provides support and structure, while membrane proteins serve many important functions. Some (not shown here) control the movement of substances into and out of a cell. Others, such as the CD4 molecule, hold one cell to another and help identify one cell to another. Still others serve as cell-surface receptors for hormones, cytokines, chemokines, and other substances. The chemokine receptors CXCR-4 and CCR-5, shown here, are used by HIV along with the CD4 molecule to enter a cell.*

bent into loops or loose folds. Some membrane proteins also have sugar molecules attached to the protruding end. These are known as "glycoproteins."

The lipids and proteins of the cell membrane serve vastly different purposes. The lipid bilayer is soft and fluid-like and protects the integrity of the membrane. For example, it does not break when punctured by a fine glass needle. Instead, when the needle is withdrawn, the lipid molecules flow together and fill the hole, as happens when poking a needle into an oil film.

Membrane proteins, on the other hand, are active molecules that serve many specific functions. Some are transport proteins that control the many substances that must pass in and out of the cell. Some membrane proteins form pores that remain open all the time, while others act like gates that open and close to let only certain substances pass.

Cells resemble peaches in another way: They are covered with fuzz, a molecular fuzz. They bristle with a variety of cell-surface molecules, some of which play an important role in enabling HIV to infect cells. These molecules are also important in that they help

What Is a Molecule?

SIMPLY PUT, a molecule is the smallest unit of a substance or compound that will still have the chemical properties of the substance.

Take one grain of salt, for example, and cut it in half. That leaves a speck of salt barely visible to the eye, but nothing has changed to take the "saltness" away from that speck. In fact, one could continue halving halves—were it physically possible—until nothing remained but one set of the atoms that make up salt. The atoms that make up salt are sodium, abbreviated Na; and chloride, abbreviated Cl. The smallest unit of salt, therefore, is one atom of sodium joined to one atom of chloride, or NaCl. This makes one molecule of salt. Chemically, those two atoms—NaCl—will behave as a chemist expects salt to behave, and it has the essence of "saltness." Cut this molecule in half, and the chemist no longer has salt. He or she would have one atom of sodium and one atom of chloride, which chemically behave entirely differently from salt.

NaCl is among the simplest examples of a molecule. An antibody molecule, a cell receptor, an adhesion protein, and a molecule of DNA are examples of molecules that are built of dozens, thousands, or tens of thousands of atoms. ■

diagnose HIV disease: Scientists use them to identify CD4 and CD8 cells, for example, which enables these cells to be counted (see "Why They Call It 'CD4': Telling Immune Cells Apart," Chapter 16).

There are three main groups of cell-surface molecules: adhesion proteins, cell-surface receptors, and recognition proteins.

■ Adhesion Proteins

Adhesion proteins are an important category of proteins that help cells selectively attach to other cells and to the fibers and other materials that surround them in the body. An example of an adhesion protein is the CD4 receptor of helper T lymphocytes. The CD4 receptor helps the helper T cell join with an antigen-presenting cell (see Chapter 16). The CD4 molecule is also the primary cell-surface molecule needed by HIV to attach to and infect helper T lymphocytes and monocytes/ macrophages, all of which are immune-system cells. The CD8 molecule on the surface of killer T lymphocytes is an adhesion protein that helps that type of cell lock onto an infected cell as a prelude to destroying it.

■ Cell-Surface Receptors

Cell-surface receptors interact with substances outside the cell to produce a signal that causes some appropriate change inside the cell. Some signals ultimately turn genes on or off, while others initiate or stop some activity within the cell. Substances that interact with cell-surface receptors include hormones, cytokines, and growth factors (which stimulate cell growth). Cell-surface receptors for chemokines, which are cytokines that activate and direct the migration of white blood cells, are now known to serve as co-receptors (i.e., they are used along with the CD4 molecule just described) for entry of HIV into helper T lymphocytes and monocytes/ macrophages (see Chapter 16). The chemokine receptors now known to be used by HIV as co-receptors during infection of immune cells are the following:

- CCR-5, and CCR-2 and CCR-3. CCR-5 is used by strains of HIV present during early infection. CCR-5 is also needed by HIV to infect monocytes and macrophages. A small number of people lack a working version of the CCR-5 receptor, and these people tend to resist initial infection by HIV and have disease that progresses more slowly to AIDS.

- CXCR-4 is a receptor on helper T lymphocytes that is used by the more virulent strains of HIV present during advanced HIV disease. The CXCR-4 receptor is also known as "fusin" because the strains of HIV that use it as a co-receptor also promote the fusion of infected lymphocytes with uninfected lymphocytes to form syncytia (see Chapter 4). There is also evidence that some strains of HIV-2, a virus that causes a slower-progressing form of AIDS (see Chapter 18), can use the CXCR-4 receptor as the primary receptor for infecting immune cells.

Many white blood cells have receptors for interleukin-2 (IL-2), a cytokine produced by helper T cells that have been stimulated by an antigen. Several kinds of white blood cells have IL-2 receptors. When molecules of IL-2 bind with those receptors, it causes the white blood cells to begin dividing and proliferating. There are many kinds of cell-surface receptors. Some bind with hormones, while others bind with small proteins known as "peptides." Receptor molecules are very specific, just as locks are matched specifically with keys. For example, an IL-2 receptor will bind only with a molecule of IL-2 or a chemical that closely imitates IL-2 (the substance that binds with a receptor is known generally as a "ligand").

Antibodies, which attack foreign substances—antigens—in the body, are produced by B lymphocytes and are first present in lymphocytes as cell-surface receptors (see Chapter 16). But when a B cell is stimulated by the presence of a matching antigen, it begins producing its antibody in large quantities and releasing it into the bloodstream (see also Chapter 16).

■ Recognition Proteins

Recognition proteins allow cells to recognize the cells around them. In this way, a cell learns whether it is in the correct location in the body during development. But recognition proteins are also used by lymphocytes and other white blood cells to recognize the cells they contact. Recognition proteins are also a kind of receptor protein because they cause the cell to react in some particular way when they contact a particular molecule on the surface of neighboring cells.

■ CELL CYTOPLASM

The cytoplasm is the region of the cell between the nucleus and the cell membrane. It contains the submicroscopic equipment—the organelles— needed by the cell to generate energy, process food and waste, produce proteins, and carry out the cell's role in the body. Much of the activity in the cytoplasm is devoted to producing proteins (described in Chapter 15) and to transmitting signals from the cell surface to the cell nucleus, where genes are switched on and off. Examples of cell organelles include the following (Figure 14.2):

- Mitochondria: bacteria-sized oval-shaped structures that combine oxygen with food molecules to produce the energy needed by the cell.

- Lysosomes: vesicles in the cell that contain enzymes for the digestion of substances taken up by the cell.

- The cytoskeleton: protein filaments and tubules that give the cell its shape and transport materials within the cell.

- Endoplasmic reticulum: a maze of sheets, sacs, and tubules. The endoplasmic reticulum is built of a lipid-bilayer membrane similar to that of the cell membrane. It is continuous with the membrane that surrounds the nucleus. The endoplasmic reticulum plays an important role in the synthesis of lipids (fats and oils), cell-surface proteins, and proteins that are secreted by the cell.

- Rough endoplasmic reticulum (RER): areas of endoplasmic reticulum that have a bumpy appearance because they are studded with ribosomes, assemblages of RNA and proteins that play an important role in protein synthesis (Chapter 15). The RER is important in the production of proteins that are either sent to the cell surface or secreted from cells. RER is also important in HIV replication. It produces the HIV gp160 protein that forms the knobs that stud the surface of the virus. This protein is then modified by enzymes in the Golgi apparatus.

- Golgi apparatus: a collection of stacked, flattened sacs and vacuoles. The Golgi apparatus modifies and packages proteins and other materials that are to be secreted by the cell or are to be transported to other organelles. It is in the membranes that make up the Golgi apparatus,

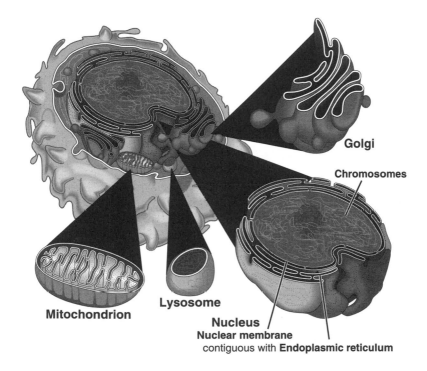

Fig. 14.2 ■ *Examples of cell organelles. Mitochondria generate chemical energy for cells. Lysosomes contain enzymes for the digestion of substances taken up by the cell. The nucleus is bounded by a porous membrane and contains the cell's chromosomes. The endoplasmic reticulum and Golgi apparatus are involved in the production of proteins.*

for example, that sugars are added to certain proteins to make them glycoproteins (see Chapter 15). The Golgi apparatus adds sugars to the glycoprotein that becomes the knobs on the surface of HIV. It also packages and transports the knobs to the cell membrane.

■ CELL NUCLEUS

The nucleus is a sphere in the center of the cell. All cells of all types—except for mature red blood cells—have a nucleus. The nucleus is covered by a lipid-bilayer membrane that is very porous. The nucleus houses the cell's chromosomes, of which there are 23 pairs in humans.

Each chromosome consists of a long, thin molecule of DNA plus a coating of proteins. The DNA is more tightly coiled than the filament in a light bulb. In one way, though, a molecule of DNA is like a stretched-out roll of paper towels. From a distance, that length of paper towels looks like one long, narrow sheet of paper. But it is actually made up of hundreds of individual sheets that are joined together. Similarly, a strand of DNA is one long, narrow string of genes. Genes, however, have different lengths, and there are several thousand genes to a chromosome (see also Chapter 19).

The proteins in a chromosome play important roles in keeping DNA tightly coiled, and in regulating the activity of genes.

■ CONCLUSIONS

This chapter opened by comparing cells to bricks in a building, but while a brick is literally a lifeless lump of clay, a cell is perhaps the most extraordinary of living things: A single cell, microscopic in size, carries out a multitude—thousands—of different chemical reactions within it in the course of daily life. Much of this activity is concerned with protein synthesis, described in the next chapter. As you read that chapter, keep in mind that everything described takes place in a speck invisible to the naked eye.

At the same time, this fleck of life is also a member of a much larger society. In addition to caring for itself, it contributes in some genetically determined, flexible, and responsive way to the functioning of the entire organism. And when the organism is threatened by an invader such as a virus, it is cells—principally those of the immune system—that respond to defend it. In the case of early HIV infection, a struggle of titanic proportions ensues: The immune system destroys billions of virus particles daily but at a cost of billions of immune-system cells. Meanwhile, the immune system also remains actively engaged with the body's day-to-day other tasks and enemies.

Chapter 15

DNA, RNA, AND PROTEIN SYNTHESIS

DNA, RNA, and protein are three fundamental constituents of living cells. They form a tightly coordinated threesome that works to maintain the life and the health of cells. DNA is the repository for the cell's genetic information; RNA transports and translates that genetic information within cells; and proteins make up enzymes and other elements necessary for life. An understanding of DNA, RNA, and proteins is helpful for understanding the life cycle and biology of HIV, for understanding the tests used to detect the presence of HIV, and for understanding how the drugs work that are used to treat HIV infection. DNA and RNA and proteins are members of two of the four major classes of molecules that make up living things. These four classes of molecules are the nucleic acids, proteins, carbohydrates, and lipids.

■ THE FOUR MAJOR CLASSES OF MOLECULES MAKING UP LIVING THINGS

■ Nucleic Acids

Nucleic acids are the family of molecules to which DNA and RNA belong. Both DNA and RNA consist of chains of units known as "nucleotides" (see "The Bases That Make Up DNA and RNA Exist in Three Chemical Forms in Cells"). DNA, found primarily in the cell nucleus in the form of chromosomes, is the genetic material of all living cells.[1] It contains the information required for the production of all proteins and, subsequently, all the other substances needed for life. For this reason, DNA is said to "encode" or "code for" the proteins needed by the cell. In almost all cases, molecules of DNA consist of a double-stranded helix (see Figure 15.1). Molecules of DNA usually take the form of filaments, although some take the shape of a circle (to picture this, think of a decorative, twisted, wrought-iron bar bent into a circle).

But while DNA has primarily one form and one function, RNA takes several forms and serves several functions, most of which relate to the production of proteins. For example, one type of RNA carries genetic messages from the nucleus to the cytoplasm and another serves as a delivery vehicle for protein-building blocks. RNA is also the genetic material of many types of viruses, including retroviruses. DNA and RNA are described in more detail later.

■ Proteins

Protein molecules are composed of chains of amino acids. The sequence of amino acids in the chains determines the final shape of a protein, and the shape is critical to the function of the protein. Proteins in the food we eat serve as a source of essential amino acids that are used by cells to produce the proteins they need. The word "protein" comes from *proteios,* the Greek word for "primary," which is appropriate because proteins are the primary component of cells, making up half their dry weight. Proteins play a variety of roles in cells.

Structural Proteins

These proteins contribute to the structure of the cell. For example, they form microtubules and microfilaments that give cells their shape in the same way poles give shape to a tent.

Regulatory Proteins

Regulatory proteins activate or deactivate genes and other proteins. Some regulatory proteins bind directly with DNA, and these are known as "DNA-binding proteins."

Enzymes

Enzymes are globular-shaped proteins that catalyze, or direct, chemical reactions in cells. To catalyze a chemical reaction, an enzyme combines with another molecule, known as its "substrate," in a lock and key fashion. Enzymes are responsible for most of the metabolic activity that takes place in cells. This includes the production, or synthesis, of proteins, nucleic acids, and other cell components such as lipids, or fats; the production of energy from nutrients; and the breakdown of unneeded cellular components. (These biochemical activities of the cell are referred to generally as "metabolism," or cellular metabolism.)

Cell-Surface Molecules

Many of the molecules found on the surface of cells (see Chapter 14) are made entirely or predominantly of protein. They include the CD8 molecule on the surface of cytotoxic T lymphocytes, and CD4 molecules on the surface of helper T lymphocytes (see Chapter 16), which are used by HIV to enter helper T cells.

Respiratory Proteins

Hemoglobin is a protein found in red blood cells that transports oxygen to cells and carries carbon dioxide away during respiration.

Proteins Released by Cells

Other proteins are produced by cells and released into the surrounding milieu. These include cytokines, many kinds of hormones, and collagen, which is a fibrous protein found in bone, skin, tendons, and cartilage.

■ Carbohydrates

This class of molecules includes the sugars and starches. Carbohydrate molecules contain primarily carbon, oxygen, and hydrogen. Sugar and starch in the diet comprise the primary source of energy for the body. Sugars are also incorporated into many other kinds of molecules. For example, they make up the "backbone" of DNA and RNA (the sugar molecule incorporated into RNA is known as ribose [pronounced ´rye-bose]; the sugar in DNA is known as deoxyribose [de-oxy-´rye-bose]). Sugar molecules are also incorporated into some proteins, forming glycoproteins (the prefix "glyco-" indicates "sugar"). The envelope proteins of HIV, gp120 and gp41 (which together make up the gp160 molecule), are glycoproteins.

■ Lipids

Lipids include the fats, oils, and steroids. Fats and oils store energy in both plants and animals. They are composed of building blocks known as "fatty acids." As components of the diet, fats and oils contain about twice as much energy (i.e., calories) as proteins or carbohydrates. Lipids known as phospholipids are a major structural component of the cell membrane and of the envelope on HIV. The high lipid content of HIV's envelope determines some of this virus's properties, such as its fragility in the environment.

■ DNA

Deoxyribonucleic acid, or DNA, is the material that carries genetic information in all forms of life other than a few groups of viruses. A molecule of DNA, plus associated proteins, makes up a chromosome. Humans have 46 chromosomes in most body cells; germ cells—eggs and sperm—contain 23 chromosomes, half the number found in all other cells. These half-sets become a full set when a sperm unites with an egg at fertilization. Thus, 23 of every person's chromosomes come from the mother and 23 from the father.

The continuous, thread-like molecule of DNA that lies at the heart of a human chromosome is really a string of genes (see Chapter 14). Each gene contains the information needed by the cell to make one protein or a subunit of a protein. Scientists estimate that there are 100,000 to 200,000 genes in the human genome (the term used to describe a complete set of an organism's genes; the human genome is the set of genes found on the 23 chromosomes of an egg or sperm). The genome of HIV, by contrast, has only nine major genes (see Chapter 18).

A molecule of DNA has the shape of a spiral ladder (Figure 15.1). The outer edges of the ladder are known as the DNA backbone (it is actually a double backbone because one is found on each side of a DNA molecule). This backbone is made up of deoxyribose sugar molecules alternating with a phosphate molecule.

The steps in the DNA "ladder" are formed by pairs of units known as "bases." There are four bases in DNA: adenine, cytosine, guanine, and thymine, abbreviated A, C, G, and T, respectively. In DNA, these bases pair off in a specific way: Adenine always pairs with thymine; cytosine always pairs with guanine.

This is an extremely important relationship in biology, and it is known as "complementary base pairing." Complementary base pairing also occurs when RNA pairs with DNA during protein synthesis (see below).

■ The Human Genome versus the HIV Genome

The DNA making up the human genome contains an estimated 3 billion base pairs (bp). Each human chromosome, that is, each of its molecules of DNA, contains from 50 million to 250 million bp. The genome of HIV-1 contains 9,700 bp. ■

■ HOW DNA REPLICATES

A cell must duplicate each of its chromosomes—its DNA—prior to cell division to ensure the transmission of all of its genetic information to its daughter cells. This process is known as "DNA replication." It begins

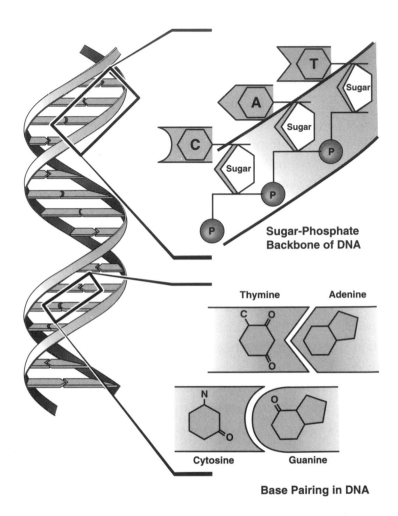

Sugar-Phosphate Backbone of DNA

Thymine   Adenine

Cytosine   Guanine

Base Pairing in DNA

Fig. 15.1 ■ *The DNA double helix. A molecule of DNA resembles a long ladder twisted to form a double helix. The sides of the ladder—the DNA backbone—consist of repeating sugar molecules joined by phosphate groups. The steps of the ladder are formed by the bases named adenine (A), cytosine (C), guanine (G), and thymine (T). Adenine always pairs with thymine, and cytosine always pairs with guanine. A gene is a length of DNA that contains the information for a particular protein. The sequence of bases along one of the two DNA strands determines the sequence of amino acids in that protein. This information is copied in the form of messenger RNA during the first phase of protein synthesis (see text and Figure 15.2). Some of the base sequences in the gene form so-called promoter and enhancer regions that regulate the copying of the gene during protein synthesis (see Figure 19.1).*

when the original double strand of DNA divides down its length—the steps of the ladder separate in the middle. This leaves a length of the molecule looking like an open zipper, with its teeth, the bases, exposed. An enzyme—DNA polymerase—then moves along the open edge of each original strand, adding new bases (in the form of nucleotides) down the length of each original strand. Which base should be added at each step is determined by complementary base pairing. A similar process occurs along the second original DNA strand. Thus, each of the two strands in the original DNA molecule serves as a pattern, or template, for construction of a new strand. This process produces two identical molecules of double-stranded DNA.

HIV also constructs a molecule of DNA shortly after it enters a host cell. HIV, however, carries its genes in the form of RNA (genomic RNA). So while the cell uses a preexisting length of DNA as a template on which to build a new strand, HIV uses its genomic RNA as a template. It assembles a DNA duplicate of its RNA genome using the viral enzyme reverse transcriptase (see Chapter 18). Anti-HIV drugs such as AZT, ddI, ddC, d4T, and 3TC work by masquerading as bases. When they are taken up by reverse transcriptase to form viral DNA, they block further construction of the viral DNA, and thus block viral replication (see Chapter 5).

■ RNA

Ribonucleic acid, or RNA, is also built of bases connected to a backbone of phosphate and sugar. Three of these bases—adenine, cytosine, and guanine—are also found in DNA. RNA, however, contains the base uracil (abbreviated as U) instead of thymine. RNA differs from DNA in other ways, too. While DNA usually comes in only one form—a long, threadlike double-stranded helix, RNA is single stranded and takes different shapes depending on its function. Most types of RNA in cells play a role in protein synthesis. Following is a description of the major types of RNA:

- Messenger RNA (mRNA). The single-stranded and thread-like molecule of mRNA is a copy of a gene. It is assembled in the nucleus and travels to the cytoplasm with its "message," the information for the construction of a particular protein.

■ Ribosomal RNA (rRNA). rRNA is an important component of ribosomes, submicroscopic structures that reside in the cell's cytoplasm
and are the engine that drives the production of proteins. Ribosomes
look like squat snowmen made from one large and one small snowball.
The "snowballs" are subunits that come together to form the ribosome. Ribosomes travel along a strand of mRNA, read its message,
and help link amino acids in the proper sequence to build a particular protein molecule. That sequence corresponds to the information
encoded by the mRNA.

■ Transfer RNA (tRNA). The single strand of this RNA takes the form of
a cloverleaf. tRNA works like taxicabs that shuttle—transfer—amino
acids to the ribosomes that assemble them into proteins.

■ Nuclear RNA, or ribozymes. This type of RNA was only recently discovered. In combination with certain proteins, ribozymes "edit" molecules of mRNA before they leave the nucleus (see "Protein Synthesis
in Cells"). Ribozymes are unusual because they are a nucleic acid that
has the properties of an enzyme, hence their name.

■ Viral RNA. This type of RNA carries genetic information for a large
group of diverse viruses known as "RNA viruses." RNA viruses include
the polio, influenza, measles, and mumps viruses, as well as HIV and
other retroviruses (see Chapter 17).

Both the cell and HIV can use the nucleoside form of each base during DNA synthesis, although the nucleosides must be converted into nucleotides before they can be added to a growing DNA strand. The drugs
AZT, ddI, ddC, d4T, and 3TC have structures that are very close to the
normal nucleoside form of each base; that is, they are "analogues" of
each base. But while the enzyme reverse transcriptase will use an analogue in place of a natural nucleoside during viral DNA synthesis, the
analogue will not fit properly in the new DNA strand and will block its
further assembly by the enzyme. This in turn prevents the virus from
building its DNA, and therefore prevents it from producing progeny vi-
rons. Because these drugs work by inhibiting reverse transcriptase, they
are known as "nucleoside analogue reverse transcriptase inhibitors" (see
also Chapter 5).

The Bases That Make Up DNA and RNA Exist in Three Chemical Forms in Cells

■ As simple, individual molecules of **adenine, cytosine, guanine, thymine,** and **uracil**. In this form, chemists classify these bases as either purines or pyrimidines. Adenine and guanine are purines; cytosine, thymine, and uracil are pyrimidines. In complementary base paring, a purine pairs with a pyrimidine.

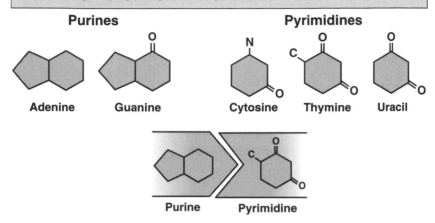

■ As a **nucleoside**. Nucleosides consist of one of the bases plus a five-sided sugar molecule. This five-sided sugar molecule is a ribose in RNA and deoxyribose in DNA.

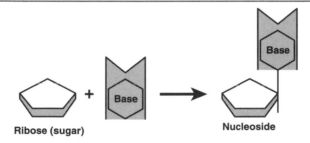

■ As a **nucleotide**. Nucleotides consist of one of the bases plus a five-sided sugar molecule plus one to three phosphate groups (a phosphate consists of an atom of phosphorus with four atoms of oxygen). Nucleotides are the building blocks of DNA and RNA.

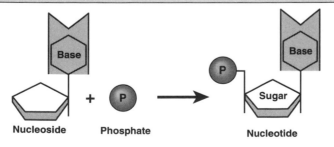

■ PROTEINS AND PROTEIN SYNTHESIS

Proteins are compounds made from one or more chains of smaller molecules known as "amino acids."[2] Proteins occur in numerous shapes and sizes, though most contain between 50 and 1,000 amino acids. Chains of amino acids smaller than this are called "peptides" (researchers also refer to fragments of proteins as peptides or polypeptides). Many types of proteins, including antibodies, cell-surface receptors, and proteins that turn genes on and off, consist of two or more subunits. Proteins with two subunits are known as "dimers"; those with three are "trimers."

■ Genes and Proteins

Genes provide the blueprint needed by cells to make proteins. But how do genes carry that information? Just as Morse code uses sequences of dots and dashes to spell out words, DNA uses sequences of adenine, cytosine, guanine, and thymine to spell out the sequence of amino acids needed to form a particular protein. Each sequence of three bases spells out a genetic "word" that represents one amino acid for the protein that is encoded by the gene. This sequence of three bases is known as a "codon." Each codon identifies one of the 20 amino acids (e.g., the mRNA base sequence cytosine, uracil, adenine—CUA—represents the amino acid leucine).

The collection of three-base sequences that specify all amino acids constitutes the "genetic code." The genetic code is universal: The DNA of all living things uses the same code words, or codons, for the same amino acids. This is why genes transferred from one species to another as done in genetic engineering can function in the recipient species.

■ PROTEIN SYNTHESIS IN CELLS

The production of proteins by cells occurs in three fundamental steps (Figure 15.2):

1. In the nucleus, a gene is "switched on," or activated (see also Chapter 19). The double-stranded DNA of the gene unzips to expose its

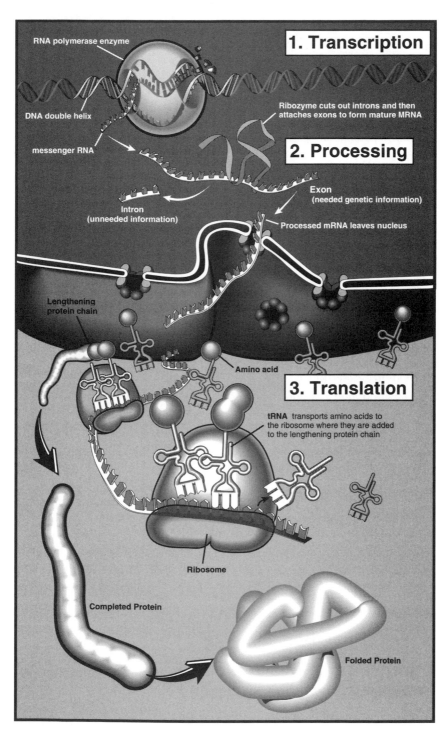

Fig. 15.2 ■ *The three steps of protein synthesis.*

bases, as in DNA replication. The cellular enzyme RNA polymerase then copies the sequence of bases along one of the two DNA strands (the information-containing strand) in the form of messenger RNA (mRNA). Because DNA is rendered or transcribed in the form of RNA, this stage of protein synthesis is known as "transcription."

2. The new molecule of mRNA needs to be processed or "edited": Unneeded lengths, known as "introns," are snipped out (introns do not contain information needed for construction of most proteins). The remaining sections, or "exons," are stitched back together to form a mature mRNA. This work is done in the nucleus by splicing enzymes, the ribozymes. The mature mRNA molecule then travels from the nucleus to the cytoplasm.

3. In the cytoplasm, the little "snowballs" of ribosomal RNA pair up to form ribosomes. Ribosomes attach to the "start" end of the mRNA and travel along its length. As they go, they read the sequence of bases in the mRNA three bases, or one codon, at a time, which specifies the order of amino acids that will make up the protein. The appropriate amino acids are delivered to the ribosome by cloverleaf-shaped molecules of transfer RNA (tRNA). The amino acids are chemically joined like snap beads in a chain to form a particular protein strand. Because the message in the mRNA is translated from a sequence of bases to a sequence of amino acids, this phase of protein synthesis is known as "translation."

When the chain of amino acids is complete, it leaves the ribosome and folds into its final shape. If the protein is produced on a ribosome that is attached to the rough endoplasmic reticulum (see Chapter 14), it may also receive further modification, such as having a sugar structure added, making it a glycoprotein.

■ MUTATIONS IN GENES CAN CAUSE CHANGES IN PROTEINS

A protein's final shape is largely determined by the number and the sequence of the amino acids that form its chain. Shape is extremely important to a protein's function—a protein that is not shaped properly

■ Where Retroviruses Got Their Name

The direction in which information flows during protein synthesis is known as the "central dogma of biology." It is represented as follows:

DNA → RNA → Protein

Of all the forms of life on Earth, the only known exceptions to this direction in the flow of genetic information occurs among a few groups of viruses, principally the retroviruses. In retroviruses, the flow of information travels this way:

RNA → DNA → RNA → Protein

Whereas most organisms produce RNA from DNA, *retro*viruses produce DNA from RNA ("retro" means "reverse"). Scientists call this "reverse transcription," and it is this unusual property that earned the retroviruses their name. Reverse transcription is accomplished by the viral enzyme reverse transcriptase. Retroviruses need reverse transcriptase to "read" RNA and make a DNA copy of their genes. That DNA copy is then incorporated into a chromosome in the host cell. There, it constitutes proviral DNA, which is transcribed by the cell's enzymes, to produce viral mRNA and viral proteins (see also Chapter 18). ■

may work only weakly, if at all. This is true because many proteins work by physically interacting with other cellular components. The shape of enzymes, antibodies, proteins that regulate genes, and of all proteins is critical. This is so because shape, in turn, determines the configuration of the "active site"—the region of the protein that most intimately interacts with other molecules. The active site of a DNA regulatory protein is the cluster of amino acids that directly binds with a certain group of bases in DNA. The active site of an antibody is the small number of amino acids that actually bind to an antigen. The active site of HIV's gp120 molecule is the region of this molecule that binds with the CD4 receptor on helper T cells.

It is the precise shape of the active site (or sites) of an enzyme that enables it to serve as a catalyst for a specific chemical reaction. If amino acids are not linked together in exactly the right sequence during the synthesis of an enzyme, the enzyme might not function well and a particular chemical reaction might not occur. If that chemical reaction is critical to life, it can mean the death of the cell, or even the death of the organism.

What could cause a change in the sequence of amino acids in a protein? The most important cause is a genetic mutation—an error or change in the sequence of bases in the DNA of the gene that codes for that particular protein.

A mutation in a gene often—though not inevitably—results in a change in the sequence of amino acids in the protein encoded by that gene. If that change makes the protein fold improperly, or if it occurs in a critical region, such as its active site, the protein may no longer be able to carry out its function.

Occasionally, though, mutations help a virus like HIV or a pathogenic bacterium to survive. Mutations in HIV genes result in the production of a spectrum of virus particles, or virions, in any one person that are genetically different in small ways from other virions in that same person. These genetic differences allow some virions to survive when a patient begins taking antiviral drugs (see Chapter 5). Such drug-resistant viruses are sometimes known as "escape" mutants because they are able to escape the otherwise toxic effects of a drug on their life cycle.

■ PROTEIN SYNTHESIS BY HIV

Once the viral DNA produced by reverse transcriptase is inserted into a chromosome in the host cell, which happens through the action of HIV's integrase enzyme, it then becomes known as "proviral DNA," or a provirus (see Chapter 18). At this point, the provirus can begin directing the production of proteins just as cellular genes do. These proteins, however, will be viral proteins, those needed to form new virions.

Protein synthesis by HIV is similar to that of the cell: First, viral genes are transcribed into mRNA; next, viral mRNAs travel to the cytoplasm; there, ribosomes translate their messages and assemble viral protein molecules with the help of cellular tRNAs; viral proteins then undergo certain changes and assemble to form new virions, completing the virus replication cycle.

Since viruses lack much of their own protein-making machinery (e.g., ribosomes and tRNA), they depend entirely on the materials and machinery of the host cell. HIV assembles its mRNA from nucleotides present in the host nucleus. In the cytoplasm, it uses ribosomes, tRNAs, and amino acids provided by the host cell. Movement of the viral proteins to the cell membrane is also accomplished using mechanisms available within the host cell.

■ Polyproteins and Other Unusual Features of HIV Protein Synthesis

(Note that the genes discussed here are described in Chapter 18.)

Despite the fundamental similarities of protein synthesis by the cell and by HIV, the two also differ in several interesting ways. These differences are important for understanding the biology and replication of HIV. For example, HIV contains nine genes, but it produces 17 proteins. Usually, one gene is responsible for one protein or one subunit of a protein. How can HIV produce more proteins than it has genes?

It happens because three of HIV's genes—the *gag, pol,* and *env* genes—produce polyproteins. Polyproteins are a string of proteins linked together. They are produced by a single long mRNA. Later, polyproteins are cleaved by HIV's protease enzyme into the individual working proteins. A protease is an enzyme that cuts other proteins into smaller pieces. (Because polyproteins must be processed to obtain working proteins, they are sometimes known as "pre-proteins.") Anti-HIV drugs known as protease inhibitors work by blocking the action of the viral protease enzyme.

The Gag polyprotein is produced by a long mRNA that leaves the nucleus unedited by mRNA splicing enzymes (i.e., no introns are eliminated from the mRNA). The mRNA leaves the nucleus and is read by ribosomes. There, the amino-acid chain is constructed with the help of tRNAs. The finished polyprotein contains four final proteins: the p17 matrix protein (MA); the major capsid protein, p24 (CA); the nucleic acid–binding protein, p9 (NC); and the p7 protein, which is important for virion assembly (this protein is referred to as the "proline-rich protein" because it is high in the amino acid proline).

Molecules of a fatty acid, myristate, affix to the amino-acid sequences for the matrix protein as they are assembled. This process is known as "myristylation." If myristylation of the Gag protein is blocked, virions cannot form. Researchers are studying ways to inhibit myristylation as a strategy for the treatment of HIV infection.

Finally, the Gag polyprotein is packaged into a new virion. At that point, the viral protease enzyme cleaves it into the four working proteins.

The *pol* gene produces a polyprotein that is still more unusual. HIV's *pol* gene carries information for three enzymes: protease, reverse transcriptase, and integrase. The mRNA produced by the *pol* gene sometimes also includes the information for these enzymes plus the matrix and capsid proteins (this occurs because the *pol* gene and the *gag* gene overlap; see Figure 18.2).

This long mRNA travels straight to the ribosome, again without any editing. There, an unusual polyprotein is produced. As a ribosome reads the mRNA, it stops at one point and jumps backward one base, then continues reading the mRNA. This is called "frame-shifting," which means that the ribosome has paused and shifted over one base, and is now "reading" a different sequence of codons.

As a result of frame-shifting, the ribosome produces two polyproteins fused together—a Gag/Pol fusion protein. The Gag/Pol fusion protein contains both the *gag*-gene polyprotein (MA, CA, NC, and p7) as well as the *pol*-gene polyprotein appended to its end (see Chapter 18). The fusion protein is also cleaved by the HIV protease. The fusion protein produces the matrix and capsid proteins from the *gag* gene, plus the protease, reverse transcriptase, and integrase enzymes encoded by the *pol* gene.

The *env* gene also produces a polyprotein, the gp160 molecule. The gp160 is cleaved by a cellular protease enzyme to produce HIV's envelope proteins, the gp120 and gp41 glycoproteins. The gp120 is the molecule in HIV that binds with host cells and begins the process of infection. The gp120 and gp41 fit together and form a mushroom-like shape, with gp41 serving as the stem that is anchored in the viral envelope, while gp120 is the mushroom's cap.

The remaining six genes in HIV's genome produce proteins that regulate the activity of other HIV genes. Some of these regulatory activities include overseeing the cleavage of polyproteins, the packaging of proteins into the virion, and the release of the virion from the cell membrane.

Why should HIV produce polyproteins? Possible advantages include the following:

- Because of gene overlapping, a maximum of genetic information is encoded in a minimum of genetic material.

- Polyproteins reduce the number of viral components that have to be synthesized and targeted to the cell membrane for self-assembly.

- Because they are packaged in the form of a nonfunctional polyprotein, viral enzymes such as reverse transcriptase and protease are prevented from becoming active prematurely.

■ THE ASSOCIATION BETWEEN VIRUSES AND CELLS MAKES DRUG DEVELOPMENT DIFFICULT

The relationship between viruses and their host cells is so intertwined—particularly in the case of retroviruses, which permanently merge their genetic material with that of host cells—that they have been called the "ultimate parasites." This intimate association makes it difficult to develop antiviral drugs because antiviral drugs must specifically target essential components of the virus's molecular machinery while leaving the machinery of the cell intact. Such agents must be designed in the laboratory.

However, development of antiviral drugs can occur only after extensive basic-research studies needed to understand the molecular details of a virus's replication cycle sort out and identify the viral and cellular enzymes involved in it. A selected viral enzyme must then be produced (viral enzymes appear to be the most vulnerable target for antiviral drugs) and purified, and its three-dimensional structure worked out. Once the detailed structure of the enzyme molecule is known, other researchers can design drugs that fit precisely into the enzyme's active site and interfere with its function.

Gaining this extraordinarily detailed knowledge requires a highly sophisticated understanding of molecular biology and advanced biotechnological capabilities. Had HIV disease emerged 50, or even 30, years ago, scientists would have lacked the know-how to discover the means to fight it with antiretroviral agents such as those now emerging from research laboratories, and HIV would have had that much longer to devastate lives.

■ The Meaning of Those Letters and Numbers

Terms such as tat, Tat, or TAT, and gp120 inevitably turn up in medical papers and scientific articles that discuss the molecular biology of HIV disease or cancer. They are a way of referring to a gene, to the protein produced by the gene, or to a protein only.

Genes are often named using lowercase letters (sometimes numbers are included, too). The genes found in HIV, for example, include *gag, pol,* and *env.*

The proteins produced by these genes often carry the same name as the gene, except that it will be spelled using an initial capital letter (as in this book) or using all capital letters. The protein produced by the *gag* gene, for example, might be spelled in other books or in medical journals as GAG or Gag. (Beware, though. These spellings represent an attempt at a convention among medical books and scientific journals, but there is still a lot of variation among them that can cause confusion even for experienced readers of the scientific literature.)

A protein may also be referred to in more than one way. HIV's capsid protein, for example, might be referred to using the abbreviation "CA" or as p24. The "p" identifies the molecule referred to as a protein; the number 24 refers to the mass of the protein molecule in kilodaltons (a kilodalton is a thousand daltons; one dalton is about the mass of one atom of hydrogen).

Sometimes the final protein produced by a gene has a sugar attached to it. It is then known as a glycoprotein and is referred to by the letters "gp" followed by the molecular mass in kilodaltons.

The *env* gene, for example, produces one large molecule that is cut into two units that then have sugars added to them. These two glycoproteins then combine loosely to form the receptor that allows HIV to attach to a host cell. These two envelope proteins are known as gp120 and gp41, indicating that they are glycoproteins with a mass of 120 and 41 kilodaltons, respectively. ■

ENDNOTES

1. A small amount of DNA is also found in mitochondria.

2. There are 20 common amino acids: alanine, arginine, asparagine, aspartate, cysteine, glutamine, glutamate, glycine, histidine,* isoleucine,* leucine,* lysine,* methionine,* phenylalanine,* proline, serine, threonine,* tryptophan,* tyrosine, and valine.* Those followed by an asterisk are the 9 essential amino acids, which must be supplied by the diet; the other 11 can be produced by the cell when necessary.

Chapter 16

THE IMMUNE SYSTEM: AN OVERVIEW

The job of the immune system is to control or eliminate viruses and other microbes that threaten the body with infection and disease. An equally important but lesser understood role of the immune system is to eliminate damaged cells that are, or might become, cancerous.

Tragically, key cells of this defense system are extremely susceptible to infection by HIV. In most people, this infection results in HIV disease, the hallmark of which is the progressive deterioration and eventual destruction of the immune system. During advanced HIV disease the deterioration of the immune system is usually accompanied by opportunistic infections, cancer, and other disorders. This aggregation of illnesses, together with the immune deficiency due to HIV infection, is known as "acquired immune deficiency syndrome," or AIDS.

Knowledge of the immune system and how it works is important for understanding the course and impact of HIV disease on the body, as well as for the diagnosis and management of HIV disease. The detection of anti-HIV antibodies in blood serum diagnoses HIV infection (see Chapters 1 and 2). Similar tests are used to determine whether HIV-infected persons are, for example, at risk of developing toxoplasmosis or tuberculosis. Physicians also monitor the numbers of CD4 lymphocytes as indicators of the progression of HIV disease, and as indicators for starting treatments that can prevent certain opportunistic infections (i.e., prophylactic therapy).

But the immune system is astonishingly complex and much more needs to be learned about it to harness it for the prevention and treatment of HIV disease. One important goal in AIDS research is the development of a vaccine to prevent HIV infection. Researchers are also examining ways to enhance the activity of immune-system cells to fight disease. This is the field of immunotherapy, another strategy being explored to improve the treatment of HIV disease (see Chapter 5).

Understanding how the immune system works begins by realizing that just as the nation's military is divided into branches specialized to combat an enemy on land, on sea, and in the air, so the immune system has one branch to cope with disease-causing microbes in the blood and another branch to deal with microbes hidden within cells.

Microbes in the blood and other body fluids are neutralized—killed or rendered harmless—by antibodies, which are produced by B lymphocytes. This is the "antibody-mediated immune response" (also known as the humoral immune response or humoral immunity).

Microbes located within cells are eliminated by specialized cytotoxic, or "killer" cells. These cells are mobilized through the "cell-mediated immune response." In addition, antibodies and certain cytotoxic cells work together to eliminate virus-infected cells through a third type of immune response" known as "antibody-dependent cell-mediated cytotoxicity," or ADCC.

The body reacts to HIV infection with both the antibody-mediated immune response and the cell-mediated immune response (see also Chapter 4). Both these immune responses, however, must be initiated by helper T lymphocytes, also known as "CD4 lymphocytes." HIV infects and destroys helper T cells, and it is the loss of these cells that leads to the collapse of the immune system and to HIV disease.

The major components of the immune system include the following:

- White blood cells. These form the immune system's front line of defense; they are the cells that are actively engaged in fighting infectious organisms. White blood cells include lymphocytes, that is, B cells,

plasma cells, T cells, and monocytes/macrophages (Figure 16.1); neutrophils; and natural killer cells.

■ Accessory cells, known as antigen-presenting cells. Antigen-presenting
cells work with lymphocytes and other white blood cells to trigger
and control an immune response. Ironically, some of these cells also
play a major role in the HIV disease progression (see below and Chapter 4).

■ Cytokines. These are substances released by certain immune cells to
influence the activity of other immune cells. Some cytokines inten-
sify an immune response, while others suppress it. This chemical
communication is essential in regulating both antibody- and cell-
mediated immunity. Cytokines include the interleukins, the interferons, and cell growth factors. Another family of cytokines that are
proving important to HIV disease are the chemokines. Chemokines
are released at sites of injured or infected tissues. They cause the redness and soreness of inflammation and help activate and attract immune cells to fight the infection and to clean up damaged cells. Recent
evidence shows that certain cell-surface receptors for chemokines are
used by HIV, along with the CD4 molecule, to enter a cell. HIV infection disrupts the production and release of cytokines by immune
cells.[1]

■ The lymphoid organs. The lymphoid organs are the sites at which the
various cells of the immune system come together and interact to produce immune responses (see "Where Immune Responses Take Place in
the Body"). They include the thymus, spleen, and lymph nodes. The
progression of HIV disease leads to the destruction of the internal
structure of these organs (see Chapter 4).

■ ANTIBODY-MEDIATED IMMUNITY

The antibody-mediated immune response reacts to foreign material in
the blood and other bodily fluids. For this reason, it is also known as the
"humoral immune response." The major components of an antibody-
mediated immune response include antibodies, B lymphocytes, and
helper T lymphocytes.

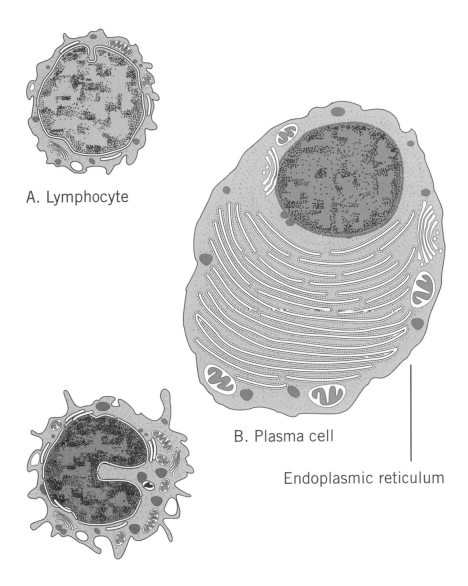

A. Lymphocyte

B. Plasma cell

Endoplasmic reticulum

C. Monocyte/macrophage

Figure 16.1 ■ A. Lymphocyte. T lymphocytes and resting B lymphocytes are identical in appearance and can be distinguished only through the use of antibodies (see "Why They Call It 'CD4': Telling Immune Cells Apart").

B. Plasma cell. Plasma cells are B lymphocytes that have been activated to produce large quantities of antibody. The additional cytoplasm of plasma cells, compared to a resting B lymphocyte (as shown in A), is needed for the high level of antibody synthesis.

C. Monocyte/macrophage. The kidney bean–shaped nucleus is characteristic of macrophages when viewed under a microscope.

■ Antibodies and Antigens

Antibodies are large protein molecules found in blood, mucus, tears, urine, saliva, breast milk, and extracellular fluid, the fluid that surrounds body cells.

Antibodies are produced in response to and interact with specific target molecules known as "antigens." An antigen is any substance, though it is usually a protein, that stimulates the formation of antibodies. In fact, the word "antigen" comes from *"anti*body *gen*erator." Antigens include bacterial toxins such as diphtheria and tetanus toxins, and proteins or glycoproteins that are constituents of microbes—bacteria, viruses, fungi—and foreign cells. Microbes and bacterial toxins infect or injure cells after first binding to a cell-surface molecule (see also Chapter 14). HIV, for example, binds with CD4 molecules and chemokine receptors on the surface of CD4 lymphocytes to gain entry into these cells.

Antibodies that arise in response to the presence of an antigen in the body combine with—bind to—the antigen. This often prevents the microbe or toxin from binding with the cell, thereby neutralizing the microbe or toxin. Antibodies that have this effect are called "neutralizing antibodies." In addition, antibodies that are bound to an antigen stimulate the activity of the complement system (see "Complement: Another Important Component of the Immune System"), and they stimulate the activity of certain immune cells to ingest the antibody-laden antigen. The process by which cells ingest microbes and other materials in the body is known as "phagocytosis," and it is conducted primarily by macrophages (see below) and white blood cells known as "neutrophils."

The presence of an antibody in the blood indicates that the immune system has responded to the presence of a particular antigen. In the case of HIV, the presence of antibodies to HIV is evidence that a person is infected by the virus. If an HIV-infected person is also given an antibody test for toxoplasmosis, and the test result is positive (indicating the presence of this antibody as well), this person has at some prior time also been infected with the *Toxoplasma* organism. Because *Toxoplasma* causes a latent infection, this person is at high risk of developing toxoplasmosis when he or she progresses to AIDS.

Characteristics of Antibodies

- Antibodies are large Y-shaped protein molecules; it is the ends of the arms of the Y that recognize an antigen.

- Antibodies in blood are found in the serum, the fluid that remains after blood is allowed to clot.

- Antibodies in the blood of a pregnant woman cross the placenta and enter the blood of the developing fetus. This includes antibodies to HIV. Thus, a baby born to an HIV-infected mother will always test HIV positive for up to 18 months after birth, even if the baby is not infected by HIV. For this reason, a positive HIV antibody test result obtained from an infant less than 18 months old does not mean that the infant is HIV infected. After 18 months, and if the child is infected, his or her own antibodies will have replaced those passed along by the mother, and a positive result on an HIV antibody test will then truly reflect the child's infected status (see also Chapter 12).

- As mentioned already, neutralizing antibodies are antibodies that prevent virus particles from infecting cells. Although the immune system produces many kinds of antibodies to HIV, only those antibodies that bind to the viral envelope protein, gp120, exhibit neutralizing activity.

- Antibodies are also sometimes referred to as "immunoglobulins" (abbreviated "Ig"). There are five families of immunoglobulins: IgA, IgD, IgE, IgG, and IgM. Each family serves a different role in immune defense.[2] See also "Where Immune Responses Take Place in the Body."

■ B Lymphocytes

B lymphocytes are the white blood cells that produce antibodies. They are also the only cells in the body that do so. Each B cell produces only one specific antibody. And that antibody binds, or reacts, with only one specific antigen. For example, an antibody that reacts with one region of the gp120 protein on the surface of HIV will react with that region of that protein and with no other part of any protein. The site on a protein at which an antibody binds is known as an "epitope."

B cells that are not producing antibodies are called "resting B cells." A resting B cell is like a nearly idle factory that is running at minimum capacity; the cell itself consists mostly of a nucleus surrounded by a small amount of cytoplasm. When a B cell is activated—stimulated to produce its antibody—it is like a factory that expands to work at high capacity. The B cell doubles or triples in size to accommodate the cellular machinery needed to produce the antibody protein. During an immune response, activated B cells can churn out ten million antibody molecules per hour! These highly activated B cells are known as "plasma cells."

■ The Antibody-Mediated Immune Response: How It Works

The antibody-mediated immune response defends the body against bacteria and viruses in the blood and extracellular fluid. It is also activated to fight such things as parasitic worms in the blood and intestines, and it helps neutralize bacterial toxins such as diphtheria and tetanus toxins. The following describes the stages of an antibody immune response, which can take five days or more to deploy.

- The antibody-mediated immune response begins with resting B cells that are being carried through the body in the blood and lymphatic fluid. Resting B lymphocytes do not release antibody molecules into the blood. Instead, they retain them and display the molecules of their antibody molecules like antennae or sensors on their surface. In other words, molecules of the antibody produced by resting B lymphocytes are used as cell-surface receptors (see Chapter 14).

- When a B cell contacts an antigen that fits its antibody, the antigen binds with the antibody on the cell surface.

- After traveling to the nearest lymph node, the B lymphocyte "presents" the bound antigen to a helper T cell. The two cells make contact, with the CD4 molecule on the helper T cell serving as an "adhesion molecule" that helps stabilize the docking between the two cells.

- The joining of the two cells stimulates the helper T cell to release cytokines that complete the activation of the B cell (activation began when the B lymphocyte contacted its antigen). These cytokines also promote the proliferation of more helper T cells that can activate other B cells. (Helper T cells are described in more detail later.)

- The fully activated B cell now divides to produce daughter B cells, which produce more of the same antibody. The original cell and its daughter cells enlarge and become antibody-producing plasma cells (see Figure 16.1 B).

- Fully activated B cells release their antibody molecules freely into the blood, mucus, or other body fluids. Free antibody is carried through the blood and binds to its antigen wherever the antigen is encountered. It is free antibodies such as these that are detected by the HIV antibody test.

- Some of the B cells produced during the immune response do not become antibody-producing plasma cells. These B cells become "memory cells." Their job is to keep a molecular record of the antigen. These long-lived cells remain in the body for years, ready to promote a quicker immune response should the antigen enter the body again.

- When the infection is brought under control, helper T cells produce cytokines that slow the production of antibodies by B cells. At this point, many of the daughter B lymphocytes produced by the first activated B cells are no longer needed. Some of these cells revert to resting B cells, but many self-destruct through a process of cell suicide known as "apoptosis."

■ CELL-MEDIATED IMMUNITY

Cell-mediated immunity detects and eliminates pathogens located within cells. These pathogens include viruses; bacteria that invade cells, such as the bacterium responsible for tuberculosis; and protozoan parasites responsible for opportunistic infections such as *Toxoplasma* and *Cryptosporidium* (described in Chapter 7).

Whereas antibody-mediated immunity occurs in response to antigens in the blood and extracellular fluid, cell-mediated immunity is triggered by the presence of antigen-like molecules on the surface of infected cells.

The major players in cell-mediated immunity are T lymphocytes, macrophages, and antigen-presenting cells.

■ T Lymphocytes

T lymphocytes were given their name because they mature in the thymus gland, a lymphoid organ that lies on the heart. T lymphocytes make up about 70% of all lymphocytes. T cells share the following characteristics:

■ Each T cell reacts with only one specific antigen.

■ T cells detect antigens using receptors on their surface. These receptors are similar to the antibody receptors on resting B cells.

■ The antigens recognized by T cells consist of fragments of proteins— bits of virus or bacteria—displayed on the surface of antigen- presenting cells.

■ T lymphocytes become activated when they are presented with an antigen on the surface of B cells, macrophages, or other antigen- presenting cells.

■ Why They Call It "CD4": Telling Immune Cells Apart

Lymphocytes are like penguins: They all look alike. Under the microscope, B cells and T cells appear identical. Fortunately, they do differ immuno- logically. Each has unique kinds of molecules on its cell surface. These are known as "cell-recognition molecules." Each class of lymphocytes (and many other types of cells, also) has several different cell-recognition mol- ecules on its surface. Cell-recognition molecules can also be used to iden- tify the cell's lineage and its stage of maturity (for example, T lymphocytes from the thymus gland and T lymphocytes from a lymph node will reveal shared but slightly different sets of recognition molecules).

Once scientists identify the unique cell-recognition molecules on a cell, they can produce antibodies in the laboratory—monoclonal antibodies— that react with only that recognition molecule. By linking the monoclonal antibody to a fluorescent dye or radioactive isotope, they can then use the antibody to identify that particular kind of cell. (For example, when fluo- rescent CD4 monoclonal antibody is added to lymphocytes in a test tube, the antibody will bind with the CD4 molecule on helper T cells, causing them to glow when viewed under a fluorescence microscope.)

Usually, several—a cluster of—cell-surface molecules and monoclonal antibodies are used to distinguish B lymphocytes, helper T lymphocytes, cytotoxic T lymphocytes (CTLs), and other cells. This has led to a system nomenclature in which each type of lymphocyte is given a "cluster of differentiation," or CD, number. Helper T cells, for example, are identified as CD4 cells because they carry the "CD4" pattern of recognition molecules:

- They display the CD3 molecule on their surface; that is, they are CD3 positive (CD3+). The presence of the CD3 molecule distinguishes T lymphocytes from other types of lymphocytes.

- They also display the CD4 molecule on their surface; that is, they are CD4 positive (CD4+).

- Last, the cells lack the CD8 molecule on their surface; that is, they are CD8 negative (CD8−).

Thus, cells that are CD3+, CD4+, and CD8− are identified as helper T lymphocytes. CTLs, on the other hand, have the "CD8" pattern of molecules on their surface. They are CD3+, CD4−, and CD8+. Macrophages, which also display the CD4 molecule but lack CD3, are CD3−, CD4+, and CD8−.

The use of monoclonal antibodies linked to fluorescent dyes is the fundamental means by which CD4 lymphocytes are counted. While several techniques can be used, they all at some point involve the application of a fluorescent antibody for the CD4 molecule to a small sample of blood. An instrument called a flow cytometer is usually used to count the number of cells displaying the antibody (i.e., the number of cells that fluoresce) as the sample of blood flows cell by cell through a narrow beam of light.

Note that cell-surface molecules are not just ornaments on the surface of cells; they are involved in the activities of the lymphocyte. The CD4 molecule, for example, is an "adhesion molecule" that helps hold a helper T cell to its antigen-presenting cell during activation. The CD8 molecules on CTLs play an important role in detecting infected cells by binding with MHC–protein fragment complexes on the surface of the body's cells. (For more information on cell-surface molecules, see Chapter 14.) More than 125 CD molecules have now been identified, many of which are found on more than one type of cell. ■

There are two varieties of T lymphocytes: helper T cells, or CD4 lymphocytes; and cytotoxic T cells, or CD8 lymphocytes. Normally, the ratio of helper T lymphocytes to cytotoxic T lymphocytes is 2:1. Changes in the ratio of CD4 to CD8 cells are sometimes used instead of, or in addition to, absolute numbers of CD4 cells to measure the progress of HIV disease.

Helper T Lymphocytes

These lymphocytes are called helper cells because they help coordinate and activate both B lymphocytes, which results in an antibody immune response (described earlier), and cell-killing cytotoxic lymphocytes, which results in a cell-mediated immune response. The activation of other immune cells by helper T lymphocytes occurs largely through the release of cytokines. Without helper T lymphocytes, it is impossible for the body to mount full-scale immune responses.

Helper T lymphocytes also go by the name of CD4 lymphocytes because they have a high number of CD4 molecules on their surface (see "Why They Call It 'CD4': Telling Immune Cells Apart"). This is the molecule (sometimes referred to as the CD4 "receptor") to which HIV binds before infecting a T cell. In addition, helper T lymphocytes display receptors for chemokines that are also needed by HIV to enter the cell. The most important chemokine receptors used by HIV as "co-receptors" for infecting helper T cells include CCR-5 and CXCR-4; the CCR-5 co-receptor used by HIV is found on monocytes/macrophages. (In older scientific literature, helper T lymphocytes were known as T4 cells or inducer T cells.)

CD4 lymphocytes are hit the hardest during HIV infection, and the gradual drop (or percent change) in the number of CD4 cells is used as a marker for the progression of HIV disease (see Appendix 2 and Chapter 4). The normal number of CD4 T cells in the body ranges from 500 to 1,500 cells per mm^3.

Cytotoxic T Lymphocytes

The job of cytotoxic T lymphocytes (CTLs) is to destroy infected cells, including HIV-infected cells. CTLs are also called CD8 lymphocytes because they display an abundance of CD8 molecules on their surface. (Other names for CTLs are killer T lymphocytes, and, in older scientific literature, T8 cells.)

Activated CTLs release substances that break down, or lyse, the membrane of infected cells. This kills the infected cell and the infecting organism. In addition, CD8 cells release cytokines that attract macrophages (see below), which help in the destruction of the invading microorganism and the cleaning up of the resulting cellular debris.

■ Macrophages

Macrophages (see Figure 16.1C) are important in controlling fungal and bacterial infections. A macrophage is the mature form of a white blood cell known as a "monocyte." When a monocyte leaves the bloodstream and enters the tissues of the body, it changes somewhat in appearance and becomes a macrophage.

Macrophages have many important functions. As mentioned earlier, they have the ability to engulf bacteria and other foreign particles, a process known as "phagocytosis." They then display pieces of the phagocytosed material on their surface. In this way, macrophages serve as antigen-presenting cells (see below) and help stimulate immune responses. Macrophages in the brain are known as "microglial cells."

Macrophages also release and respond to cytokines. A helper T cell can release cytokines that activate macrophages, enabling them to destroy infected cells with greater efficiency. In this way, activated macrophages contribute to cell-mediated immunity.

Monocytes and macrophages play important roles in HIV disease. Both cells have CD4 receptors and the co-receptor CCR-5 and can be infected by HIV. But it appears they are not killed as readily as helper T cells by HIV, leading many scientists to suspect that macrophages serve as reservoirs of HIV infection and as vehicles that carry HIV to tissues throughout the body, including the brain. The immune functions of macrophages are impaired during HIV disease, possibly because cytokine signals from helper T cells become disrupted.

■ Antigen-Presenting Cells

Antigen-presenting cells play an important role in initiating and maintaining an immune response. These cells take up antigen molecules, break them into fragments, and display them on their surface. There, the antigen fragments can be detected by helper T lymphocytes, which initiate either an antibody-mediated immune response, a cell-mediated immune response, or both.

Note that a helper T cell itself becomes activated when it encounters an antigen on an antigen-presenting cell. An activated helper T cell then begins dividing and producing daughter cells. It also releases cytokines, including the growth-stimulating cytokine interleukin-2, which stimulates nearby activated helper T cells and cytotoxic T cells, causing them to divide and produce daughter cells. In this way, the intensity of an immune response grows and spreads through the body. There are four main types of antigen-presenting cells:

- B lymphocytes must present their antigen to helper T cells. This fully activates the B cell and initiates the antibody immune response.

- Macrophages that contact antigen travel to nearby lymph nodes and display the antigen on their surface to helper T cells. They thereby play an important role in stimulating B lymphocytes and T lymphocytes.

- Dendritic cells act as sentinels and couriers for the immune system. They are antigen-presenting cells that are found in skin and the mucous membranes. This places them at the two most common sites of infection, and they are often the first to make contact with an antigen. When dendritic cells contact an antigen, they leave their location and travel to nearby lymph nodes. In the lymph nodes, they display the antigen to helper T lymphocytes. Dendritic cells in the skin are also known as "Langerhans' cells."

- Follicular dendritic cells (FDCs) are also antigen-presenting cells, but they are unrelated to the dendritic cells just described. FDCs are stationed in lymph nodes and have long filament-like strands that filter antigens from the lymphatic fluid passing through the node. They serve to concentrate and monitor the presence of an antigen. When much antigen is present, many lymphocytes in the lymph node will be activated by FDCs; when antigen is nearly cleared, the amount of antigen filtered out by the FDC will be much less and the number of lymphocytes that are activated will be correspondingly fewer. FDCs display their antigen to passing helper T lymphocytes to amplify immune responses.

The roles of FDCs as efficient filters and antigen-presenting cells have tragic consequences during HIV disease. Along with other antigens, FDCs also assiduously filter free HIV particles from the lymphatic fluid, thereby helping to concentrate HIV virions in the lymph nodes. As the virus particles cling to the filaments of the FDCs, they infect many of the helper T cells that contact the FDCs; the FDCs themselves do not become infected, however. (For more about the role of FDCs in HIV disease, see Chapter 4.)

Paradoxically, then, a mechanism that normally increases the effectiveness of the immune system helps sow the seeds of its destruction.

■ ACTIVATION OF CELL-MEDIATED IMMUNITY

Cell-mediated immunity depends on the presence of antigens on the surface of infected body cells and on the surface of antigen-presenting cells. These antigens arrive there with the help of proteins known as "class I" and "class II MHC molecules."[3]

■ Class I MHC Molecules

Class I MHC molecules are produced by all cells in the body except red blood cells (mature red blood cells lack a nucleus and therefore cannot produce proteins). After a class I MHC molecule is assembled inside a cell, it travels to the cell membrane where it is displayed on the cell surface. During the journey to the cell membrane, however, each class I MHC protein is linked to a sample of a protein found within the cell.

In this way, samples of proteins produced in the cell—including pieces of any virus or bacteria present—end up on the cell surface attached to a class I MHC molecule. Like department-store display windows, class I MHC molecules exhibit to the world outside a sample of the goods contained inside. In this way, antigens from pathogens hidden within the cell can be detected by CTLs, which use MHC–protein fragment complexes on the cell surface to identify infected cells. When an infected cell is detected, the CTL is activated to kill the cell by lysing it.

■ Class II MHC Molecules

Class II MHC molecules are found only on antigen-presenting cells. Following the assembly of class II molecules inside a cell, they too are sent to the cell surface. And on the way there, they too are linked with fragments of proteins. But these proteins come from outside the cell rather than from inside.

Antigen-presenting cells have the job of sampling materials that lie outside the cells. For example, dendritic cells in the mucous membrane lining the throat, the airway, or the intestines take up samples of the molecules in the fluid surrounding the cells. These samples of molecules are brought into the cells and broken down into fragments. The fragments are combined with class II MHC molecules and taken to the cell surface where they can be examined by helper T lymphocytes. Dendritic cells can also travel to a lymph node to present antigen there.

B lymphocytes also use class II MHC molecules to present an antigen to helper T cells (see above). After an antigen binds to the B cell's antibody receptor, the B cell brings the receptor and the antigen into the cell. It then breaks the antigen into fragments, combines the fragments with class II MHC molecules, and displays the MHC–protein fragment complex on the cell surface for presentation to helper T cells.

■ WHERE IMMUNE RESPONSES TAKE PLACE IN THE BODY

Both antibody-mediated and cell-mediated immune responses require contact between antigen-presenting cells—B lymphocytes, macrophages, dendritic cells, and FDCs—and helper T cells. Most of these contacts occur in the following places.

■ Lymph Nodes

Lymph nodes are rounded capsules of lymphatic tissue located throughout the body, although clusters of them occur in the neck, in the armpits, along the back wall of the abdomen, and in the groin. Lymph nodes normaly range in size from a pinhead to the size of an olive. Together with the spleen, they contain about 95% of the body's two trillion lymphocytes. Lymph nodes are connected by thin-walled lymphatic vessels that carry lymphatic fluid, or lymph. Lymph is a clear yellowish fluid that is nearly identical to blood serum in composition. It is collected from the body's tissues by lymphatic vessels and passes through a series of lymph nodes. Lymph eventually re-enters the bloodstream near the heart through an opening called the "thoracic duct." Lymphocytes and antigen-presenting cells use both blood and lymph to travel through the body. The circulation of the lymph occurs as follows:

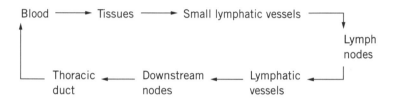

Lymph nodes are the sites at which most immunologically important events occur. The outer regions of lymph nodes contain germinal centers. These are dense aggregates of B lymphocytes that are proliferating and producing antibodies. Other regions of the node contain concentrations of T lymphocytes, antigen-presenting cells, and FDCs that filter the lymphatic fluid as it passes through the node. This internal structure of the lymph node deteriorates over the course of HIV disease.

■ Spleen

The spleen is a soft, spongy organ that lies on the left side of the body somewhat behind the stomach. Blood, rather than lymph, flows through the spleen, and it is the primary site of immune responses to antigens that occur in the bloodstream. Like lymph nodes, the spleen contains dividing B lymphocytes organized into germinal centers. Other areas of the spleen contain concentrations of T lymphocytes interacting with B cells and antigen-presenting cells.

■ Skin

The skin is a tough, multilayered barrier (Figure 16.2A) that separates and protects the body from the outside world. Two percent to 4% of the cells in the skin are antigen-presenting dendritic cells (also known historically as Langerhans' cells). These cells are thought to present antigens from fungi and other pathogens to helper T cells, thereby initiating an immune response. HIV infection weakens immune reactions in the skin, allowing the development of infections by bacteria, fungi, and even the mites responsible for scabies.

■ Mucous Membranes and Mucosal Immunity

In contrast to skin, mucous membranes are thin, delicate tissues (Figure 16.2B). Mucous membranes line the digestive, respiratory, reproductive, and urinary tracts; the eyes; and even the base of the fingernails. The respiratory system and the digestive system are the major sites at which viruses, bacteria, fungi, and infectious protozoa enter the body. Dense aggregates of lymphocytes collect in groups near the surface of many mucous membranes. These collections are known as "diffuse lymphoid tissues." Their sites in the digestive system include the tonsils and adenoids, the appendix, and Peyer's patches in the small intestine.

The body uses a certain family of antibodies, called IgA, to fight infectious agents entering through mucous membranes. The B cells that make these antibodies, as well as the T lymphocytes in mucous membranes, are said to be responsible for mucosal immunity.

An immune reaction in the mucous membrane of the digestive tract is thought to work as follows. Certain cells—M cells—in the lining of the small intestine sample material in the intestinal canal by engulfing small particles. These particles can include bits of food, bacteria, viruses, or material from parasites. The particles are passed along to antigen-presenting cells—B lymphocytes and macrophages—in the underlying diffuse lymphoid tissue. Antigens displayed by antigen-presenting cells activate helper T cells. They in turn activate local B cells to produce antibodies (principally IgA antibodies) against the antigen. They can also activate CTLs and macrophages.

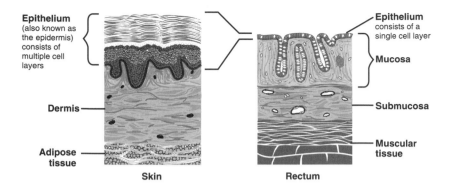

Figure 16.2. ■ A. *A section of hairless skin and mucous membrane. The epidermis is built of multiple layers of epithelial cells topped by a thick layer of protective keratin. Skin is an effective barrier against invasion of the body by viruses and microbes.*

B. *Mucous membrane. Compared with skin, a mucous membrane is a delicate tissue: Only a single layer of epithelial cells (top layer of mucosa) protects the underlying tissue. Thus, a mucous membrane is more easily damaged by physical trauma and is more readily invaded by viruses and bacteria. For this reason, high numbers of lymphocytes (not shown) are often present in the mucosal and submucosal layers of a mucous membrane.*

The antibodies end up in the mucus and nearby extracellular fluid. Some antigen-laden B lymphocytes and antigen-presenting cells from the mucous membrane also enter the circulation to trigger the antibody production by B cells in lymph nodes. In this way, antibodies to an intestinal pathogen also end up in the lymphatic system and bloodstream.

Because sexually transmitted HIV must penetrate the mucous membrane of the vagina or rectum, researchers think that mucosal immunity could play an important role during early HIV infection. This also leads to the question of whether a vaccine for HIV infection should also be designed to stimulate a stronger mucosal immune response (see Chapter 10). A weakening of mucosal immunity during HIV disease probably contributes to the development of candidiasis in the mouth, throat, esophagus, and vagina, and to the many opportunistic infections that begin in the lungs.

■ ANTIBODY-DEPENDENT CELL-MEDIATED CYTOTOXICITY

A third kind of immune response, ADCC, involves the lysing of infected cells that are precoated with antibodies. In ADCC, infected cells are destroyed not by CTLs, but by other types of white blood cells, including natural killer (NK) cells, neutrophils, and monocytes/macrophages. (NK cells make up about 5% of white blood cells in the blood. They inhibit the growth of cancer cells and help fight bacterial and fungal infections.)

ADCC can occur during HIV infection when anti-HIV antibodies bind with HIV proteins present on the surface of infected cells. The HIV gp120 protein, for example, is present on the surface of infected helper T lymphocytes. Anti-gp120 antibodies can bind with gp120, and ADCC cells (primarily NK cells) in turn can bind with the antibody and destroy the infected cells. Sometimes, however, gp120 molecules floating freely in the bloodstream—after being released by dead HIV-infected cells—will bind with the CD4 receptor of uninfected helper T cells. If anti-gp120 antibodies bind with these gp120 molecules, they can lead to the destruction of uninfected helper T lymphocytes by ADCC cells, further damaging the immune system.

■ COMPLEMENT: ANOTHER IMPORTANT COMPONENT OF THE IMMUNE SYSTEM

Complement is an important part of the immune system that helps defend the body against bacteria. Complement is a system of 20 proteins in the blood that work sometimes on their own and sometimes in conjunction with antibodies. Complement proteins work by way of a chain reaction that is triggered by the presence of infecting bacteria or by the presence of antibodies attached to the cell wall of bacteria. In this way, the proteins *complement* the action of antibodies, and it is this activity that gives them their name.

After complement proteins attach to bacteria, they form "membrane attack complexes" that produce holes in the cell wall of bacteria, destroying them. The presence of complement proteins on bacteria also attracts neutrophils and macrophages that engulf the bacteria. In addition, complement proteins make nearby blood vessels more porous. This admits more antibodies and white blood cells to the site of infection and intensifies the immune defense response.

Whether HIV infection disrupts the complement system is not well studied, but the infections acquired by people with HIV are not characteristic of a complement deficiency.

∎ CONCLUSIONS

Clearly, the immune system provides an elegant, extraordinarily complex, dynamic, and wonderfully coordinated defense system against the myriad of pathogens that would otherwise colonize the human body. And AIDS has demonstrated the tragic consequences of this system's destruction. The emergence of HIV disease, however, also triggered an explosion of research on the immune system. Not only has it revealed much about HIV disease itself, but this work is also leading to many advances against other immune-related diseases, ranging from cancer to autoimmune diseases such as multiple sclerosis and rheumatoid arthritis.

Yet, much work needs to be done to gain the critical understanding required to help the human immune system defeat HIV and to restore immunity in people with advanced disease who may have responded well to antiviral treatment but remain vulnerable to opportunistic diseases because of continuing immune impairment. It is also critical to learn how the immune system interacts with HIV to bring virus levels down during acute infection. This could lead to a better understanding of the so-called correlates of immunity that need to be known for the development of an anti-HIV vaccine (see Chapter 10), which is the key to truly defeating the epidemic worldwide.

■ The Names of Cells in the Immune System

The immune system is made up of white blood cells. These cells are referred to by many names in the medical literature. Many of the cells were named first by scientists who had only killed and stained cells to study under the microscope. Later when immunologists categorized the cells based on their function, new names came to be used. The various types of immune cells are grouped below in categories that are often referred to in medical books and in the scientific literature. They are presented here to help readers make sense of the many ways researchers can refer to the same white blood cell (in certain contexts, B cells, for example, can be referred to as antigen-presenting cells, effector cells, and mononuclear cells).

- The term "antigen-presenting cells" refers to B lymphocytes, dendritic cells (those that occur in the skin are sometimes called Langerhans' cells), and follicular dendritic cells, all of which "present" antigens to helper T cells.

- "Effector cells" is a general term for immune cells that neutralize antigens or destroy infected cells. These cells include cytotoxic lymphocytes, B lymphocytes, macrophages, and natural killer cells.

- Granulocytes are white blood cells that when killed, stained, and viewed under the microscope are seen to contain granules in their cytoplasm. These cells are known as neutrophils, basophils, and eosinophils. Granulocytes are the most numerous nucleus-containing cells in the body; only red blood cells, which do not contain a nucleus, are more numerous.

- "Leukocyte" is another name for a white blood cell.

- Lymphocytes are the cells responsible for antibody-mediated immunity and cell-mediated immunity. There are about two trillion lymphocytes in the human body. In terms of numbers of cells, the number of lymphocytes in the immune system is equivalent to the number of all the cells making up the brain or liver. Most lymphocytes fall into one of two categories: B lymphocytes and T lymphocytes. A plasma cell is a mature B cell that is producing antibodies.

- Mononuclear leukocytes are cells with nuclei that appear smooth and round under the microscope, in contrast to the appearance of polymorphonuclear leukocytes (see below). Mononuclear leukocytes include lymphocytes, monocytes/macrophages, and natural killer cells.

- The term "phagocytes" refers to neutrophils and macrophages, which engulf bacteria and cellular debris in the body. The process by which cells engulf material is known as "phagocytosis."

- The term "peripheral blood mononuclear cells" (PBMCs) refers to lymphocytes, monocytes, natural killer cells, and other cell types found in circulating blood (as opposed to those in lymphatic organs). PBMCs constitute about 3% of all lymphocytes in the body; the remaining 97% is found in the organs of the lymphatic system.

- "Polymorphonuclear leukocytes" is another name for neutrophils, basophils, and eosinophils because the nucleus of these cells has many lobes and can take many shapes (i.e., it is polymorphic).

- "Regulatory cell" is a general term sometimes used to refer to helper T lymphocytes, which regulate immune responses. ■

ENDNOTES

1. A particularly important cytokine that is released in response to viral infections is interferon (IFN). There are several categories of interferons, but IFN-alpha and IFN-beta (known together as type-I IFN) are both released by all nucleated cells in the body as an early response to viral infection. The action of type-I IFN is to inhibit viral replication, stimulate the activity of natural killer (NK) cells, and increase the production of molecules (class I MHC molecules) that display viral antigens on the surface of infected cells (both NK cells and MHC molecules are described in this chapter). Interestingly, the fevers that occur during a viral infection are often due to the IFN that is released to fight the infection.

2. IgA is the kind of antibody found primarily in mucus, tears, saliva, and breast milk; it is the type of antibody produced to fight microbes in mucous membranes. IgD is the category of antibody present in small amounts in human serum; its function is unknown. IgE is active during allergies; it stimulates cells that release histamine. IgG is the major category of immunoglobulin in the blood; it is most often present during bacterial and viral infections and attracts macrophages and other components of the immune system to the site of infection. IgM is present during early immune responses; it attracts macrophages and complement proteins and promotes the binding of antigens to B cells.

3. "MHC" stands for "major histocompatibility complex." This is the name given to the set of genes that codes for MHC molecules. In older scientific literature, MHC molecules were called "human leukocyte-associated antigen," or HLA.

■ *Chapter 17*

VIRUSES: AN OVERVIEW

This chapter outlines the similarities and differences among medically important viruses. It also briefly shows how retroviruses, particularly HIV, compare with other viruses. All organisms—vertebrate and invertebrate animals, plants, fungi, protozoa, and bacteria—can be infected by one type of virus or another. Not all viral infections result in disease, however. Furthermore, many viruses may perform a beneficial role in the evolution of plants and animals by transferring genetic material from one host to another.

■ CHARACTERISTICS OF VIRUSES

Viruses are infectious particles that are too small to be seen through an ordinary light microscope. They are dozens to hundreds of times smaller than the average cell and far simpler in structure. Virus particles contain none of the organelles such as ribosomes and mitochondria that cells or bacteria contain and that carry out the complex biochemical activities needed to sustain life. Consequently, virus particles cannot produce energy from food or synthesize proteins on their own. They neither grow nor divide as do animal cells, bacteria, and fungi. They multiply only after invading a host cell and do so using the host cell's energy and protein-producing machinery to synthesize viral proteins and copies of the viral genetic material. These molecules then assemble themselves into new free virus particles, or virions.

The virions of many viruses, such as herpesviruses, accumulate in the cell until the infected cell bursts open, releasing new virions and killing the cell. Other types of viruses, such as retroviruses, bud from the cells. Budding can leave cells undamaged when virions are released in low numbers; when virions are present in high numbers, their budding can also kill cells. Newly released virions are shed into the fluid surrounding cells (i.e., extracellular fluid) and into other body fluids and secretions through which they can reach other cells, other parts of the body, or even other hosts. The effects of a virus on its host cells and the immune system's response to the virus determine the course of the infection and the symptoms the host experiences.

Inside cells, the ability of viruses to multiply and grow their own kind suggests that they are living things; outside of cells, they are small packages of inert substances that bear little resemblance to a living organism. Therefore, viruses are considered to be entities that are at the very frontier of life.

■ THE THREE MAIN COMPONENTS OF VIRIONS

Virus particles, or virions, have three main components:

- A collection of genes—a genome—that is made of either RNA or DNA. For this reason, virologists divide viruses into two main groups: DNA viruses and RNA viruses.

- A protein coat, or capsid, that surrounds and protects the genome.

- An outer envelope. Viruses that bud from cells, including retroviruses, also have an outer envelope that surrounds the capsid. This envelope consists of a membrane that is similar in composition to the cell membrane but, in addition, contains certain viral proteins.

Some viruses, including HIV, carry a variety of proteins within their capsid in addition to their genome. Most of these proteins are viral enzymes needed for outer replication. The outer envelope that surrounds the capsid of budding viruses consists of a bit of cell membrane that newly formed virions take with them as they leave the host cell.

The most distinguishing characteristics of viruses are the shape of their capsid, the presence or absence of an outer envelope, the type and size of the genome, and their method of replication. These traits influence the way different viruses infect cells, how and where in the cell they replicate, and how readily their genome mutates.

■ VIRAL CAPSIDS

The capsid protects the viral genome from the environment and is important for the attachment of virions to their host cells. The capsid also gives the virions their shape. A capsid is usually made up of repeating protein units—capsomers—that fit together like bricks in a building. The capsid plus the DNA or RNA genome is known as the "nucleocapsid." Capsids of most viruses fall into one of three categories according to their shape: helical, icosahedral, and complex.

- Helical viruses. The capsids of helical viruses are formed of repeating protein subunits stacked in a spiraling fashion to form a cylinder. The hollow core houses the DNA or RNA genome. All animal viruses with a helical capsid also have envelopes. Examples include the viruses responsible for mumps and measles.

- Icosahedral viruses. An icosahedron is a sphere-like structure composed of 20 identical triangular faces. This produces a strong shell that encloses a nearly maximum volume (a sphere encloses a maximum volume). The geodesic dome is an icosahedron. Many viruses, including HIV, have icosahedral capsids.

- Complex viruses. These viruses have capsids that contain many different proteins. Poxviruses, such as smallpox and vaccinia, are among the most complex known. The brick- or oval-shaped capsid can be very large—up to 400 nanometers (nm) long, or four times the size of HIV—and contain more than 100 different proteins.

■ VIRAL ENVELOPES

The outer membrane of cells (see Chapter 14) is fragile, and so are most viral envelopes. Both are damaged by heat, freezing, and drying. They are also damaged by acids and bases, fat solvents, detergents, soaps, and disinfectants such as chlorine, phenol, and hydrogen peroxide. This is why HIV, an enveloped virus, cannot survive drying or be transmitted on dry toilet seats, doorknobs, and countertops. It is also why HIV is easy to kill with common disinfectants. Many nonenveloped viruses, on the other hand, can resist harsh conditions.

A number of proteins are found in viral envelopes, and two of them are of major importance. They are the glycoproteins that project from the envelope like spikes ending with knobs. They recognize and attach to specific molecules on the host cell. In HIV, the gp120 forms the knobs; it attaches the virus to the CD4 molecule on host cells. The gp41 glycoprotein is rooted in the envelope and forms the stem of the spike; it is important for fusion of the virions with cells. Other proteins can be found in the envelope, but they play no role in the life cycle of the virus. They are derived from the host cell, being acquired by accident when virions bud from cells.

Another protein associated with the viral envelope is the matrix protein. It lies between the envelope's lipid layer and the capsid and gives rigidity to the virion.

■ THE VIRAL GENOME

Viral genomes can be composed of either DNA or RNA, and their composition determines how the virus replicates. Most viruses carry only a single copy of their genome per virion. Retroviruses are an exception to this; they carry two copies of their genome on two molecules of RNA.

■ Four Important Characteristics of Viral Genomes

Shape
Viral genomes can form a straight string (i.e., a linear molecule) or a circle. Some RNA viruses, such as influenza viruses, have a genome that is

segmented into several short RNA molecules. Each short string encodes a different set of viral genes. HIV's genome consists of two identical RNA molecules, which means that it contains two copies of each viral gene.

Structure

DNA in plants and animals resembles a ladder twisted into a spiral. This shape is known as a double-stranded helix (see Chapter 15). Many DNA viruses also have genomes made of double-stranded DNA (dsDNA). Others have DNA that consists of only a single strand—their DNA would look more like a comb with stubby teeth. These viruses are known as single-stranded DNA (ssDNA) viruses. Likewise, some RNA viruses have genomes that consist of double-stranded RNA (dsRNA), while other RNA viruses have genomes made of single-stranded RNA (ssRNA). As mentioned already, HIV's genome consists of two molecules of ssRNA.

Size

The size of a genome is measured in terms of its length in nucleotides, the basic building blocks of RNA and DNA (see Chapter 15). Viruses with longer genomes tend to have more genes and produce more proteins than do viruses with smaller genomes. The length of ssRNA or ssDNA viral genomes is measured in terms of thousands of bases—in kilobases (kb). Genomes consisting of dsDNA or dsRNA are measured in thousands of base pairs, or kilobase pairs (kbp). DNA viruses often have longer genomes than do RNA viruses. This is because large molecules of RNA are more fragile and more likely to fragment than are large, double-stranded molecules of DNA.

The genomes of DNA viruses range in size from 3,200 base pairs (or 3.2 kbp) in hepatitis viruses to some 250,000 base pairs (250 kbp) for the largest DNA herpesviruses and for poxviruses. The human genome, by contrast, consists of about 3 billion base pairs.

RNA viruses with dsRNA genomes range from 18,000 to 27,000 base pairs (18 to 27 kbp). The ssRNA viruses have genomes ranging from 1,700 to 21,000 bases (1.7 to 21 kb) in length. The genome of HIV, a ssRNA virus, has a length of 9,700 bases (9.7 kb). Two of these strands are present in each virion.

Sense

Sense is a property that belongs only to ssRNA viruses. It refers to whether the single strand can by itself produce viral proteins in host cells. That is, sense refers to whether or not the genome of a RNA virus can behave as if it were a messenger RNA (mRNA). The sense of a ssRNA virus can be positive (+) or negative (−). When a genome with positive sense is experimentally injected into a cell, it will infect the cell and produce new virions as if a complete virus particle had entered the cell. The cell "reads" the ssRNA as it would "read" mRNA and translates it directly into protein (see Chapter 15).

When a genome with negative sense is injected into a cell, however, it must first make a positive-sense copy of itself (i.e., a second RNA molecule that is the mirror image of the first). The positive RNA copy then becomes the mRNA used for the production of new viral proteins. However, the enzyme that makes this copy is in the capsid and is missing when the genome only is injected experimentally into cells. Such an experiment cannot result in infection and the production of viral proteins. Some ssRNA viruses are ambisense—part of the genome has positive sense and part has negative sense—and they have a more complicated replication mechanism.

The genome of most dsDNA viruses can by itself be infectious when experimentally injected into host cells. This is because dsDNA is made of two strands, one of which has positive sense, and because the cell provides the enzymes needed for viral protein synthesis (see Chapter 15).

■ INFECTION OF CELLS AND VIRAL REPLICATION

Viruses multiply by infecting cells and replicating in them. In the course of their replication, viruses can cause diseases that range from the innocuous (e.g., the common cold) to the deadly (e.g., hemorrhagic fever and AIDS).

Viral replication occurs through complex interactions between the virus and its host's cells. Some viruses replicate in cell nuclei and some in cytoplasm. In general, the replication cycle of viruses consists of **eight** steps (for the specific steps in HIV replication, see Chapter 18): attachment, penetration, uncoating, production of viral proteins, replication of the viral genome, assembly, release, and maturation.

1. Attachment. Infection begins when one or more virions attach to a host cell. This occurs when a protein on the surface of the virions binds with one or more molecules on the surface of a cell. If a cell lacks the correct surface molecule, the virus usually will not infect it (although there are exceptions to this). HIV's attachment molecule is the gp120 molecule, which protrudes from the viral envelope; the gp120 molecule binds with the CD4 molecule found on the surface of helper T lymphocytes and on macrophages. HIV also uses one or more co-receptors to enter cells. These co-receptors include three chemokine receptors known as CCR-2, CCR-5, and CXCR-4 (see Chapter 18).

2. Penetration. After attachment, the virions enter the cell, usually either by fusion or by being engulfed by cells capable of phagocytosis or endocytosis. Enveloped viruses (including HIV) enter cells by fusion: The viral envelope fuses with the cell membrane, thereby delivering the naked capsid into the cytoplasm. Nonenveloped viruses, and some enveloped viruses, enter cells when they are engulfed by the cell and brought into the cytoplasm in vesicles.

3. Uncoating. Immediately after penetration, the virions' capsids completely or partially disintegrate. This "uncoating" exposes the viral genome to the interior of the cell. In enveloped viruses such as retroviruses, the process of uncoating starts with the fusion of their outer envelope with the cell membrane.

4. Production of viral proteins. The goals of viral replication are the production of new viral proteins and of viral DNA or RNA, and the assembly of these components into new infectious virus particles. In the course of replication, viral genomes direct the production of several classes of proteins, including the following:

   ■ Structural proteins, which make up the capsid and the viral components of the envelope.

   ■ Viral enzymes needed for replication.

   ■ Viral regulatory proteins, which control the timing and rate of replication.

- Viral proteins that interfere with protein production by the cell, thereby hijacking cellular materials and machinery for the production of viral proteins.

- Virokines, which are virus-produced proteins that subvert the body's immune response to the virus. Virokines inhibit the release of cytokines by immune cells, reduce the production of MHC molecules, and block the chain reaction of complement proteins (described in Chapter 16).

5. Production of viral genome, or viral genome replication. Viruses must replicate their genome for incorporation into progeny virions. This is done by both DNA and RNA viruses, and they do so using a variety of mechanisms.

6. Assembly of new virus particles. As viral proteins and new genomes are produced, they accumulate separately in particular locations in the cell. At some point, the components come together and assemble themselves into new virus particles. The site of viral assembly varies with the type of virus. It also depends on whether the virus replicates itself in the nucleus or cytoplasm and by what mechanism the virus is released from the cell. For example, herpesviruses assemble in the nucleus, while HIV and most other retroviruses assemble at the cell's surface membrane. Still other viruses assemble at membranes that line vacuoles in the cell.

7. Release from the cell. Most nonenveloped and some enveloped viruses lyse, or break cells open, when they are released from infected cells. Such viruses are referred to as "cytocidal" (i.e., cell killing) viruses; those that do not usually kill the cell are called "noncytocidal" viruses. Lytic viruses include herpesviruses and adenoviruses. Enveloped viruses, like HIV, bud from cells, but they can also lyse cells when large numbers of virions bud simultaneously.

8. Maturing of virions. The maturing of new virions often involves changes in the proteins that make up the capsid or in proteins contained inside the capsid. For example, progeny HIV particles become mature—and infectious—when their protease enzyme cuts up their long Pol polyprotein. This cleavage produces active versions of the viral reverse transcriptase, protease, and integrase enzymes

(see Chapter 18). Protease inhibitors, a class of anti-HIV drugs, block the protease enzyme from carrying out this step (see Chapter 5). In some viruses, assembly and maturation occur in quick succession inside the cell; in other viruses, including HIV, maturation occurs after new virions have left the host cell.

■ VIRUS SHEDDING

Virus shedding is the release of virions in an area of the body that enables them to spread from one person to another. Viruses are usually shed from the same areas of the body that they use to enter it. For example, HIV, cytomegalovirus, and hepatitis B virus are shed into saliva, semen, and cervical secretions. The amount of virus in each of these secretions varies, however. Infectious HIV is abundant in genital secretions but is present in such small amounts in saliva that it does not lead to transmission through ordinary kissing. In addition, there are natural inhibitors in saliva (proteolytic enzymes and certain glycoproteins that are currently under study) that inactivate the virus. Major sites of viral shedding include the following:

- Genital tracts. Semen and vaginal secretions are important in the transmission of sexually transmitted disease viruses such as HIV, HTLV, papillomavirus, hepatitis viruses, and several herpesviruses (particularly herpes simplex virus type 2).

- Respiratory tract. Respiratory viruses are usually shed in mucus or saliva. They are then expelled from an infected person in droplets produced by coughing, sneezing, and talking. Large droplets leave the air quickly, but microdroplets evaporate to produce droplet nuclei—aerosols—that are smaller than a red blood cell. Aerosols remain in the air for long periods and can travel great distances. (Note that HIV is not a respiratory virus and is not transmitted by aerosols.)

- Intestinal and urinary tracts. Intestinal viruses are shed into the feces and are spread particularly well by the diarrhea that they cause. Some viruses—such as cytomegalovirus—are shed into the urine. Shedding of virus into urine is usually not an important route of transmission in humans, although it is for some animal viruses.

■ TRANSMISSION OF VIRUSES

After a virion is shed from the host cell, it becomes free to infect other cells in the body or other hosts. Viruses infect other hosts through horizontal transmission or vertical transmission. Horizontal transmission occurs when a virus is transmitted from one person to another. Vertical transmission occurs when a virus is passed from mother to child before, during, or shortly after birth, such as during breast-feeding. Vertical transmission can occur with HIV, rubella virus, cytomegalovirus, herpes simplex virus type 2, and hepatitis B viruses. (See also Chapter 3.)

■ ROUTES OF VIRAL INFECTION

A number of factors determine the course of a viral infection. One of the most important is the site—or route—through which the virus enters the body. The skin, with its outer layer of dead, dry cells, is an extremely effective barrier against viral infection. Viruses can enter the body through skin only if it has fresh cuts, abrasions, deep scratches, or punctures such as those caused by animal bites.

The moist surface provided by mucous membranes, on the other hand, is the most important portal of entry for viruses into the body. Mucous membranes consist of a thin layer of live epithelial cells covered by a thin blanket of mucus (see Figure 16.2). The mucus is produced by mucus-producing cells found among the epithelial cells. Because mucous membranes provide an inviting entry for viruses (some of which, like cold viruses, flourish there), they are protected by a particular group of antibodies—immunoglobulin A (IgA)—and by a number of underlying lymphoid organs (see also Chapter 15). Mucous membranes are components of the following organ systems:

- The reproductive system. The cavities and channels—various tubes and tubules—of the genital and urinary systems are lined by mucous membranes and are breeding grounds for microbes that cause sexually transmitted diseases. Among viruses, herpesviruses, papillomaviruses, and HIV and other retroviruses are transmitted through sexual contacts because the mucosal cells of the genital system shed these viruses.

- The gastrointestinal (GI) system. The mouth, throat, esophagus, stomach, small and large intestines, rectum, and anus constitute the GI system, and all are lined by mucous membranes. Microbes enter the GI system along with foods, liquids, or any object or material placed in the mouth. Herpesviruses often infect the mouth and throat; other viruses infect the cells lining the intestines. Most do not survive the highly acidic conditions of the stomach or the bile and proteolytic enzymes of the small intestine. The walls of the intestines—including those of the rectum—are also well endowed with underlying dense concentrations of lymphocytes and monocytes/macrophages. These cells are there for defense but they can become infected by HIV during anal intercourse, particularly if it tears the mucous membrane of the rectum, bringing infected semen into direct contact with blood (see Chapter 3).

- The respiratory system. This is the most common site of viral entry to the body. Mucous membranes line the nose, throat, and airways to the lungs. The respiratory tract is protected to some extent from infection by the adenoids and tonsils, which are rich in lymphocytes and monocytes/macrophages.

- The eyes. The conjunctiva is a mucous membrane that covers the eyeball and lines the eyelids. The eyes are an unusual route of infection, though, because they are constantly washed by tears and wiped by the eyelids. Nevertheless, some herpesviruses, adenoviruses, and enteroviruses infect the conjunctiva of the eyes.

■ VIRUS SPREAD IN THE HOST ORGANISM

Once beyond the barrier of a mucous membrane and into the body, a virus usually attaches to cells that have a cell-surface molecule appropriate for that type of virus, and the viral replication cycle begins (see "Infection of Cells and Viral Replication," above). The specificity of the virus for particular cell types is known as "viral tropism." Some viruses, once they have infected groups of cells in a tissue, remain in that tissue as a local infection. Rhinoviruses, which cause colds, and influenza viruses are examples of viruses that cause localized infections.

Other viruses, such as the measles virus, infect an initial site in the respiratory tract and then spread throughout the body, producing a systemic infection. Some viruses, including HIV, infect white blood cells and use the bloodstream to spread to other parts of the body (laboratory experiments also indicate that HIV may spread from one cell to another when an infected cell contacts an uninfected one; see Chapter 4). Viruses such as the herpesvirus that causes chickenpox spread through the body by traveling the lengths of nerve fibers.

■ COURSE OF INFECTION

A viral infection can have several outcomes: It can be nonproductive, acute, or chronic. Chronic infections in turn can be persistent, latent, or progressive.

- Nonproductive, or abortive, infection is an infection that is stopped by first-line (and nonspecific) immune defenses, which includes interferon produced by the infected cells within hours, and by the complement system (described in Chapter 16).

- Acute infection is an infection that is usually brief because it is effectively brought under control by the immune system. Often, the immune system eliminates the virus entirely from the body. Examples are colds, flu, and measles.

- Chronic infection means that once in the body, the virus always remains there to some degree. HIV, for example, produces a chronic infection. Chronic infections in turn are usually either persistent or latent. A persistent infection begins with an acute infection phase that is brought under control by the immune system. A few virus particles escape, however, and cause long-term illness. In a latent infection, some virus particles escape the body's immune defenses and establish a lifelong infection that usually remains asymptomatic. Under certain circumstances, however, the virus can become reactivated. This results in a renewed acute infection until the immune system again brings the virus under control. The herpes simplex viruses type 1 and 2, for example, can infect nerve cells latently, producing no symptoms until certain conditions (stress, fatigue) activate these viruses to produce cold sores or genital ulcers. Varicella-zoster virus, the herpesvirus that causes chickenpox, can first produce an acute infection—chicken-pox—then establish a latent lifelong infection that may break out later in life as shingles (which is an acute infection until the immune system again brings this herpesvirus under control).

HIV infection (and infections by related viruses in animals) is a rare example of a chronic, persistent, *and progressive* infection. At no time can the immune system overcome it completely, and it ultimately over-whelms the body's immune defenses.

■ VIRAL DAMAGE CAUSES DISEASE

Viruses can affect host cells in many ways, depending on how compatible the virus's replication needs are with the survival of its host cells. A replicating virus consumes much of the energy and many of the substances needed by cells for their own growth and maintenance. A well-adapted virus exists like smoldering embers, active enough to produce new virions but at levels low enough to avoid causing illness in the host; a poorly adapted virus burns like a skyrocket with explosive replication that kills the host. An example of a smoldering, well-adapted virus is varicella-zoster virus. In many people, it produces an acute chickenpox infection that is so mild it almost remains unnoticed. The virus then enters a long latent phase during which it ceases to produce new virions except under special circumstances when it flares up and causes shingles. The Ebola virus, on the other hand, can readily infect a human host and grow wildly out of control. It kills cells throughout the body, including those that line the blood vessels, and rapidly destroys its host.

In addition to HIV and related animal viruses, some herpesviruses also infect cells of the immune system. Epstein-Barr virus (EBV), for example, infects B lymphocytes and may influence the immune system by altering the production of cytokines, the chemical messengers needed for a well-functioning immune system.

Some viruses also contribute to the development of cancer. This happens when a virus disrupts the control of cell proliferation. Usually other conditions, known as cofactors, must also be present for viruses to cause cancer. Cancer-causing viruses include EBV, which is linked to certain types of lymphoma, and human papillomavirus (HPV), implicated in cervical cancer. In addition, a new herpesvirus, human herpesvirus type 8 (HHV-8), has been associated with Kaposi's sarcoma. HIV probably plays an indirect role in cancer development in patients with HIV disease (see Chapter 8).

■ RETROVIRUSES

HIV and other retroviruses are unique among viruses in that they carry two copies of their genome on separate single strands of RNA. Both these strands have positive sense, and both are used to produce the DNA copy of the genome that becomes incorporated into the host cell's genome as a provirus (see Chapter 18). The family of retroviruses contains the following subfamilies:

- Oncoviruses: the RNA tumor viruses. Examples include the human viruses HTLV-I, HTLV-II, the chicken Rous sarcoma virus, and the murine and feline leukemia viruses.

- Spumaviruses (also known as "foamy viruses" for the foamy-like appearance they give cultured monkey kidney cells). Examples include the human and simian foamy viruses, and the bovine and syncytial viruses.

- Lentiviruses. Examples include HIV-1, HIV-2, simian immunodeficiency virus (SIV), feline and bovine immunodeficiency viruses (FIV and BIV).

■ Lentiviruses

Lentiviruses such as HIV stand apart from other retroviruses in that they have more complex genomes. All retroviruses have three major genes that code for polyproteins. These are the *gag, pol,* and *env* genes. All retroviruses also have two regulatory genes in common, the *tat* and *rev* genes, which regulate virus replication. Lentiviruses, however, also have four so-called auxiliary genes: *nef, vif, vpu,* and *vpr.* The proteins produced by these genes are thought to influence the rate of viral replication and virulence. In HIV, the roles of *vif, vpu,* and *vpr* remain uncertain, and they are the object of ongoing research.

Chapter 18

THE HUMAN IMMUNODEFICIENCY VIRUS

The human immunodeficiency virus (HIV) is by now probably the most thoroughly studied virus in history. HIV was identified as the cause of AIDS in 1984, and soon after, as a lentivirus, one of three subfamilies of retroviruses (see Chapter 17). The discovery of HIV then enabled researchers to devise tests needed to detect HIV infection in people, protect the nation's blood supply, screen existing drugs for anti-HIV effectiveness, and, later, design drugs to treat HIV infection.

Today it is known that the AIDS virus exists as two separate types, HIV-1 and HIV-2. They are very similar in structure and genome, although HIV-2 appears to cause disease less frequently and after a longer period of time.

A single HIV particle, or virion, looks something like a rubber ball covered with suction cups. Toss the ball against a wall, and the suction cups cause it to stick there; bring HIV into contact with certain human cells, and it sticks to them—not by suction cups, but chemically, using knob-like structures that stud its surface. The knobs, made up of molecules known as gp120, are extremely important in HIV disease and vaccine research.

HIV is thousands of times smaller than the cells it infects. A single virion of HIV is about 100 nanometers (nm) in diameter, about the average size for a virus; a red blood cell, on the other hand, is about 7,000 nm in diameter. It would take 10,000 HIV particles to span a millimeter, and 250,000 to extend to an inch.

To imagine dissecting an HIV particle is to imagine stripping away the layers of an onion. The outside layer of HIV is the viral envelope, which is studded with the gp120 knobs (Figure 18.1). Peel back the envelope and uncover a second layer, the matrix. Peel back the matrix and find a tapered cylinder. This is the hollow core, or capsid, of HIV. Peel back the wall of the capsid, and the heart of the virus—its genetic material, in two strands of RNA—is exposed. The RNA carries the virus's genome, its small but powerful catalog of genetic instructions, nine genes in all. Also packed within the core are several protein molecules, the virus's own enzymes. They include reverse transcriptase, integrase, and protease, all essential to HIV's ability to reproduce itself after invading a cell.

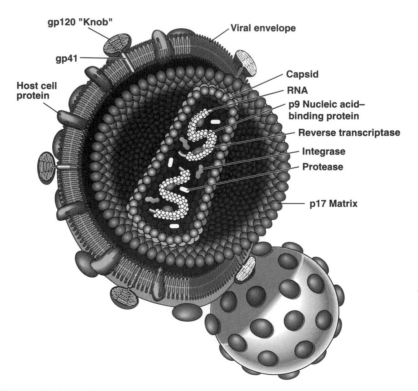

Figure 18.1. ■ *The structure of HIV-1.*

■ A CLOSER LOOK AT THE COMPONENTS OF HIV-1

■ The Viral Envelope

The outer layer—the viral envelope—of HIV consists of material resembling a cell membrane. The cell membrane is a double layer of lipid molecules, or fat, that can be easily damaged by drying, detergents, and disinfectants. The presence of this envelope makes HIV a rather fragile virus, unlike the polio virus or the virus that causes the common cold. Viruses such as the cold virus do not have such an envelope and can tolerate harsher environmental conditions (see Chapter 17).

■ gp120 Molecule

As mentioned already, the envelope of HIV is studded with knobs—72 in all. Each projects from the envelope like a flattened sphere on a short stem. The knobs consist of the gp120 molecule. The stem is composed of a second envelope glycoprotein, gp41.

The knobs enable HIV virions to attach to and enter certain cells—those, for example, that have the CD4 receptor and co-receptors on their surface (for more on cell-surface receptors, see Chapter 14). The CD4 receptor is found in greatest numbers on helper T cells and monocytes/macrophages, both of which are important immune-system cells (see Chapter 16).

It is interesting to note, however, that the link between gp120 and gp41 is fragile, and that the gp120 molecule is frequently lost from the virion. Since HIV cannot infect cells without gp120, this results in high numbers of noninfectious HIV virions in the body. It also results in non-infected CD4 cells carrying gp120 on their surface and being killed by misguided natural killer (NK) cells (see Chapter 16 for descriptions of NK cells).

The gp120 molecule is also important to HIV disease in another way. It is the molecule most readily recognized by the immune system. A number of antibodies react with different regions of the gp120 molecule. When antibodies attach to these sites, they can disable—neutralize—the virus by preventing gp120 from binding with the CD4 receptor. One of

the most important sites on the gp120 molecule for antibody neutral-
ization is an area known as the "third variable region," or V3 loop (this
region of the molecule changes so often as a result of genetic mutations
from one viral generation to the next that it is known as a "hypervariable
region"). The V3 loop plays an important role in the fusion of HIV's envelope with the cell membrane when the virus infects a cell (see "How
HIV Replicates"). Another important antibody-neutralization site on
gp120 is the area on the molecule that binds with the CD4 molecule on
lymphocytes (this site on the gp120 molecule is officially known as the
"CD4-binding domain").

■ Viral Matrix

The viral matrix lies just below the viral envelope and is needed to maintain the structure of the HIV virion; it also enables the DNA copy of the
viral genome to pass into the cell nucleus (also described later under
"How HIV Replicates"). It is made up of the p17 matrix (MA) protein.
The matrix protein is linked with the viral envelope through a fatty acid
that is added to the protein molecule shortly after it is produced in the
cell during viral replication. The fatty acid that is added to the protein is
myristic acid, and the process through which it is added is known as
"myristylation" (see also Chapter 15).

■ Capsid

The capsid, or central core of HIV, is made up primarily of an estimated 1,200 molecules of the p24 capsid (CA) protein. Inside the capsid are two identical strands of RNA. This is HIV's genetic material.
Each strand contains a complete set of viral genes; that is, each strand
represents an HIV genome. Bound to the RNA strands is the p9 nucleic
acid–binding protein (NC). As mentioned earlier, also found in the
capsid are molecules of the enzymes integrase, protease, and reverse
transcriptase.

Table 18.1. ■ *The Genes of HIV and the Function of Their Protein Products*

Gene	Designation of Protein according to Size (in kilodaltons)	Function of Protein
STRUCTURAL GENES		
env	gp120*	Surface glycoprotein (SU)— binds with CD4 receptor
	gp41*	Transmembrane glycoprotein (TM)— anchors p120 to envelope
gag	p24*	Capsid protein (CA)
	p17*	Matrix protein (MA)
	p9	Nucleic acid–binding protein (NC)
	p7	Proline-rich protein
pol	p66*	Reverse transcriptase (RT)
	p51*	RNase H—breaks down viral RNA after DNA copy is made
	p32	Integrase (IN) enzyme
	p10	Protease (PR) enzyme
REGULATORY GENES		
tat	p14	Transactivation factor— activates transcription
rev	p19	Regulates production of viral protein
nef	p27	Role uncertain; may be necessary for disease progression
vif	p23	Viral infectivity factor— role uncertain; may increase viral infectivity
vpu	p16	Viral protein U—necessary for virion budding from the cell
AUXILIARY GENES		
vpr	p15	Viral protein R—improves efficiency of replication
vpx	p15	Found only in HIV-2—increases viral infectivity

Proteins that result in antibodies detected by ELISA and Western blot tests and used in the diagnosis of HIV. Adapted from Levy JA. HIV and the Pathogenesis of AIDS. Washington, DC: ASM Press, 1994.

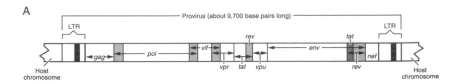

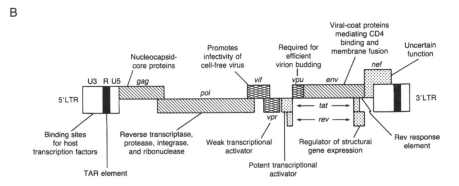

Figure 18.2 ■ *The genome of HIV.*

A. *A schematic showing how HIV's genes are organized in the provirus. Gray areas show where genes overlap.*

B. *The proviral genome as often diagrammed in scientific journals. Each rectangle represents a gene. Overlapping rectangles show areas of overlapping genes. Parts of the tat and rev genes are separated by portions of the vpu and env genes. When tat and rev are transcribed, the intervening genetic material is cut out and the necessary pieces are spliced together. This produces the mature messenger RNA (mRNA), which travels to the cytoplasm. There it is translated by ribosomes to produce the Tat and Rev proteins. (In some instances, tat and rev mRNAs are spliced to produce what is known as the Tev protein, which may help regulate tat and rev.)*

Long terminal repeat (LTR) regions are found at either end of the HIV genome. They are essential for integrating the provirus into a host chromosome, and they contain promoter and enhancer sites that are important for regulating viral protein production. When regulatory proteins, which can be produced by the cell or by the provirus, bind to the regulatory sites, they stimulate or inhibit protein synthesis by the provirus (see Chapter 19). (From Greene WC. Mechanisms of Disease: The Molecular Biology of Human Immunodeficiency Virus Type 1 Infection. Copyright 1991 Massachusetts Medical Society. All rights reserved. New England Journal of Medicine 1991;324:308.)

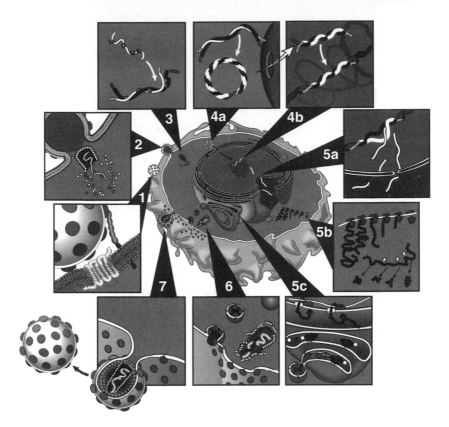

Figure 18.3. ■ *The replication cycle of HIV.*

1. Attachment: The HIV particle binds to the surface of cells bearing the CD4 molecule. A co-receptor CXCR-4 (see also Figure 14.1) is present in the membrane nearby.

2. Penetration and uncoating: With the help of one or more co-receptors (such as CXCR-4) on the cell surface, the viral envelope fuses with the cell membrane. The naked viral capsid now enters the cell cytoplasm.

3. Reverse transcription: The reverse transcriptase enzyme copies the RNA genome in the form of double-stranded DNA.

4. Integration: 4a. The DNA version of the HIV genome forms a circle and along with certain viral proteins, travels to the nucleus. 4b. There the viral enzyme integrase inserts it into a chromosome of the host cell. The DNA viral genome is now known as a provirus.

5. The activated provirus begins producing the components of new virions: 5a. Proviral genes are transcribed, and viral messenger RNAs (mRNAs) move from the nucleus to the cytoplasm. Long mRNAs form the genome of new virions. 5b. Shorter lengths are "read" by ribosomes for synthesis of viral proteins. 5c. Synthesis of viral envelope glycoprotein gp160 involves the rough endoplasmic reticulum and Golgi apparatus (see Chapter 14).

6. Assembly of new virus particles: Viral components—the proteins and copies of the RNA genome—collect below the cell membrane where they assemble themselves into complete capsids surrounded by the matrix. The envelope glycoprotein gp160 is transported to the cell membrane.

7. Release from the cell: As the new virions bud from the cell membrane, a bit of the cell membrane clings to them and becomes the viral envelope. During or shortly after budding, the viral protease enzyme cleaves the Pol polyprotein. The HIV particle is now a mature, free infectious virion.

■ THE GENOME OF HIV-1

While we can marvel at the amount of information stored by a personal computer, the amount of genetic information stored in the HIV genome is an equal wonder of compactness. Scientists have identified nine genes in HIV. From these nine genes, HIV produces its 16 proteins (Table 18.1). HIV can produce more proteins than it has genes because several genes serve double duty—the end portion of one gene will also serve as the beginning portion of another; or the beginning of one will serve as the end of another (Figure 18.2). This use of overlapping genes is not found in animal cells. The entire HIV genome consists of a little more than 9,700 nucleotides (the building blocks of DNA), making it 100,000 times smaller than the human genome. It is also likely that more products of HIV genes will eventually be discovered.

■ HOW HIV REPLICATES

Knowing how HIV replicates is important for understanding how HIV causes disease and how anti-HIV drugs work. There are two aspects of HIV's replication that are helpful to understand: first, the specific steps involved, which are described here and shown in Figure 18.3; second, how HIV replication is controlled, which is discussed in Chapter 19. (For an overview of viral replication in general, see Chapter 17.)

Attachment

Attachment of HIV occurs when the glycoprotein knobs that project from the viral envelope—the gp120 protein—bind with the CD4 molecule and the CCR-2, CXCR-4, or CCR-5 co-receptors on the surface of immune-system cells. The gp41 molecule, which anchors gp120 to the envelope, then plays an important role in promoting the fusion of the viral envelope with cell membranes.

CCR-2, CCR-5, and CXCR-4 (the latter is also known as fusin or LESTR/fusin) normally function as receptors for chemokines, which are a class of cytokines (described in Chapter 16); in terms of their interaction with HIV, these molecules are often referred to as co-receptors for HIV. A lack of these chemokine receptors on CD4 cells can also help keep

HIV out: Evidence indicates that people who inherit two mutated genes for the CCR-5 receptor (one mutated gene from the mother and one from the father) may be highly resistant to HIV infection; people who inherit only one mutated form of the receptor (either from the mother or the father) tend to be long-term nonprogressors (see Chapter 4).

Penetration and Uncoating

The outer layer of the virus—the viral envelope—fuses with the cell membrane, thereby plunging the HIV capsid into the cell cytoplasm. The capsid is partially removed; that is, the virion is uncoated, which exposes the viral RNA genome to the cell's cytoplasm, setting the stage for the next step.

Reverse Transcription

Reverse transcriptase, a viral enzyme carried in HIV's capsid, now comes into play. There are two identical strands of the RNA genome in each HIV virion. Reverse transcriptase uses both of these strands as a template to copy the RNA genome into the form of a double-stranded DNA molecule. Reverse transcriptase begins copying one of the RNA genome strands, then it copies a little of the second strand. It continues jumping back and forth this way as it assembles the DNA version. The construction is accomplished using nucleotide-building blocks commandeered from the host cell. A single-stranded DNA molecule—half of the DNA molecule lengthwise—is produced first; the second and matching DNA strand is assembled through complementary base pairing (see Chapter 15).

Before its job is done, reverse transcriptase also extends each end of the viral DNA molecule. These extensions become the long-terminal repeats (LTRs). The LTRs are important in two ways: They enable the viral DNA to be inserted into a chromosome in the host cell, which is a crucial step in retroviral infection, and they play a major role in regulating the production of viral proteins. When the DNA copy is finished, the enzyme RNase H, which is part of the reverse transcription enzyme, degrades the virus's original RNA genome.

A major class of anti-HIV drugs works by blocking the process of reverse transcription. These drugs, the reverse transcriptase inhibitors, include AZT, ddI, ddC, d4T, 3TC, delavirdine, loviride, and nevirapine (see Chapter 5).

Insertion

When the reverse transcription is completed, the viral DNA curls to form a circle that is almost closed; that is, the LTRs at each end of the viral DNA nearly touch. This circular viral DNA now migrates into the cell nucleus (it passes through pores in the nuclear membrane with the help of a chemical "signal" on the matrix protein). In the nucleus, the ends of the viral DNA—the LTRs—fuse with one of the 46 chromosomes in the host cell. The circular viral DNA now straightens and is incorporated into a host chromosome in a random location. This fusion of viral and host DNA occurs with the help of integrase, another viral enzyme carried in HIV's capsid. The viral genome is now a dsDNA provirus.

From now on, the provirus is a permanent part of the host chromosome. If the host cell divides, the proviral DNA is duplicated and passed to the two daughter cells, as is the cell's normal DNA. This permanent integration of the virus into host cells is a characteristic of retroviruses and makes it impossible, for the time being, to conceive of a treatment that would eliminate the virus from the body. For this to happen, all the infected cells themselves must be eliminated.

Production of Viral Proteins and Viral Genomes

The provirus can remain latent indefinitely in resting helper T cells. If the infected cell is activated, however, the genes in the provirus are activated as well. It takes command of the host cell's protein-producing machinery. This process weakens the cell by reducing its capacity to produce the proteins it needs for its own survival. The production of viral proteins occurs in a manner similar to that of cellular proteins: First, viral genes are copied—transcribed—as messenger RNA (mRNA). Second, the mRNA travels to the cell's cytoplasm where ribosomes bind to it. Third, ribosomes travel along the mRNA, reading its genetic instructions and translating them into viral proteins (see Chapter 15). However, the control of *viral* protein production is very different from the control of *cellular* protein production (see Chapter 19).

HIV produces three kinds of proteins: proteins that regulate the production of new virus particles (regulatory proteins), proteins that go into the structure of new virus particles (structural proteins, which include the three viral enzymes), and proteins that serve other functions (auxiliary proteins) (see Table 18.1).

Three genes in HIV—the *env, pol,* and *gag* genes—are responsible for the production of ten structural proteins. Each of these genes actually produces large polyproteins that are later chopped into a number of smaller separate proteins (for a description of how polyproteins are produced, see Chapter 15):

- The *env* gene produces a polyprotein—the gp160 molecule—that is cleaved by a cellular protease enzyme to form the gp120 and the gp41 molecules. (The glycoproteins gp120 and gp41 form the knobs that project from HIV's envelope.)

- The *gag* gene produces a polyprotein that is cleaved by the viral protease to produce four mature proteins: the capsid protein (CA, forms the "case" that surrounds viral genomic RNA and the viral enzymes), the matrix protein (MA, important for structural stability of the virion), the nucleic acid–binding protein (NC, important for packaging RNA inside the capsid), and the proline-rich protein (important for virion assembly and release).

- The *pol* gene produces a polyprotein that is cleaved by the HIV protease to produce the enzymes reverse transcriptase, RNase H, integrase, and protease.

To end up in the viral envelope, the gp120 and gp41 molecules first become part of the host cell's membrane. For this to happen, the mRNA produced from the envelope gene *(env)* follows a path through the cell that is different from that of other HIV proteins. The path is the same as that followed by cellular secretory proteins. While the mRNAs for most HIV proteins are read by ribosomes that are free in the cytoplasm, the mRNA for the envelope gene is read by ribosomes that are part of the rough endoplasmic reticulum (RER), a series of channels that wind through the cell (see Chapter 14).

As the new gp160 polyprotein leaves the ribosomes of the RER, it is anchored in the membrane that forms the walls of the RER. The molecule moves from the RER and into the Golgi complex. The Golgi complex is the cellular organelle that packages materials produced by the cell into vesicles.

As the gp160 moves through this process, it is folded and sugars are added to it, thereby converting it to a glycoprotein. This process of adding sugar to a protein is known as "glycosylation." Along the way, the gp160 is cleaved by a protease enzyme belonging to the cell (i.e., a cellular protease). This produces the gp120 and gp41 molecules. The two subunits now take on the form of HIV's knobs, with the gp41 molecule implanted in the wall of the Golgi complex. Next, they bud from the Golgi complex as vesicles that move to the cell membrane (Figure 18.3, 5c). The vesicles then fuse with cell membrane, placing the anchored knobs on the outside of the cell, ready to become part of the envelope of budding virions.

Copies of the viral genome are produced when an accumulation of the Rev protein, a regulatory protein, triggers the transcription of the whole length of proviral DNA to form long mRNAs. These single-stranded RNAs then become the genomes of progeny virions (see also Chapter 19).

Assembly of New Virus Particles

All other viral proteins produced during viral replication accumulate in the cell's cytoplasm. There, the *gag* gene proteins assemble themselves into new capsids. As each capsid forms, it encapsulates the RNA genome, as well as the large polyprotein produced by the *pol* gene. The process of formation of the capsid and the materials it contains is known as "encapsidation." Also during assembly, matrix proteins unite to enclose the capsid.

Release from the Cell

As the new virions pinch off, or bud, from the cell, they take a bit of the cell's lipid-bilayer membrane with them. This fragment becomes the outer envelope of the retrovirus. It includes the knobs produced by the envelope gene, and a few proteins that belong to the cell membrane itself (these are not made use of by the virus).

Maturing of the Virions

Inside the capsid, either during or shortly after budding, HIV's protease enzyme cleaves the long Pol polyprotein. This step produces the working copies of the reverse transcriptase, integrase, and protease enzymes, and makes the HIV particle fully capable of infecting other cells and starting a new replication cycle.

The production of new virions by a provirus takes from 8 to 12 hours, and each provirus can produce thousands of progeny.

For a description of how HIV replication is regulated at the gene level, see Chapter 19.

■ HIV IS A HIGHLY CHANGEABLE VIRUS

At one time, people played a game called telephone in which someone whispered a story to one person, that person told it to the next, and so on through a circle of people. By the time the story reached the last person, it usually proved strikingly different from the way it began. So it is with HIV in an infected person: The virus has an extraordinary tendency to change genetically—to mutate—during the period of infection. This tendency is known as "genetic variability" or "genetic drift."

The mutations in HIV are believed to arise largely because the enzyme reverse transcriptase is prone to making errors as it makes the DNA copy of the virus's RNA genome. These errors usually occur when reverse transcriptase uses a wrong base during construction of the DNA copy. The rate of these errors—these mutations—by reverse transcriptase is estimated to be 1 wrong DNA base for each 1,000 to 10,000 bases added. Since HIV's genome contains some 9,700 DNA bases, that means almost every HIV particle produced is likely to have from one to ten genetic mutations.

Genetic variation can also arise in HIV if virions from two genetically different virus strains infect a cell simultaneously, as could happen if a person is infected by two different sexual partners. The reverse transcriptase from one of these strains might then use an RNA strand from each of the two genomes to construct its DNA molecule. The resulting "hybrid" provirus will be a combination of the genomes of the two HIV strains. Such mixing of genes is known as "genetic recombination."

HIV's high mutation rate, together with the high rate of virion production during HIV infection, results in a mix of genetically different virions in any one individual with HIV disease. Genetic variation in HIV helps explain why genetically and biologically different forms of HIV can be isolated not only from two HIV-infected persons but also, over time, from the same person. Genetic variability has several implications:

■ It explains why viral resistance to drugs readily arises in patients treated with AZT or other antiretroviral drug given as monotherapy: Of the mix of genetically different virus strains in a patient, by chance some will be more resistant to the drug. When a patient begins taking a drug, the majority of virus particles will be killed by it, leaving only those that are resistant. The resistant strains then come to predominate in the patient, and the treatment becomes ineffective.

■ It might explain in part why HIV infects certain cells more readily than others. For example, HIV isolated from brain cells has an easier time infecting macrophages but it cannot infect intestinal cells. The tendency for a virus strain to prefer some types of cells over others is called "cell tropism." Some isolates of HIV, for example, are much more efficient at infecting macrophages than are others. (New research also suggests that the phenomenon of cell tropism may also be due, in part or principally, to the particular mix of cell-membrane co-receptors needed by different HIV strains to enter a particular type of cell.)

■ It can affect HIV's relative ability not only to replicate, but also to induce helper T lymphocytes to fuse and to form syncytia, and kill cells. This might help explain why HIV disease can progress differently in different people. For example, a switch from non-syncytium- to syncytium-inducing viral strains appears to correlate with faster progression to advanced disease. Syncytium-inducing viral strains replicate more rapidly and kill cells more readily than do non-syncytium-inducing strains (see also Chapter 4).

■ Types and Subtypes of HIV

Over the course of the epidemic of HIV/AIDS, enough genetic mutations in HIV have accumulated that distinct HIV classes or subtypes have arisen. So far, scientists recognize 11 distinct subtypes—also known as "clades" or "genotypes"—of HIV-1. They also have identified subtypes of HIV-2. Subtypes are distinguished by differences in DNA base sequences for the envelope protein gp120 and for the Gag protein. Amino-acid sequences in the gp120 molecule differ by 20% to 40% between subtypes and those in the Gag protein differ by 15%. Within each subtype, *env* sequences can differ by 10%; *gag* sequences can differ by up to 8%.

HIV-1 subtypes are designated by the letters of the alphabet. Subtypes A to J and O have been described so far, and more are likely to be added in the future. Subtypes A through J constitute the major subtypes of HIV, and these have been gathered into one major group, group M (for major). Viruses with sequences that do not fit into one of the A to J subtypes are placed in group O (for outliers or out group). All HIV-1 subtypes have been identified in Africa and Sweden. Specific countries and regions in which they predominate are listed in Table 18.2.

Table 18.2. ■ *Predominant HIV Subtypes in Various Countries and Regions*

HIV Subtype	Region or Country of Predominance
Group M	
A	Central and East Africa
B	Americas, Europe, Thailand, Japan
C	Southern Africa, India
D	Central, East, and South Africa
E	Thailand, Japan, India
F	Romania, Brazil, Zaire
G	West Africa
H	West Africa, Taiwan
I	Cyprus
J	Zaire
Group O	Unusual or recently identified subtypes that do not fit into the categories in group M

The study and tracking of subtypes is important because subtypes may respond differently to a given anti-HIV treatment. Moreover, they might not all be detected by present diagnostic tests. This is particularly true for subtypes in group O. Antibodies to these viruses can be missed in blood when one is using the presently available screening and confirmatory tests, which are based primarily on the strains of subtype B found in North America and Europe. The subtyping of HIV can be important as well for tracking the spread of HIV from various regions of the world and from one individual to another.

■ HIV-2

In early 1986 a form of HIV that differed substantially in its genetic makeup from other HIV viral strains was isolated during a study of Senegalese sex workers. More than half—55%—of the DNA base sequences in its proviral genome were different from those of HIV-1. Furthermore, most antibodies that reacted with the more familiar form of HIV did not react with the new virus. That is, the new virus presented the immune system with a new set of antigens. This meant that a different test would be needed to detect antibodies to the new virus in patients and in the blood supply (see Chapter 2). Scientists designated this virus as a new type of HIV, and named it HIV-2.

Interestingly, antibodies to HIV-2 envelope proteins also react, or cross-react, with envelope proteins from some strains of the simian immunodeficiency virus (SIV). For this reason, some scientists believe HIV-2 evolved from a strain of SIV (see "The Origin of HIV").

HIV-2 also differs from HIV-1 in its distribution and in the disease it causes. HIV-2 is found primarily in West Africa: Senegal, Gambia, Ivory Coast, and Cape Verde Islands. In fact, evidence of HIV-2 infection in West Africa goes back to the early 1960s. Recently, its spread through India has raised major concern for its control.

HIV-2 produces an immunodeficiency that is ultimately similar to advanced HIV disease (AIDS), but people infected with HIV-2 often maintain higher levels of CD4 cells for a longer period and so have a longer disease-free period. For example, a study of Senegalese sex workers followed a group of women infected with HIV-2 and a group infected with HIV-1.[1] The study found that women infected with HIV-1 had only a 67% chance of not developing advanced disease (AIDS) after five years; women infected with HIV-2 had a 100% probability of being AIDS free after five years.

Other evidence suggests that HIV-2 is much less infectious than HIV-1 per sexual act. It is also estimated to be less likely to be transmitted perinatally than HIV-1. For all these reasons, HIV-2 is considered less virulent than HIV-1. This difference in virulence could be due to a lower rate of replication of HIV-2, resulting in a lesser concentration of virions in blood and genital fluids.

Another study of Senegalese sex workers found, through a risk-assessment analysis, that women infected with HIV-2 had a nearly 70% lowered risk of infection with HIV-1.[2] This does not mean that people should try to get infected with HIV-2 to fend off HIV-1, but it does suggest that with help—that is, if first confronted by a less virulent but antigenically related virus—the immune system can fend off HIV-1 infection. This lends support to the notion that it should be possible to develop an anti-HIV vaccine.

■ THE ORIGIN OF HIV

The illness caused by HIV, AIDS, is unprecedented. Never before has medical science confronted a virus that destroyed the very cells that coordinate the body's immune defenses against infection and cancer. Scientists still can only speculate about the origin of HIV, but generally a new infectious agent in humans has one of three origins:

- It could be a virus that previously existed harmlessly in people, and then mutated to become harmful.

- It could be a virus that existed in an isolated population of humans, which may or may not have been resistant to it, and then broke out into the general population.

- It could be a virus that was present in animals and became transmissible to humans through a series of mutations.

Many scientists believe the third possibility now best explains the origin of HIV. They suggest that HIV-2 evolved from a strain of SIV that occurs harmlessly in an African monkey, the sooty mangabey (SIVmm). When rhesus monkeys, which are Asian, are infected with SIVmm, they develop an AIDS-like disease. Several lines of evidence suggest a link between SIV and HIV-2. For example, SIVmm is genetically very similar to HIV-2, much more so than to HIV-1. Antibodies to HIV-2 envelope proteins react with envelope proteins from several strains of SIV. Furthermore, a laboratory worker who accidentally became infected in 1994 with a strain of SIV from macaques (SIVmac) has not yet developed signs of disease but did develop antibodies to several SIV proteins, which is an indication of true infection. Last, a strain of HIV-2 that was nearly identical to SIVmm was detected in a person in Liberia.

The origin of HIV-1 is an even deeper mystery. It is known that chimpanzees harbor a strain of SIV, SIVcpz, that is closely related to HIV-1. According to the animal-infection scenario, a remote and isolated tribe of Africans who hunted, trapped, or ate chimpanzees could have become infected through their hunting or eating activities by a strain of SIVcpz that had become genetically capable of infecting humans. Expansion of African cities in the 1950s, which attracted people from remote parts of the country, could have introduced the virus to larger population centers. By the 1970s, the virus was transmitted to travelers in those cities, who carried it to other parts of the world, where it subsequently became known as HIV-1.

The origin of SIVcpz in chimpanzees is open to question, however. To date, SIVcpz has been found in only three African chimpanzees, and it remains unknown whether the virus is widespread in wild chimpanzee populations.

Researchers are looking for other retroviruses that infect nonhuman primates in the hope that additional HIV-1 progenitor viruses will be found. Such viruses could provide the clues needed to better explain the origin of HIV-1.

ENDNOTES

1. Marlink R, et al. Reduced rate of disease development after HIV-2 infection as compared to HIV-1. *Science* 1994;265:1587–1590.

2. Travers K, et al. Natural protection against HIV-1 infection provided by HIV-2. *Science* 1995;268:1612–1615.

Chapter 19

GENES AND GENE REGULATION IN HIV

Each of the 46 chromosomes in a human cell consists of a long helical molecule of double-stranded DNA that is covered by a variety of proteins. All 46 DNA molecules are highly condensed, tightly curling over themselves, which enables them to fit inside the cell nucleus. The proteins covering the DNA molecule serve several functions. Some help maintain DNA's complex, coiled structure, while others are involved in turning genes on and off.

A stretched-out molecule of DNA consists of a long series of individual genes. It might contain several thousand contiguous genes. Genes come in different lengths. A short gene might be 5,000 base pairs long; a large gene can be as long as 100,000 base pairs. (For a description of bases and base pairing, see Chapter 15.)

■ GENES SERVE TWO PURPOSES IN LIFE

The entire complement of human genes is present in all nucleated human cells.

- In germ cells—eggs and sperm—genes pass parental characteristics to offspring.

- In the cells of the body—the somatic cells—genes "express" the information for making proteins needed by the cell and the organism as a whole. Scientists often use the words "gene product" as a generic name for protein because the product of a gene's expression is a protein.

■ HOW GENES ARE ORGANIZED

Genes have two main segments: a structural segment and a regulatory segment (Figure 19.1). The structural segment contains the information that describes the structure of a protein. That is, the sequence of base pairs in the structural segment of the gene spells out, in the language of the genetic code, the sequence of amino acids that make up a protein or part of a protein. The structural region of a gene in turn is divided into exons and introns. Exons are DNA sequences that contain the actual information needed to build the protein. Introns are lengths of genetic information that are not needed for the structure of the protein. In some genes, introns play a role in gene regulation, but in most, their function is unknown. Introns are transcribed as messenger RNA (mRNA) during transcription, but the intron segments are cut out of the mRNA before it leaves the cell nucleus (see Chapter 15).

A gene's regulatory region controls whether the gene is turned on, or activated, and to what degree it is to be active. An activated gene is ready to be transcribed into mRNA (see also Chapter 15).

The regulatory region of a gene has two segments, a promoter and an enhancer. The promoter is the primary on-off switch for a gene. A gene is activated when certain small regulatory proteins bind to the promoter. The promoter is also the point at which mRNA begins forming at the start of gene transcription; that is, it is the transcription start site.

The enhancer also plays an important role in gene activation and transcription. The binding of regulatory proteins to the enhancer improves the efficiency of the process of transcription.

The regulatory proteins that bind to the promoter and enhancers are known by several names, including DNA-binding proteins, activation proteins, and transactivation proteins.

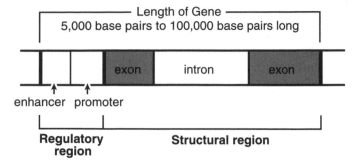

Figure 19.1. ■ *A simplified diagram of a gene from an animal cell. The regulatory region contains enhancer and promoter segments. The promoter is a gene's on-off switch; the enhancer determines how efficiently the gene is transcribed. The structural region is divided into exons and introns (see Chapter 15), the length and number of which vary with the gene.*

■ GENE REGULATION AND CONTROL OF PROTEIN PRODUCTION IN HIV-1

The regulation of HIV genes is similar in certain respects to the regulation of cellular genes. As in cellular genes, the promoter and enhancer play an important role in viral gene activation and rate of transcription. An important difference is that whereas cellular genes usually each have their own promoter and enhancer regions, the HIV proviral DNA has promoter and enhancer regions that trigger the activation and transcription of the entire HIV-1 genome. When the provirus is activated, it begins producing new virus particles through the production of viral proteins and copies of the whole viral genome (see Chapter 18).

Activation of the provirus is triggered by DNA-binding proteins that are produced *by the cell.* These cellular regulatory proteins bind to promoter and enhancer elements in the provirus, triggering the transcription of all viral genes. DNA-binding proteins produced by other viruses infecting the same cell can also activate the HIV provirus.

Here is an overview of how scientists think the production of new virus particles is controlled:

1. First of all, the HIV-infected resting helper T cell must be activated to multiply for new virions to be produced. As long as the infected T

cell is resting, the provirus remains inactive—latent. However, activation of the infected cell also activates the provirus. T-cell activation occurs through contact with an antigen-presenting cell or in response to cytokines such as interleukin-1 (IL-1) or tumor necrosis factor (TNF). (These and other cytokines are released by a variety of other cells.) A helper T cell can also be activated by another infecting virus, including HTLV-I, herpes simplex virus, Epstein-Barr virus, cytomegalovirus, human herpesvirus 6, and hepatitis B virus. For this reason, cells coinfected with one of these viruses and with HIV can display increased HIV replication. (Also for this reason, HIV-infected people must protect themselves to any extent possible from infection with other viruses.)

2. Antigen-presenting cells, cytokines, and other viruses activate the helper T cell by triggering the production of DNA-binding proteins by the cell. One important example of such a cellular DNA-binding protein is nuclear factor kappa B, or NF-κB. NF-κB helps regulate the production of proteins needed by the activated T cell for cell growth, cell division, and the production of cytokines. Protein synthesis by the cell begins when regulatory proteins such as NF-κB bind with promoters and enhancers on cellular genes.

3. NF-κB, it turns out, also binds with the promoter of the provirus. The promoter and enhancer regions of the HIV proviral DNA are located in the long terminal repeat (LTR) segments at each end of the proviral genome (see Figure 18.2). When NF-κB or other cellular activation proteins bind with proviral promoter and enhancer, they activate the provirus. The proviral genes now undergo transcription—that is, they are now copied as mRNA. At this point, transcription still occurs at a very low level.

4. All the genes are transcribed, but most of the resulting mRNAs remain in the nucleus. The only mRNAs that travel to the cytoplasm are those for three regulatory proteins encoded by the provirus. These HIV regulatory proteins—Tat, Rev, and Nef—are the first proteins to be produced by viral genes. These viral regulatory proteins will determine how fast or slowly all other viral proteins—and, therefore, new virions—will be produced.

5. The Tat protein binds to a site known as the Tat-responsive element, or TAR, present on all mRNAs produced by the provirus. When high levels

of Tat are present in the infected cell, it can increase the rate of transcription of all HIV genes up to 1,000-fold—including that of the *tat* gene itself. For this reason, high levels of Tat result in high levels of virus production.

6. The Rev protein, upon reaching a certain amount in the cell, activates the transcription of structural viral proteins, and the production of mRNAs that extend the length of the entire HIV genome. These become the single-stranded RNA genomes of the progeny virions. These long mRNAs actually do double duty because when they reach the cytoplasm, they are translated to produce the Gag and Pol polyproteins. The Rev protein also chemically stabilizes these long "genome" mRNAs and other long viral mRNAs. It does this by attaching to a special binding site—the Rev-responsive element (RRE)—which is present on all mRNAs produced by the provirus (except for the mRNAs for the Tat, Rev, and Nef proteins). When Rev reaches a certain concentration in the cell nucleus, it attaches to the RRE on the mRNAs produced by the provirus and is held there. This enables these mRNAs to then move to the cytoplasm where they are translated into viral proteins.

7. The Nef protein is the third important HIV regulatory protein. Its role in HIV replication is not clearly defined. In the simian immunodeficiency virus, Nef appears to be important to the development of simian AIDS.

■ *Chapter 20*

THE EMERGENCE AND EARLY YEARS
OF THE HIV/AIDS EPIDEMIC*

Between October 1980 and May 1981, five young gay men in Los Angeles were treated for *Pneumocystis carinii* pneumonia, or PCP. Until then, PCP had occurred almost exclusively—and only rarely—in elderly people, transplant recipients, cancer patients, or others who had needed treatment with powerfully immunosuppressive drugs. The five gay men had, in addition to PCP, other diseases characteristic of immune deficiency. Yet, they were young—aged 29 to 36—and had no history of immune impairment.

Physicians are expected to report cases of unusual health problems to the Centers for Disease Control and Prevention (CDC) in Atlanta, Georgia. The CDC issues the *Morbidity and Mortality Weekly Report (MMWR),* a weekly publication that regularly updates physicians and public-health officials on disease outbreaks and other causes of illness and death, nationally. The five puzzling cases of PCP were reported in the *MMWR* issue of June 4, 1981.

A month later, *MMWR* reported 26 cases of Kaposi's sarcoma (KS) in young homosexual men in New York and California. KS is a rare form of

* *This chapter was coauthored with Mathilde Krim, Ph.D.*

cancer in the United States; in 1981, its incidence was estimated to have been two to six cases per 10 million people per year. It had usually occurred in elderly men, although it had been seen in people who had been recipients of organ transplants and in other patients with profoundly suppressed immune systems. However, the gay males who were the subject of the second report had an average age of 39 and no history of immune suppression. In addition to KS, many of them also had PCP and candidiasis, and one had cryptococcal meningitis and severe, recurrent herpes simplex infection. Eight of the gay men with KS died within 24 months of their KS diagnosis. This second report also mentioned that ten additional cases of PCP had been identified, four in Los Angeles and six in San Francisco.

To try to make sense of what they were seeing, officials at the U.S. Public Health Service and at the CDC looked at what all these patients had in common: Most were gay men, and many had various unusual infections generally associated with severe immune suppression. (These infections are called "opportunistic" because they cause disease only when a weak immune defense system gives them an opportunity to do so.)

The occurrence of this high number of KS cases during a 30-month period was unprecedented. The report concluded that although it was not certain that the increase in KS, PCP, and immune deficiency was restricted to homosexual men, the vast majority of cases had been reported in this population. As a result, the media began referring to the condition as "Gay-Related Immunodeficiency Disease," or GRID; others called it "gay cancer." The CDC, however, referred to the syndrome initially and more carefully as "Kaposi's sarcoma and opportunistic infections in previously healthy persons."

By the end of August 1981, the CDC had received 107 reports of KS, PCP, or both in 95 gay men, 6 heterosexual males, 5 men whose sexual orientation was not known, and 1 woman. Autopsies on some of those who had died revealed that most of their organs had been damaged by bacterial, viral, and fungal opportunistic infections. The microbes identified were not of a kind that usually poses a threat to people in reasonably good health. All indications pointed to a disastrous underlying collapse of the immune system in the deceased. But what could have caused it?

Speculation ran wild: perhaps a new and highly virulent strain of cytomegalovirus (CMV), or hepatitis virus, or Epstein-Barr virus (a virus of the herpes family); a combination thereof; the use, in parts of the gay community, of sexual stimulants, or "poppers"; or a burnout of the immune system due to an "overload" of sexually transmitted diseases that were common in the gay community. Two of the suggestions—the use of "poppers" and burnout theories—soon became unlikely because the new syndrome began showing up in people who were not users of "poppers" but injection drug users, and in women who were not drug users but who had been sexual partners of drug users. By early 1982, 159 cases of the new syndrome had been reported from 15 states, the District of Columbia, and two foreign countries.

"Many of the doctors who were seeing patients with what became known as AIDS were also seeing people with persistently swollen lymph nodes and other unusual conditions," said James Curran, now Dean of the School of Public Health at Emory University, but who at that time headed the Task Force on Kaposi's Sarcoma and Opportunistic Infections at the CDC. "These were often doctors who were seeing gay men, and, eventually, doctors seeing people with hemophilia, and they felt that maybe this was part of the same epidemic." The reports of persistently swollen lymph nodes, a condition known as "generalized lymphadenopathy," were also coming from several cities. The patients had an average age of 33, and most experienced other general symptoms as well, including fatigue, fever, night sweats, and weight loss. One of the patients with lymphadenopathy also developed KS.

The clinical significance of the lymphadenopathy, and whether it was related to the KS and opportunistic infections occurring in gay men, was uncertain. But suspicions ran strong that it was indeed related because the condition seemed to occur in gay men of the same age and cities of residence as the men who were developing KS and PCP.

"We were very confused in the early 1980s by reports of people who had only enlarged lymph nodes or an enlarged spleen, sometimes with a fever; sometimes with no fever," said Mathilde Krim, cofounder of AmFAR. "It took quite a while to learn that all these people represented different stages of the same disease. We didn't know yet that people with mild symptoms were all going to progress to the serious fatal syndrome."

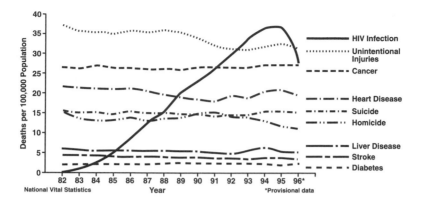

Figure 20.1. ■ *Death rates from leading causes of death in persons aged 25 to 44 years, United States, 1982–96. The rapid rise in deaths due to AIDS is clearly evident. (Data from the Centers for Disease Control and Prevention.)*

Then in June 1982, a cluster of 19 cases of KS or PCP in a group of 15 homosexual men in California and other states were studied by the CDC and linked by sexual contact. This strongly suggested that an infectious agent not yet identified as the cause of the immunodeficiency was at the root of the cases of both KS and PCP.

By May 1982, the CDC had received reports of 355 cases of KS, PCP, or other opportunistic infections in previously healthy persons between the ages of 15 and 60 years. Nearly 80% of the cases had occurred in homosexual or bisexual men; the remainder were diagnosed in injection drug users and heterosexual women. The death rate from AIDS was beginning its 15-year-long climb (Figure 20.1) and its rapid spread across the United States (Figure 20.2).

A number of practicing physicians and researchers had been closely following the events reported by the CDC in the unraveling of the medical mystery. Several of them were trying to help accumulate case study reports, that is, detailed descriptions of individual cases and their follow-up. In addition, they were managing disease symptoms in their patients as best they could. Some started calling for sexual abstinence or the use of condoms, advice that was often neither well received nor heeded. Except for people in the gay community, however, few others paid any attention at all. It was not until May 11, 1982, that the *New York Times* carried its first article on the "gay cancer." The gay communities of New York and San Francisco were profoundly alarmed because a stigma was already being attached to AIDS. Besides, while a cumulative total of a few hundred cases could appear as a "rare disease" of little public-health significance to society at large, it was already a catastrophe to groups of men who were hearing of or seeing with increasing frequency friends falling prey to or dying of the "gay cancer."

The mystery broadened further in July 1982 when 34 cases of opportunistic infections and KS were reported among Haitian immigrants in five states. Laboratory tests had revealed dysfunction of their immune systems and a marked decrease in the patients' number of helper T lymphocytes. The pattern of opportunistic infections, KS, immune suppression, and the high mortality rate—about half of these individuals had died—was similar to that reported in homosexual males and injection drug users, but none of the 23 Haitians questioned acknowledged homosexual activity, and only 1 Haitian out of the 26 who had been extensively questioned reported injection drug use. It was also learned that 11 cases of KS had been diagnosed in Port-au-Prince, Haiti, during the past two and a half years. When the media subsequently reported the designation of all Haitian immigrants as one more "risk group" for acquired immunodeficiency, it had dire consequences for that community: Thousands of Haitians in the United States were to suffer great hardships, the loss of jobs, suspicion, and insults, as well as seeing their children taunted in schools.

News of the disease took another ominous turn that July when three hemophiliacs developed PCP, weight loss, and a depletion of their helper T cells. The three men were unrelated in any way and were neither gay nor injection drug users, but they had all received clotting factor concentrates as treatment for their bleeding disorder. (Infusions of clotting factor concentrates to prevent uncontrolled bleeding are needed from several to over 100 times per year by people with severe hemophilia. The concentrates are made by pooling clotting factors extracted from the plasma of thousands of blood donors.) The sick hemophiliacs represented the first suggestive evidence that the syndrome could be spread by blood products and, hence, blood itself. This conclusion had frightening implications for hemophiliacs and for anyone requiring transfused blood.

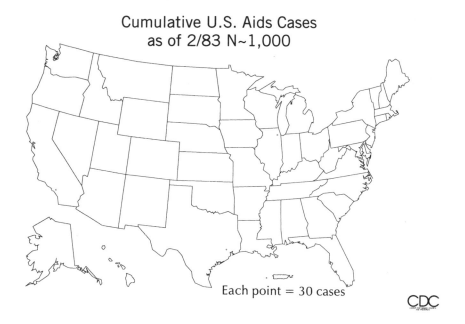

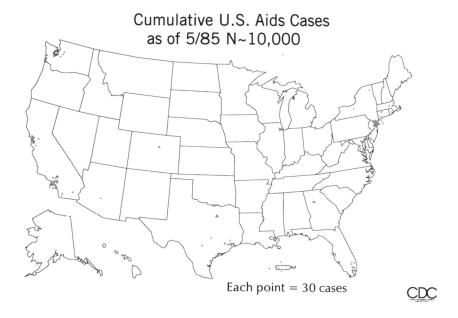

Figure 20.2. The spread of AIDS across the United States, 1983–97. (Data from the Centers for Disease Control and Prevention.)

U.S. AIDS Cases Reported through December 1988
30 Cases per Dot

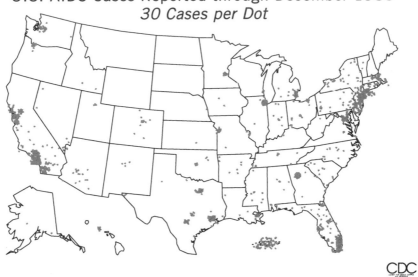

CDC

U.S. AIDS Cases Reported through December 1991
30 Cases per Dot

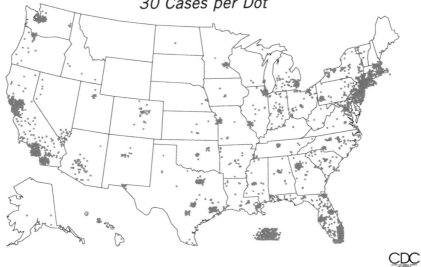

CDC

U.S. AIDS Cases Reported through December 1994
30 Cases per Dot

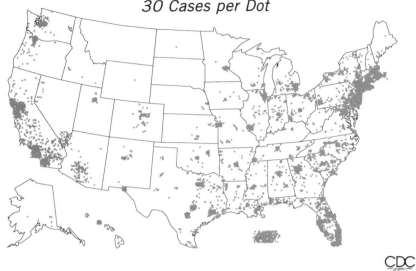

CDC

U.S. AIDS Cases Reported through September 1997
30 Cases per Dot

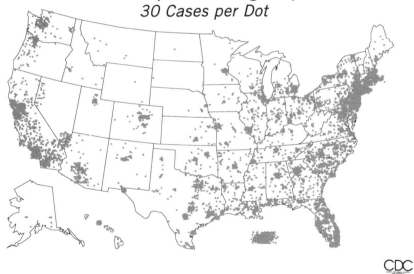

CDC

In late September 1982, the *MMWR* used for the first time the term "acquired immune deficiency syndrome," and its acronym, AIDS, to refer to the new condition, noting that 593 cases had been reported by then. It also provided details on the "case definition of AIDS." A "surveillance case definition" describes the signs and symptoms of a reportable disease so that physicians can accurately identify and report cases of such a disease to their public-health department, which in turn reports them to the CDC. These reports allow the CDC to establish "epidemic surveillance," that is, an effective way to monitor an epidemic and its growth, as well as geographic spread. The information collected is important to public-health policy making, and the case definition is of value for the accurate classification of patients in hospital disease-coding and recording systems.

The 1982 case definition of AIDS included the presence of an underlying immune deficiency in persons for whom there is no known cause for it, and certain diseases such as KS, PCP, toxoplasmosis, candidiasis, and several other opportunistic infections that became "AIDS-defining conditions."

In early December 1982, the *MMWR* reported that a 20-month-old infant developed an unexplained immune deficiency and opportunistic infections. The parents had none of the typical risk factors for AIDS, and the infant had had no personal contact with an AIDS patient. A month after birth, however, the infant had needed a blood transfusion, and one of the 19 donors of the blood used in that transfusion subsequently developed AIDS. It was the first report of AIDS transmission by blood transfusion, and this, together with reports of AIDS in people with hemophilia, raised serious concerns about the safety of donated blood and the products made from it.

December 1982 also brought four more cases of AIDS in people with hemophilia and, for the first time, four in infants, as well as the identification of 18 immunodeficient children who were being followed. "None of the four infants . . . was known to have received blood or blood products before onset of illness," the *MMWR* report noted. This suggested that the causative agent could be transferred from a pregnant woman to her infant.

In January 1983, a connection emerged between AIDS and persistent, generalized lymphadenopathy. Early that month, it was reported that two women with generalized lymphadenopathy and immune deficiency, who had been sexual partners of males with AIDS, had developed AIDS themselves. These cases strengthened the notion that AIDS was caused by an infectious agent that could be transmitted not only through blood and from mother to infant, but also through sexual intercourse. By this time, 43 females with AIDS had been reported to the CDC since June 1981.

By March 1983, the CDC had reported 1,200 cases of AIDS in the United States. It still described AIDS in cautious terms, terms that were, however, remarkably accurate: None of the statements made then by the CDC proved incorrect later, and none of its recommendations were unwarranted. These terms are summarized here:

■ Several groups of people were at high risk for developing AIDS, including homosexual men with multiple sex partners, injection drug users, and Haitians, although, the CDC noted, there were probably many individuals within these groups who were at low risk of acquiring the disease.

■ Cases of AIDS had also been diagnosed among hemophiliacs.

■ The agent responsible for the immune dysfunction in people with AIDS could be transmitted by homosexual *and* heterosexual sex, by the sharing of contaminated needles and syringes, by contaminated blood and blood products, and by pregnant women to their infants.

■ No AIDS cases had been reported in health-care workers caring for AIDS patients.

The pool of individuals capable of transmitting the agent was probably considerably larger than the number of known AIDS cases. Some gay men and hemophiliacs who did not fit the case definition for AIDS nevertheless showed nonspecific symptoms and poor immune function. This indicated that identifying individuals at risk of transmitting AIDS would be difficult until the agent responsible for AIDS was identified and a test was available to detect it.

A period of at least several months to two years after exposure to the still unidentified infectious agent seemed necessary before recognizable symptoms appeared. This raised the warning that AIDS could be transmitted by people before obvious signs of disease appeared in them.

The CDC's March 1983 report also included general guidelines for the prevention of AIDS. They were developed by the U.S. Public Health Service, with similar suggestions promulgated by the National Gay Task Force, the National Hemophilia Foundation, the American Red Cross, the American Association of Blood Banks, the Council of Community Blood Centers, and the American Association of Physicians for Human Rights. The guidelines recommended avoiding sexual contact with a person who is known or suspected of having AIDS, noting also that having multiple partners increases the risk of acquiring AIDS. The guidelines also recommended that members of groups at high risk for AIDS refrain from donating blood or plasma. In addition, the CDC's 1983 report called for studies to evaluate screening procedures used to identify and exclude blood donors who had a high probability of transmitting AIDS, since fear was justifiably growing that the nation's blood supply was contaminated with the agent responsible for AIDS.

Therefore, by early 1983 there was evidence that AIDS was caused by a presumably novel blood-borne infectious agent transmissible through blood and blood products, perinatally, and through homosexual and heterosexual sexual contact—but *not* to health-care personnel who had daily, unprotected contacts with people with AIDS. Nonetheless, there was silence and inaction on the part of the political, spiritual, and even public-health leadership of this country regarding the potential risk to all.

As a result, much of the American public reacted irrationally to press reports about AIDS with either panic or, more often, self-righteous indifference. Police in San Francisco and elsewhere demanded special masks and gloves for the handling of "potentially dangerous citizens"; in New York and Los Angeles, people feared sharing laundry facilities with gay men, or feared catching AIDS from eating salad in restaurants or touching subway railings and public toilet seats. And the obsession with AIDS as a "gay disease" endured, despite the fact that the first reports from Africa in 1983 clearly showed that its transmission there was predominantly through heterosexual contacts and that women were affected as often as men.

Lack of leadership in high places resulted in minimal funding for research on AIDS from the beginning of the outbreak until the mid-1980s, primarily because many people saw AIDS as affecting only the most marginal members of society, those who were already ostracized by much of that society; as such, they were also people who had no effective lobby representing their interests. Compared to the flurry of activity and generous spending allocated to other emerging diseases, such as legionnaires' disease, swine flu, or toxic shock syndrome, AIDS research was gravely neglected.

An "AIDS community" was forming, though. In late 1982, the Gay Men's Health Crisis (GMHC) of New York, and the KS (for Kaposi's sarcoma) Foundation of San Francisco were founded as the first nonprofit AIDS support and service organizations. (The latter is now the San Francisco AIDS Foundation.) In April 1983, the AIDS Medical Foundation (AMF) was incorporated in New York. It was the first private organization entirely dedicated to fostering and funding AIDS medical research through voluntary contributions as well as to carry out advocacy work. (AMF became one of AmFAR's two predecessor organizations.) One of AMF's early advocacy successes was the removal of the stigmatizing designation by the New York City Health Department and the CDC of Haitians as an ethnic group at high risk for AIDS.

Despite the dismal levels of federal funding for AIDS research in these early years of the epidemic, progress in unmasking the agent responsible for AIDS was made at long last by scientists in France and the United States. In April 1983, a research group headed by virologist Luc Montagnier of the Pasteur Institute in Paris discovered reverse transcriptase activity in cells from lymph nodes removed from a French AIDS patient, and saw, using an electron microscope, images of a retrovirus with a novel shape in these cells. (Reverse transcriptase is an enzyme characteristic of retroviruses that is not found in healthy human cells.)

At that time, only two rare human retroviruses were known to exist: HTLV-I and HTLV-II. Both had been discovered and studied by Dr. Robert Gallo of the National Institutes of Health (NIH) in Bethesda, Maryland, starting in the late 1970s. In May, a group of papers published by the American and French researchers in the journal *Science* linked a retrovirus to patients with AIDS. At first, Dr. Gallo was convinced that the virus was HTLV-I; Montagnier and colleague Françoise Barré-Sinoussi had isolated a virus with different characteristics.

In September 1983, at a virology meeting held at the Cold Spring Harbor Laboratory in New York, Montagnier announced further evidence about the virus discovered by his group, which had been isolated from people with swollen lymph nodes. They had named the virus "lymphadenopathy-associated virus," or LAV. It was a retrovirus, but it was not a member of the HTLV family of viruses, said Montagnier, it was a lentivirus. Furthermore, the French scientists had laboratory evidence that LAV had an affinity for and could kill helper T cells, which are identified by the presence of CD4 molecules on their surface (see also Chapter 16). Details of Montagnier's additional findings were published in the scientific literature in April 1984. That same month, Gallo announced that his research group had identified a retrovirus isolated from AIDS patients. They called it HTLV-III. And later that year, Dr. Jay Levy, a researcher at the University of California at San Francisco, and his team also isolated a retrovirus from American gay men with AIDS. They called it the "AIDS-associated retrovirus" (ARV). Furthermore, Levy's laboratory found their virus also in asymptomatic people, providing clear evidence that such apparently healthy people could be carriers of the AIDS-associated retrovirus. Researchers from the CDC, meanwhile, also isolated a virus identical to LAV and published their findings in *Science*. "All four groups shared information, learned from one another, and ended up isolating the same virus," said Curran.

Gallo's work included another important advance: His group could grow the AIDS virus continuously in a laboratory cell-culture system. This was important to further studies of the virus itself and to the production of viral proteins in the laboratory setting. Indeed, this ability would be essential for the development and widespread use of a diagnostic test for screening donated blood and for diagnosing infection in individuals. By November 1984, an experimental version of the screening test, an enzyme-linked immunosorbent assay, or ELISA, was being put through its paces by researchers. In March 1985, the Food and Drug Administration (FDA) approved the first ELISA test kit for the detection of antibodies to the virus in blood samples.

A controversy arose, eagerly fanned by the press, between the Pasteur Institute and the NIH, about who—either Dr. Montagnier or Dr. Gallo— deserved credit for discovering the virus. There was also the important but less-publicized question of which institution would benefit from the royalties derived from the licensing of the first test kit to be sold commercially. The controversy was resolved through a binational agreement. It allowed that both scientists would receive equal credit for the discovery, and that royalties would be payable to a nonprofit foundation entrusted to scientists from both countries for the advancement of AIDS research in the developing world, of which the region in greatest need was, at that time, Africa.

The discovery of the virus, the ability to propagate it in large amounts, and the development of an antibody test to detect the infection in human blood were milestones in the history of the epidemic. But the new ability to identify individuals carrying the virus also raised a host of social, ethical, and public-policy issues.[1] These were first discussed at length during the winter of 1984–85 at a series of meetings in Washington, D.C., attended by representatives of the nonprofit and industrial blood banking community; representatives of gay and hemophilia organizations; and various scientists, physicians, and public-health officials from government and private agencies. These questions had arisen: In addition to blood donors, who should be tested? Where? By whom? And what should be done with test results?

It was assumed (erroneously, as it turned out) that if testing was to be available only at blood-collection centers, people at risk would flood such centers to find out whether they carried the virus or not. This would overburden blood centers and endanger the blood supply because those who had been very recently infected would test negative on an antibody test despite their infection (why this is so is described in Chapter 2).

Many people with AIDS and the gay community as a whole were already suffering greatly from stigma and rampant discrimination that people and institutions justified by a real or alleged fear of AIDS. At the Washington, D.C., meetings, representatives of the AIDS community expressed deep concern that if testing were to be made mandatory for gay men or anyone else, and the results were to be reported to authorities, their hardships would become much worse and the right to the privacy of medical information destroyed. They were reacting to pronouncements by certain individuals and their followers who held that AIDS was due to willfully sinful behavior in defiance of "values" of which they had appointed themselves the virtuous defenders and champions. These same people called for the mandatory testing of all people at risk for AIDS (at the time, a euphemism for gay men) and the isolation, or worse, of those people found to be "AIDS-infected."

These problems were resolved when everyone attending the Washington, D.C., meetings agreed that all those who belonged to CDC-defined "risk groups" should continue to voluntarily abstain from offering to donate or sell blood. In addition, blood donors would be screened through interviews for absence of risk factors and, of course, they would have to agree that their donated blood would be tested. All others would be able to avail themselves of "anonymous testing sites."

Anonymous testing sites were to be organized and managed by state and city health departments; at such sites, testing as well as pretest and post-test counseling would be offered at no cost and without requesting the names and addresses of those tested. To the great relief of gay men and all those at risk for AIDS, it was also decided that only cases of AIDS, as defined by the CDC, along with the individual's name and address would continue to be reported to local health departments, but such cases would be reported to the CDC without identifiers. Individuals with only a positive test result would not be reportable because the significance of a positive result was still uncertain in 1985. Indeed, because of the slow rate of disease progression and the relatively short period of time during which patients had been followed, it was still not clear that HIV infection virtually always led to CDC-defined AIDS. It was still widely believed that infection could lead to either a latent, asymptomatic condition, or only to lymphadenopathy, or only to "AIDS-related complex" (ARC), and only sometimes to AIDS. This belief was soon dispelled, however. The results of long-term epidemiological studies that measured seroconversion rates among cohorts of seropositve gay men showed that the percentage of those who converted from asymptomatic to symptomatic each year did not decrease with time.[2] This allowed researchers to conclude by extrapolation that most seropositive people were likely to develop AIDS after some 15 to 18 years. Today we sadly know that with the possible exception of "long-term nonprogressors," this is essentially true.

The decisions regarding testing, counseling, and reporting, made in the early days of 1985, became the basis of AIDS-related public policies that have been followed for more than ten years.

The "period of emergence" of the epidemic of HIV/AIDS ended with the discovery of its cause, HIV. The experience with HIV/AIDS represents a classic example of the application of the epidemiological method to the understanding of a new epidemic disease: first, the identification of groups at high risk for the disease; then, the identification of one or more risk factors shared by people at risk (which created suspicion of a blood-borne infectious agent as the cause of the disease); last, the determination of the agent's routes of transmission, and therefore, also of ways to prevent its transmission. All this was learned by epidemiologists between 1981 and 1983, before HIV itself was discovered. It was a fine example of deductive research.

Starting in 1986–87, virologists, immunologists, and molecular biologists could start applying their different, inductive experimental approaches to the study of HIV/AIDS. Numerous questions had to be answered: How is HIV constituted? How does it replicate? How does it cause disease? What drugs can be selected or designed against HIV? How should they be tested? And finally, how can a safe and effective vaccine be designed, prepared, and tested to prevent HIV's further epidemic spread?

Answers to some of these questions have been forthcoming from a biomedical research effort that, though starting late, has been outstandingly productive and that holds great promise for the future.

■ WHY GAY MEN?

Why did HIV/AIDS strike the gay community so severely early on, and why is that community still so heavily burdened by it?[3]

The epidemiology of any disease is determined by multiple factors. In the case of AIDS, two factors played a major role: the regenerative ability of the immune system, which masks HIV infection for many years; and the coincidental convergence of the "sexual revolution" with the arrival of HIV in this country.

The immune system has an extraordinary capacity to regenerate itself, that is, to replace lost immune cells by the production of new ones. Thus, it can unobtrusively fight a destructive invader such as HIV for years before exhausting its cell resources, collapsing, and leaving the body vulnerable to highly symptomatic, AIDS-defining diseases. People with HIV infection remain symptom free, appearing and feeling healthy for an average of ten years after acquiring HIV infection. During all that time, however, they are infectious to others.

The second factor is of a historic nature. The 1960s' "feminist revolution" (largely made possible by effective contraception and, thanks to antibiotics, a loss of fear of sexually transmitted diseases) offered new sexual freedom not only to women but to all who felt constrained by earlier social conventions, including homosexuals.

Homosexuals are born to heterosexuals, and wherever they are born, they usually represent a minority of one within their family and immediate social environment. As they grow up, they find themselves living among people who are often profoundly disappointed in and uncomprehending of them. More often, the family and its social circle are outright hostile.

Homosexuals, therefore, seek to live in a community made of like people, within a more tolerant, broader environment, a combination found in large cities.

In the late 1960s, and throughout the 1970s, large numbers of homosexuals, particularly male homosexuals, uprooted themselves and flocked to cities. They were mainly young adults and the gay communities that sprang up in the large cities came to include relatively few older men, virtually no children, and a few adolescents in their late teens (more often than not, these were "throw-away kids," young people who had been rejected by their families because of their sexual orientation). Gay communities therefore became demographically quite different from ethnic communities. They remain much more homogeneous, not only with regard to gender but also with regard to age, with a high proportion of their constituents being in the most sexually active stage of their lives. On the other hand, these gay communities became real communities, with their own communal institutions. Some of these were cultural, some charitable (legal defense groups are particularly important to people often denied their civil rights), educational (even high schools were established for abandoned gay adolescents), political, religious, and recreational. Because what separates homosexuals from the rest of society is principally their lack of equal opportunity to express affection and sexual interest in others, gay communities established their own meeting places, clubs, bars, bookstores, bathhouses, and the like where these feelings and interests could be freely expressed.

Twenty years ago, the gay social scene included large groups of young adult males who had no need to be concerned about contraception and who held a belief (widely shared by the rest of society) that antibiotics could easily cure sexually transmitted diseases. Given that the expression of homosexuality could be seen as avenging centuries of intimidation, humiliation, and even hate and cruel persecution—not only for behavior but also for the mere expression of genuine feelings—unfettered sexual freedom became for these men emblematic of their "revolution." It was to be indulged in joyfully, defiantly, with pride, and with little or no social restraint. So it was in the gay community of the 1970s, and it was difficult to abandon in the early 1980s. In those years, the gay life and gay sex scene reached unprecedented exuberance.

It was also in the late 1960s or early 1970s—as we now know from hospital records and the testing for HIV of samples of blood and human tissue retrieved from laboratory freezers—that HIV found its way to our shores and into that community. Whether that happened through Belgian or French visitors who had left their former African colonies in the early 1960s, or through people from the Caribbean who had served in Angola and Guinea at about the same time, or through American travelers to Haiti, or through "patient zero," a ubiquitous flight attendant, as speculated by the writer Randy Shilts, no one will ever know, and it does not matter. What does matter is that 15 years before anyone knew of its existence, HIV had slipped silently into the gay communities of New York and San Francisco, where it found the means to spread from man to man, unnoticed and unimpeded for over ten years.

By the late 1970s, there were a few isolated, unexplained deaths due to "pneumonia," among gay men and others. But without special tests, these cases could not be recognized for what they were: early cases of the AIDS-defining pneumonia, PCP. Because they went unrecognized, they also went unreported. By the time clusters of cases of PCP, KS, and persistent lymphadenopathy were reported and so began to alert the medical world in 1981, countless young gay men had already become HIV infected. Since nobody was in a position to know what was going on—a silent epidemic of HIV infection—the infection continued to spread among gay men in the 1980s.

It took another two years before the CDC knew enough to issue its first cautious 1983 suggestions regarding risk reduction for AIDS. And it took three more years, until 1986, for Dr. C. Everett Koop, then Surgeon General of the United States, to issue and distribute to 150 million American families a copy of his important pamphlet on HIV/AIDS and its possible prevention. (He was, however, refused funding for the pamphlet's translation into Spanish.)

By 1984–85, the gay community was already organizing its own extensive education for prevention programs. However, as there were no funds for that purpose forthcoming from the federal government, the community had to raise the necessary resources from the public, mostly among its own members. Its educational programs proved highly effective in the second half of the 1980s. Yet they came too late to save perhaps as many as half of all gay men in the cities hardest hit by HIV, and by then, it was also too late for many others nationwide.

Gay men who became infected in the 1970s and early 1980s died of AIDS throughout the 1980s and 1990s in numbers disproportionate to their percentage in the total population. With the exception of injection drug users, they still remain at higher risk than others because the prevalence of HIV infection still is much higher in the gay community than in the rest of the American population.

HIV/AIDS is *not* a "gay disease." HIV does not have, and never had, a predilection for gay men. It simply struck their community first, without warning and without causing clinical disease for some ten years—throughout the 1970s—during which it could spread and doom half its population *before* the immune impairment it was causing became noticeable through symptoms of its most advanced stage, AIDS. Today, the HIV epidemic is growing fastest among injection drug users because they have no legal access to sterile needles, and among women of color. But anyone who is sexually active is at some risk of acquiring HIV infection unless he or she follows the precautions described in Chapter 9.

ENDNOTES

1. For a detailed account of these issues, see Bayer R. *Private Acts, Social Consequences: AIDS and the Politics of Public Health.* New York: The Free Press, 1989.

2. Kaplan JE, et al. Lymphadenopathy syndrome in homosexual men: evidence for continuing risk of developing the acquired immunodeficiency syndrome. *Journal of the American Medical Association* 1987;257: 335–337.

3. For a more detailed explanation of this topic, see Shilts R. *And the Band Played On: Politics, People, and the AIDS Epidemic.* New York: Viking-Penguin, 1993.

■ *Chapter 21*

EVIDENCE THAT HIV IS THE CAUSE OF AIDS

Since the mid-1980s, the vast majority of the medical community has held that HIV is the cause of AIDS. How do scientists determine cause and effect—that some agent causes a disease? In reality, proving cause and effect can be difficult to do. It is often tentative at first, and ultimately determined by scientific consensus. Researchers arrive at this consensus using evidence gained through epidemiological studies, laboratory experiments, and tests in animals.

■ EPIDEMIOLOGICAL STUDIES

Epidemiological studies link a disease to some risk factor or agent in the environment; the stronger the studies (e.g., the larger the number of people studied and the closer the statistical correlation between the risk factors, or possible causative agent, with the disease), the higher the probability that the cause of the disease has been found. Other important evidence used to establish cause includes answering questions like the following:

- Is the suspected cause found consistently in different populations under different circumstances?

- Is presence of the suspected cause closely correlated with the effect (e.g., does exposure to the agent usually precede onset of the disease)?

- Is the suspected cause scientifically plausible?

- Is the suspected cause compatible with the scientific understanding of the biology and natural history of the disease?

The clearest epidemiological evidence that HIV causes AIDS comes from Thailand. At the beginning of 1988, blood tests of nearly 200,000 Thais from HIV risk groups revealed fewer than 100 cases of HIV infection; by 1994, more than 700,000 Thais were estimated to be HIV positive. Waves of HIV infection were followed moving through different populations: prostitutes, gays, injection drug users, and military personnel. It then hit wives and children. This was followed later by growing numbers of AIDS cases among HIV-infected members of these populations.

Other strong epidemiological evidence that HIV causes AIDS came from studies of the following:

- People with hemophilia. Hemophilia is a group of blood diseases that result in abnormal bleeding from even minor wounds. The disease is caused by an inadequate amount, or the absence of, blood proteins known as "clotting factors." Hemophilia A, which occurs in 80% of hemophiliacs, is treated with infusions of a blood product called factor VIII. Factor VIII contains a clotting factor derived from the plasma of donated blood, usually from pooling thousands of units of donated blood. Between 1978 and 1985, an estimated 80% of all hemophiliacs with severe disease who had been treated with factor VIII became infected with HIV. From 1983 to 1989 the age at death for all hemophiliacs in the United States dropped from 63 to 38 years as the death rate due to AIDS rose in them from 20% in 1983–85 to 55% in 1987–89. Since 1985, heat treatment has been used in the preparation of clotting factors to inactivate HIV and eliminate this cause of HIV transmission: As of early 1997, the National Hemophilia Foundation knew of no new case of HIV infection due to contaminated clotting factors since heat treatment began.

■ Recipients of blood transfusions. Even before HIV was discovered, the fact that AIDS arose in recipients of blood donated by people with AIDS provided strong evidence that the syndrome was caused by a blood-borne infectious agent. In addition, when the blood test for antibodies to HIV was introduced in 1985 (and all donations that yielded a positive test result were discarded), the number of cases of HIV/AIDS in blood transfusion recipients plunged dramatically.

■ LABORATORY AND ANIMAL RESEARCH

Laboratory (i.e., cellular) and animal research studies provide additional evidence that helps establish the cause of a disease. Laboratory research seeks to identify the mechanism through which the agent causes the disease, something that cannot be determined by epidemiological studies. Laboratory studies of HIV, for example, revealed that the virus infected and destroyed cell types having the CD4 molecule on their surface. Such laboratory observations linked HIV to the immune deficiency and loss of CD4 cells seen in people with AIDS. Animal studies then helped confirm that the agent does in fact give rise to the disease.

In the case of an infectious disease, an important goal of laboratory and animal research is to fulfill criteria known as "Koch's postulates." These principles were developed by the nineteenth-century German bacteriologist Robert Koch as the necessary base of evidence that a particular microbe causes a particular disease. Koch's postulates require the following:

■ A microbe must be isolated from the organism that has developed the disease.

■ The microbe must be given to a healthy host in which it causes the same disease.

■ The microbe must be reisolated from the second host.

HIV has been isolated from virtually all patients with AIDS, which fulfills the first postulate; conversely, there is no overriding evidence that AIDS occurs in the absence of HIV infection. This strongly suggests that HIV is necessary to the development of AIDS.

(There are two conditions, however, in which certain clinical symptoms of AIDS, along with low CD4 lymphocyte counts, occur in the absence of HIV. The first case is the appearance of Kaposi's sarcoma in gay men and others at risk for HIV, but in the absence of HIV. These individuals may have low or normal CD4 counts, but all are invariably infected with the Kaposi's sarcoma-associated herpesvirus [KSHV], also known as human herpesvirus type 8 [HHV-8]. For more on KSHV, see Chapter 8. The second case is that of idiopathic CD4-positive T lymphocytopenia [ICL], which is popularly known as "AIDS without HIV." This is a rare syndrome of unknown origin in which affected individuals have CD4 lymphocyte counts below 300, have a low CD4/CD8 cell ratio [i.e., a low ratio of helper T lymphocytes to cytotoxic T lymphocytes], and often have an AIDS-defining illness such as *Pneumocystis carinii* pneumonia or cryptococcal meningitis, but have no evidence of HIV infection. ICL was first described in 1992. There is no evidence that it is transmitted from person to person. The World Health Organization and the Centers for Disease Control and Prevention have identified about 200 individuals in the United States and about 600 people worldwide with ICL.)

As yet, the requirements for the second and third postulates have not been directly fulfilled for HIV. Research is ongoing with chimpanzees, but it takes the animals approximately ten years after having been exposed to HIV to develop the disease. However, the second and third postulates have been fulfilled for a retrovirus of monkeys that is closely related to HIV. The simian immunodeficiency virus (SIV) has been recovered from animals that developed an AIDS-like immunodeficiency, and transferred to other monkeys in which it caused the same disease and from which the virus could be reisolated.

Last, the well-established observation that anti-HIV drugs can dramatically decrease viral load, halt disease progression, and allow an increase in CD4 lymphocyte counts has provided striking clinical evidence in support of HIV as the cause of AIDS.

In spite of all this evidence, some people remain unconvinced that HIV causes AIDS. The doubters do agree that infection by HIV is *correlated* with AIDS, but they claim that the evidence is insufficient to call HIV the *cause* of AIDS. A chief critic of the HIV/AIDS theory is Peter Duesberg, a retrovirologist at the University of California, Berkeley. Duesberg claims that HIV is harmless and that AIDS is caused by factors such as sexual practices, the use of illicit "hard" drugs, the use of certain recreational drugs (especially nitrite inhalers known as "poppers," believed to be aphrodisiacs), and even the use of certain antiretroviral drugs such as AZT. Duesberg, however, is widely regarded as someone who reads the scientific literature selectively, ignores evidence that does not support his views, and dismisses sound studies for trivial reasons.

Since the advent of AIDS in the early 1980s, medical science has come a long way in understanding the natural history of HIV and the course of HIV infection in the body. It is now clear that after HIV enters the body, it establishes an infection that progresses through several well-established stages: a period of acute infection, a gradual decade-long attack on and exhaustion of the immune system, followed by the development of severe opportunistic diseases and death.

Once clinical disease is present, the person is referred to as having HIV disease; prior to the development of clinical disease, the person is said to be HIV positive or HIV infected. What has been called AIDS is actually advanced HIV disease. Many people would like to discontinue use of the acronym AIDS and replace it with "advanced HIV disease." This could accomplish two things: It would help people with HIV avoid the stigma that often goes along with having "AIDS," and it would emphasize that the syndrome called AIDS is really the last stage of a disease that begins when a person becomes infected by HIV.

A final thought on establishing cause and effect in disease and on the responsibility to act in spite of incomplete understanding comes from A. B. Hill, who reminds us:

> All scientific work is incomplete—whether it be observational or experimental. All scientific work is liable to be upset or modified by advancing knowledge. That does not confer upon us a freedom to ignore the knowledge we already have, or to postpone the action that it appears to demand at a given time.[1]

ENDNOTE

1. Hill AB. The environment and disease: associaton or causation? *Proceedings of the Royal Society of Medicine* 1965;58:295–300

GLOSSARY

abortive infection ■ An infection that is stopped by the immune system before it causes disease.

accelerated approval ■ An FDA drug-approval process that involves approving a drug based on an improvement in a SURROGATE MARKER rather than on a clinical marker such as increased survival. This allows drugs to be approved for marketing in less time (although their manufacturers are required to continue clinical testing until true benefit is established).

active disease ■ An infection that shows clinical signs of disease or is transmissible to others. A person can be infected by the tuberculosis bacillus, for example, but if the infection is contained by the immune system, the person will not develop TUBERCULOSIS and will not transmit the bacillus. A person with active tuberculosis, however, shows signs of illness and can transmit the infection to others.

acute illness ■ An illness or infection that is brief or has a sudden onset; not chronic. Sometimes loosely used to mean severe.

acute HIV infection ■ The first stage of HIV infection, which begins when the virus enters the body. During acute infection, the virus replicates rapidly and spreads widely in the body.

ADCC ■ See ANTIBODY-DEPENDENT CELLULAR CYTOTOXICITY.

adenocarcinoma ■ A type of carcinoma that develops in glandular cells located in epithelial tissue.

adenopathy ■ Swelling of the lymph nodes.

adenovirus ■ Any virus that belongs to the family Adenoviridae. In humans, adenoviruses cause problems that include the common cold and other upper respiratory tract infections, conjunctivitis, and gastrointestinal illness.

adhesion proteins ■ A category of RECOGNITION PROTEINS on the surface of cells. Adhesion proteins help cells attach to other cells and materials that surround them in the body.

adjuvant ■ In vaccine technology, an adjuvant is a substance that is used to increase the antigenicity or potency of a vaccine. An adjuvant makes the vaccine seem more "foreign" to the immune system and thereby increases the reaction of the immune system to the ANTIGEN in the vaccine. In therapy, an adjuvant is a drug that is used to increase or improve the action of the principal treatment. In cancer chemotherapy, for example, adjuvant treatment is given to destroy cancer cells that might remain in the body following the surgical removal of a tumor.

advanced directives ■ Legal documents that specify a person's preference regarding the use of resuscitation, life support, and other types of medical care employed to maintain life when the person is unable to make that decision for himself or herself.

advanced HIV disease ■ Same as AIDS, that is, a phase of HIV disease marked by characteristic OPPORTUNISTIC INFECTIONS and malignancies, or by a drop in the number of HELPER T LYMPHOCYTES (i.e., CD4 lymphocytes) below 200 cells per mm^3.

Agency for Health Care Policy and Research (AHCPR) ■ An agency of the U.S. Public Health Service established in 1989 that conducts and supports health-care research and recommends guidelines for the diagnosis, management, and treatment of disease, including HIV disease.

AIDS ■ Abbreviation for acquired immunodeficiency syndrome. AIDS is the advanced stage of HIV disease. It is marked by characteristic OPPORTUNISTIC INFECTIONS and malignancies, and by a loss of HELPER T LYMPHOCYTES, or CD4 lymphocytes to less than 200 of the cells per mm^3.

AIDS Clinical Trials Group (ACTG) ■ A nationwide network of medical research centers that conduct studies on the safety and effectiveness of experimental treatments for HIV/AIDS with funding from the National Institutes of Health.

AIDS dementia complex ■ A neurological complication of AIDS that results in mild to severe mental impairment. Antiretroviral therapy has reduced the incidence of AIDS dementia complex and often slows its progress. Also known as HIV encephalopathy.

AIDS-related complex (ARC) ■ A term at one time used to refer to symptoms of disease that precede AIDS. These symptoms included swollen LYMPH NODES, night sweats, unexplained weight loss, ORAL CANDIDIASIS, and ORAL HAIRY LEUKO-PLAKIA. Same as early HIV disease (the term ARC is no longer officially recognized by the CDC).

alveoli ■ The air spaces of the lung.

ambisense ■ A property of certain viral RNA genomes in which part of the RNA strand has positive SENSE and part has negative sense.

analogue ■ A MOLECULE with a structure that resembles that of another molecule. An analogue can often be substituted for the original molecule. For example, the drug AZT is an analogue for the NUCLEOSIDE thymine.

anergy ■ The loss of T-lymphocyte function, as demonstrated by a loss of DELAYED-TYPE HYPERSENSITIVITY to common antigens such as antigens.

animal model ■ An example of a disease in an animal species that is similar enough to a human disease to enable scientists to study the development and treatment of the disease in the animal and apply the conclusions to humans.

anorexia ■ Loss of appetite.

antibiotics ■ Drugs that are usually used to treat diseases caused by infectious agents other than viruses.

antibody ■ A class of large protein MOLECULES that are produced in response to, and interacts with, specific target molecules known as ANTIGENS. Antibodies are produced by activated B lymphocytes known as PLASMA CELLS. Antibodies are found in blood, mucus, tears, saliva, breast milk, and the fluid that surrounds body cells, the extracellular fluid. Also known as IMMUNO-GLOBULINS.

antibody-dependent cellular cytotoxicity (ADCC), or antibody-dependent cell-mediated cytotoxicity ■ An IMMUNE RESPONSE that is triggered when antibodies attach to ANTIGENS on the surface of cells or parasites. In ADCC, the antibody-covered cell is destroyed by WHITE BLOOD CELLS (WBCs) other than CYTOTOXIC T LYMPHOCYTES. These WBCs include NATURAL KILLER CELLS, MACROPHAGES, NEUTROPHILS, and EOSINOPHILS.

antibody-mediated immune response ■ The IMMUNE RESPONSE that involves the activation of B LYMPHOCYTES to produce ANTIBODIES. The response results in antibody-mediated immunity.

antigen ■ A substance that can induce the production of ANTIBODY and to which an antibody will bind. Almost any biological molecule can serve as an antigen. The word antigen comes from *anti*body *gen*erator.

antigenemia ■ The persistence of ANTIGENS in the blood.

antigenic/antigenicity ■ Having the properties of an ANTIGEN, that is, the ability to induce an IMMUNE RESPONSE.

antigenic determinant ■ See EPITOPE.

antigen-presenting cell (APC) ■ A cell of the immune system that takes up ANTIGENS and displays them on its surface. The antigens can then be detected by helper T cells, which stimulate an IMMUNE RESPONSE to the antigen. Antigen-presenting cells include B lymphocytes, MACROPHAGES, Langerhans' cells in the skin, dendritic cells in lymph nodes, and epithelial cells (see EPITHELIUM) in the THYMUS.

antiretroviral ■ A substance, drug, or process that destroys a retrovirus or inhibits its replication. Often used to describe drugs active against HIV, since HIV is the most important retrovirus causing human disease.

aphthous ulcers ■ Painful sores in the mouth or esophagus that occur commonly in people with HIV. The cause of aphthous ulcers is unknown.

apoptosis ■ Programmed cell death. It is a natural biochemical pathway that causes a cell's DNA to break up and the cell to die. The body uses apoptosis to eliminate damaged and unneeded cells, such as superfluous lymphocytes upon completion of an immune response.

ARC ■ See AIDS-RELATED COMPLEX.

-ase ■ A suffix added to the name of a substance to indicate it is an ENZYME.

aspergillosis ■ An infection caused by the fungus *Aspergillus* seen in some people with AIDS. Aspergillosis usually occurs in the lungs.

asymptomatic ■ Literally means "without symptoms."

asymptomatic HIV disease ■ Stage of HIV disease during which a person shows no outward signs or symptoms of disease.

attenuated live-HIV vaccine ■ A vaccine that uses an ATTENUATED VIRUS to elicit an IMMUNE RESPONSE. Also known as live-virus vaccine. The Sabin vaccine is an example.

attenuated virus ■ A virus that has been made nonvirulent or less virulent by manipulations in the laboratory such as growing it for many generations in laboratory cells or by genetic engineering. Attenuated viruses are used in live-virus vaccines.

avirulent virus ■ A non-disease-causing virus.

azidothymidine (AZT) ■ An ANTIRETROVIRAL drug and NUCLEOSIDE ANALOGUE REVERSE TRANSCRIPTASE INHIBITOR. It is an ANALOGUE of thymidine. Also known as ZIDOVUDINE (ZDV).

bacteremia ■ Presence of bacteria in circulating blood.

base ■ In molecular biology, "base" usually refers to components of DNA and RNA. The bases in DNA are adenine, cytosine, guanine, and thymidine. The bases in RNA are adenine, cytosine, guanine, and uracil.

base pair (bp) ■ The pair of bases that form one crosspiece in a molecule of DOUBLE-STRANDED DNA. The number of base pairs (usually in terms of thousands, or kilobase pairs) is used as a measure of length of a DNA molecule or of a gene.

basophil ■ A type of WHITE BLOOD CELL that has blue and purple (or basophilic) granules in the CYTOPLASM when stained and viewed under a microscope. Basophils are a type of GRANULOCYTE.

bind ■ To join together. Examples: an antibody binds with its antigen; hormones and cytokines bind to receptors on cells; HIV's gp120 protein binds with CD4 molecules on helper T lymphocytes.

biopsy ■ The removal of small pieces of tissue for microscopic examination. Biopsies are usually done to help establish a diagnosis.

blood-brain barrier ■ A feature of the capillaries of the brain that protects it from harmful materials circulating in the blood. The cells making up these capillaries fit together extremely tightly, thereby preventing water-soluble molecules—including ANTIRETROVIRAL drugs—from passing out of the blood and into the tissues of the brain unless the capillary cells actively transport them there.

B lymphocytes ■ LYMPHOCYTES that produce ANTIBODIES.

body fluids ■ Fluids manufactured within the body. Usually refers to blood, urine, saliva, semen, and vaginal fluid.

bone marrow ■ The soft tissue that occupies the cavities inside bone. Yellow bone marrow, which consists of fat cells and connective tissue, fills the cavities of long bones. Red bone marrow occupies the spongy cavities of the pelvis, ribs, sternum, vertebrae, skull, collarbones, and shoulder blades. Red marrow is where hemoglobin and red and WHITE BLOOD CELLS are produced.

branched-chain DNA amplification (bDNA) ■ A VIRAL GENOME TEST that detects copies of viral RNA or DNA in blood or LYMPHOCYTES.

brand name ■ One of at least three names that can be used when referring to a drug. A brand name is the name given to a drug by its manufacturer after the drug receives FDA approval. Brand names are registered and the first letter is always capitalized when spelled. For example, Retrovir is the brand name for AZT. Compare with GENERIC NAME and CHEMICAL NAME.

cachexia ■ See WASTING.

cancer ■ Common name for a malignant tumor, that is, a tumor that spreads by invading neighboring tissues and by metastasizing to other locations in the body (see METASTATIC TUMOR). Cancers can be divided into solid tumors, and leukemias, LYMPHOMAS, and myelomas. Solid tumors, in turn, are divided into CARCINOMAS and SARCOMAS.

candidiasis ■ An infection of mucous membranes usually caused by the yeast *Candida albicans.* Candidiasis can occur in the mouth (oral candidiasis, or thrush), esophagus (esophageal candidiasis), and vagina (often referred to as a yeast infection). Oral candidiasis can also occur as roughened red patches on the tongue or lining of the mouth (erythematous candidiasis) and as cracks and fissures on the corners of the mouth (angular cheilitis).

capsid ■ The protein capsule that encloses the genetic material of a virus particle, or virion. The capsid gives the virion its shape, and is important for its attachment to its host cell. The capsid of HIV is made up primarily of an estimated 1,200 molecules of the p24 capsid (CA) protein.

capsomers ■ The repeating units of protein that make up a virion's CAPSID.

carcinoma ■ A CANCER that arises in epithelial tissue (see EPITHELIUM).

carcinoma in situ ■ An early-stage CARCINOMA, when it is still confined to the epithelial tissues in which it originated. A stage in the development of cervical cancer (which is a carcinoma). Also referred to as "CIS."

case ■ A set of conditions, symptoms, and situations that must exist for a disease to become reportable in a particular health SURVEILLANCE SYSTEM.

case manager ■ A person who coordinates the various kinds of assistance and resources that may be needed by someone with a disease, usually when it is chronic or serious.

catalyst ■ A substance that speeds up the rate of a chemical reaction without itself being consumed or permanently changed by the reaction. ENZYMES are catalysts made by living organisms.

catalyze ■ To speed up the rate of a chemical reaction using a CATALYST.

catheter ■ A tube placed into a vein or body cavity to allow the passage of a fluid out of or into the body.

CD ■ Abbreviation for cluster designation (also called cluster of differentiation). It refers to an international system of nomenclature for LYMPHOCYTES and other WHITE BLOOD CELLS (e.g., CD4 cells). The CD classification helps identify the function and degree of maturity of white blood cells.

CD4 cell ■ See HELPER T LYMPHOCYTE.

CD8 cell ■ See CYTOTOXIC T LYMPHOCYTE.

cell-mediated immune response ■ The IMMUNE RESPONSE that mobilizes CD8 cells (also known as CYTOTOXIC T LYMPHOCYTES or killer T cells) to destroy cells infected by a PATHOGEN. Also known as cell-mediated immunity.

cell membrane ■ The membrane that covers the cell. It consists of a double layer (a bilayer) of lipid molecules that has a number of proteins associated with it.

cell-surface receptor ■ MOLECULES on the surface of cells that bind with substances such as hormones, drugs, neurotransmitters, and growth factors. Contact between a molecule and a receptor triggers a change in the activity or behavior of the cell. Antibodies on the surface of B lymphocytes serve as receptors for the detection of antigens. When an antigen binds to its antibody receptor on a B cell, it triggers the B cell to divide and to produce antibodies that are released into the bloodstream.

cell tropism ■ See TROPISM.

Centers for Disease Control and Prevention (CDC) ■ The agency of the U.S. Public Health Service responsible for identifying, monitoring, preventing, and controlling disease, injury, disability, and premature death in the United States. The CDC, in conjunction with physicians and other specialists in HIV disease and in public health, develops recommendations for preventing and controlling HIV disease and the opportunistic infections associated with AIDS.

central nervous system (CNS) ■ The brain and spinal cord.

cerebral ■ Relating to the brain.

cerebrospinal fluid (CSF) ■ The fluid that bathes the brain and spinal cord.

certified laboratory ■ A medical testing laboratory approved by the health department because it meets requirements for training, expertise, and accuracy.

cervix ■ The rounded, conical opening of the uterus.

chancroid ■ A highly infectious, painful, venereal ulcer caused by the bacterium *Hemophilus ducreyi*.

chemical name ■ One of at least three names that can be used when referring to a drug. The chemical name of a drug is derived from its chemical structure. The chemical name for AZT, for example, is 3´-azido-3´-deoxythymidine.

chemokines ■ CYTOKINES that activate and direct the migration of WHITE BLOOD CELLS. There are two subfamilies of chemokines, the CXC and the CC chemokines. CELL-SURFACE RECEPTORS for chemokines are used by HIV, along with the CD4 molecule, to enter the cells it infects.

chemoprophylaxis ■ The use of drugs to prevent disease.

chemotherapy ■ The use of drugs to treat disease.

chlamydia ■ A sexually transmitted infection of the urogenital tract caused by bacteria belonging to the genus *Chlamydia*.

chromosome ■ Thread-like structures in the nucleus of cells that consist of a molecule of DNA plus a number of proteins. Chromosomal DNA bears genetic information in the form of a string of genes. There are 46 chromosomes in human SOMATIC CELLS and 23 in human GERM CELLS.

chronic infection ■ An infection in which a virus or other PATHOGEN is always present to some extent in the body. Chronic infections can be a PERSISTENT INFECTION or a LATENT INFECTION.

clade ■ A name for genetic subtypes or major GENOTYPES of HIV.

class I MHC molecules ■ See MAJOR HISTOCOMPATIBILITY COMPLEX (MHC) MOLECULES.

class II MHC molecules ■ See MAJOR HISTOCOMPATIBILITY COMPLEX (MHC) MOLECULES.

clinical ■ Involving human patients.

clinically latent ■ Without outward signs or symptoms of disease despite underlying disease. The asymptomatic phase of HIV disease is an example of a clinically LATENT INFECTION.

clinical trial ■ Scientific study of the safety and effectiveness of a new drug or treatment in humans. Clinical trials are usually done in three phases, known as PHASE I, PHASE II, and PHASE III CLINICAL TRIALS.

clotting factors ■ PROTEINS that are needed for blood to clot. Clotting factors obtained by pooling many units of donated blood plasma are used to treat HEMOPHILIA.

CMV colitis ■ An infection of the intestines by CYTOMEGALOVIRUS that produces fever, weight loss, anorexia, malaise, abdominal pain, and severe diarrhea. It can also produce hemorrhaging and perforation of the intestine, both of which are life-threatening conditions.

CMV esophagitis ■ Inflammation of the lower esophagus due to infection by CYTOMEGALOVIRUS. CMV esophagitis more typically occurs in patients with a CD4 count below 50 cells per mm³ and produces large, shallow ulcers in the region of the esophagus that joins the stomach.

CMV retinitis ■ Infection of the eyes by CYTOMEGALOVIRUS that causes progressive, irreversible loss of sight when untreated. CMV retinitis occurs in up to 40% of people with advanced HIV disease. Antiviral treatment can halt progression of CMV retinitis, and it should be sought immediately when signs or symptoms are noticed.

coccidioidomycosis ■ An OPPORTUNISTIC INFECTION of the lungs caused by the fungus *Coccidioides immitis*.

colitis ■ Inflammation or infection of the colon that has a variety of causes.

colposcopy ■ Examination of the tissues of the cervix and vagina with a colposcope, an instrument with a magnifying lens. Colposcopy helps detect abnormal growths suggested by a PAP TEST and select tissues for BIOPSY.

combination therapy ■ The use of two or more drugs to treat a disease. Antiretroviral drugs are best used in combination to treat HIV disease.

compassionate use ■ A program of the Food and Drug Administration that makes individual experimental drugs available to very sick patients who have no other treatment options at the request of the patient's physician to the drug's manufacturer.

complementary base pairing ■ The matching, or pairing, of BASES in DNA and the pairing of bases between MESSENGER RNA (mRNA) and DNA during PROTEIN SYNTHESIS.

complex viruses ■ Viruses with CAPSIDS that contain many different PROTEINS.

computed tomography (CT) ■ A diagnostic test that produces multiple X-ray–like images of organs, muscles, and other soft tissues.

confirmatory test ■ A test with high SPECIFICITY and SENSITIVITY that is used to verify the results of an HIV ENZYME-LINKED IMMUNOSORBENT ASSAY (ELISA).

contagious ■ A property of disease-causing microorganisms that are transmissible from person to person by direct or indirect contact. See also INFECTIOUS DISEASE.

correlates of immunity ■ The specific aspects of an immune response to an infectious agent that must occur to achieve protective immunity against that agent. Identifying correlates of immunity is necessary for the design of protective vaccines against certain pathogens, HIV in particular. Also known as CORRELATES OF PROTECTION.

correlates of protection ■ See CORRELATES OF IMMUNITY.

cross-resistance ■ Resistance to one drug that results in resistance to other drugs in the same class. For example, when resistance to a drug such as AZT also produces resistance to a related drug such as ddI.

cryptococcosis ■ An OPPORTUNISTIC INFECTION caused by the fungus *Cryptococcus neoformans*. Cryptococcosis is the most common cause of meningitis in people with AIDS.

cryptosporidiosis ■ An OPPORTUNISTIC INFECTION of cells in the digestive tract by the protozoan *Cryptosporidium parvum*. It is a common cause of diarrhea in persons with HIV disease.

cytokine ■ Chemicals produced by cells that influence the activity and behavior of other cells. Some cytokines increase the intensity of an IMMUNE RESPONSE, while others suppress it. Still other cytokines regulate the development of immune cells in the bone marrow. Examples of cytokines are the INTERLEUKINS and INTERFERONS.

cytomegalovirus (CMV) ■ A herpesvirus, also known as herpesvirus 5, that can infect a variety of organs. In people with AIDS, CMV can infect the eyes, causing CMV RETINITIS; the esophagus, causing CMV ESOPHAGITIS; and the intestines, causing CMV COLITIS.

cytoplasm ■ The region of the cell outside the NUCLEUS. The cytoplasm contains the cell's ORGANELLES.

cytotoxic T lymphocyte (CTL) ■ A T lymphocyte that is activated by the CELL-MEDIATED IMMUNE RESPONSE. CTLs destroy cells infected by viruses, bacteria, or protozoan parasites. Also known as killer T cells, and as CD8 lymphocytes because they display large numbers of CD8 cell-surface molecules (they are also referred to as T8 cells in older scientific literature).

delayed-type hypersensitivity ■ A type of CELL-MEDIATED IMMUNE RESPONSE. Delayed-type hypersensitivity involves the accumulation of MACROPHAGES and CYTOTOXIC T LYMPHOCYTES (CTLs) at a site in the body where an ANTIGEN is present. Because this reaction takes time to develop, the response is called delayed-type hypersensitivity. It occurs, for example, during a PPD skin test for tuberculosis. A positive test produces a swelling and hardness of the skin about 18 hours later. Loss of delayed-type hypersensitivity to common antigens (such as those for the yeast *Candida albicans*) indicates weakened cell-mediated immunity.

dendritic cell ■ A type of ANTIGEN-PRESENTING CELL that is found in skin and mucous membranes.

deoxyribonucleic acid (DNA) ■ A MOLECULE (specifically, a nucleic acid) that primarily serves as the carrier of genetic information in cells and in many viruses.

didanosine (ddI) ■ An ANTIRETROVIRAL drug and NUCLEOSIDE ANALOGUE REVERSE TRANSCRIPTASE INHIBITOR. ddI is an analogue of the nucleoside adenosine.

discordant couple ■ In AIDS research literature, a couple in which one person is HIV infected and the other is not.

disseminated ■ Occurring widely in the body. Disseminated disease is disease that has spread from an initial site of infection to other areas of the body.

DNA ■ See DEOXYRIBONUCLEIC ACID.

DNA-binding proteins ■ Proteins that bind to DNA to activate or deactivate genes by binding to PROMOTER and ENHANCER regions of genes. They are a type of REGULATORY PROTEIN. Also known as activation proteins and transactivation proteins.

DNA probe ■ Short segment of single-stranded DNA that is designed to pair and attach to (i.e., hybridize with) a specific place on another DNA strand.

DNA vaccine ■ A VACCINE that involves injecting noninfectious fragments of viral DNA into the body.

dot blot ■ A variety of ENZYME-LINKED IMMUNOSORBENT ASSAY that uses drops of blood or serum placed on a special paper to be treated in a way that produces a color if the sample contains certain antibodies. This technique is used in HIV tests that involve HOME SPECIMEN-COLLECTION KITS.

double-stranded DNA (dsDNA) ■ The usual structure of DNA molecules in living things. Each strand of dsDNA consists of a backbone, which is a chain of sugar molecules linked together by phosphate groups. Double-stranded DNA consists of two of these chains. The two chains are linked along their length by the complementary pairing of the BASES that extend from each sugar molecule (see COMPLEMENTARY BASE PAIRING). Double-stranded DNA molecules are helically twisted, poducing a shape known as the "DNA double helix."

double-stranded RNA (dsRNA) ■ RNA that consists of two strands of RNA joined along their length by the complementary pairing of their BASES. (See COMPLEMENTARY BASE PAIRING.) Many RNA viruses have a genome that consists of dsRNA.

dysplasia ■ An abnormal growth of cells that is often precancerous.

dyspnea ■ Shortness of breath or difficulty breathing.

early HIV disease ■ The stage of HIV disease that follows the ASYMPTOMATIC phase. It is characterized by the development of one or more characteristic OP-PORTUNISTIC INFECTIONS that include ORAL CANDIDIASIS, herpes simplex disease, SHINGLES, and ORAL HAIRY LEUKOPLAKIA.

effector cell ■ General term for immune cells that actively participate in elim-inating or neutralizing antigens or destroying infected cells. Effector cells include CYTOTOXIC T LYMPHOCYTES, B LYMPHOCYTES, MACROPHAGES, and NATURAL KILLER CELLS.

ELISA ■ See ENZYME-LINKED IMMUNOSORBENT ASSAY.

-emia ■ Suffix indicating that the specified thing is in the blood or is a condi-tion of the blood.

encephalopathy ■ General term for any disease of the brain.

enhancer ■ A region of a gene that helps regulate the activity of the gene. The binding of REGULATORY PROTEINS to the enhancer region of a gene improves the efficiency of MESSENGER RNA (mRNA) formation during TRANSCRIPTION, the first phase of PROTEIN SYNTHESIS.

***env* gene** ■ The gene in HIV that encodes information for the production of the GP160 POLYPROTEIN. The gp160 polyprotein is later cleaved to form the GP120 and GP41 envelope proteins.

enzyme ■ A MOLECULE that greatly accelerates a chemical reaction in living things without itself being consumed in the process. The names of enzymes usually end with the suffix -ASE.

enzyme immunoassay (EIA) ■ See ENZYME-LINKED IMMUNOSORBENT ASSAY.

enzyme-linked immunosorbent assay (ELISA) ■ A test for the detection of in-fections in blood or other body fluids by revealing the presence of antibodies to the infectious agent. It is commonly used as a screening test for HIV infection.

eosinophil ■ A type of WHITE BLOOD CELL and a PHAGOCYTE that has yellow and orange (eosinophilic) granules in its CYTOPLASM when treated with certain stains and viewed under a microscope. Eosinophils are a type of GRANULOCYTE.

epidemic ■ A outbreak of an infectious desease or other condition that affects a large number of people at the same time in the same community or geographic area.

epithelium ■ A tissue that covers the body and lines its cavities and internal organs. It is composed of single or multiple layers of epithelial cells.

epitope ■ The specific site on an ANTIGEN molecule to which a single ANTIBODY binds. Also known as an antigenic determinant.

Epstein-Barr virus (EBV) ■ A HERPESVIRUS associated with infectious mononucleosis, NON-HODGKIN'S LYMPHOMA, Burkitt's lymphoma, and ORAL HAIRY LEUKOPLAKIA. EBV is also known as human herpesvirus 4.

escape virus/escape mutant ■ A virus or other PATHOGEN that has mutated in a way that makes it resistant to one or more drugs. Escape mutants can avoid or escape the otherwise toxic effect of the drug(s) used to treat the infection they cause and continue to replicate.

erythematous candidiasis ■ See CANDIDIASIS.

expanded-access programs ■ FDA-approved programs that authorize the use of experimental drugs for people who cannot participate in CLINICAL TRIALS.

exposure ■ In a public-health sense, the act or condition of being brought into direct contact with a PATHOGEN (a virus, bacteria, or other infectious agent). Exposure to a pathogen does not mean one is infected with the pathogen.

extracellular ■ The area outside of or surrounding cells. Extracellular fluid, for example, is the fluid that occupies the fine spaces between cells.

follicular dendritic cells (FDCs) ■ ANTIGEN-PRESENTING CELLS found in LYMPH NODES. FDCs have long filament-like strands that filter ANTIGENS from the lymphatic fluid passing through the node.

Food and Drug Administration (FDA) ■ The federal agency responsible for regulating (i.e., approving, licensing, and overseeing) the testing of drugs, vaccines, biological agents, and medical devices for use in humans.

frame-shifting ■ An event that sometimes occurs during the synthesis of some HIV proteins. Frame-shifting occurs when a ribosome that is reading a molecule of MESSENGER RNA (mRNA) pauses, jumps backward one base, then continues reading the mRNA (i.e., the ribosome's "reading frame" is thus shifted by one base). Frame-shifting results in the production of HIV FUSION PROTEINS.

full-blown AIDS ■ Late stage of HIV infection with manifestations of AIDS-defining diseases such as OPPORTUNISTIC INFECTIONS or certain CANCERS.

fungus (plural: fungi) ■ Primitive plant-like organisms that include the yeasts. A number of OPPORTUNISTIC INFECTIONS are caused by fungi.

fusin ■ A CHEMOKINE receptor. Also known as CXC-chemokine receptor-4, or CXCR-4. HIV binds with fusin, along with the CD4 molecule, to successfully infect helper T cells.

fusion protein ■ A POLYPROTEIN that results from FRAME-SHIFTING. A fusion protein is produced by one long MESSENGER RNA that carries information from two different genes.

***gag* gene** ■ The HIV gene that contains information for the production of the capsid protein (see CAPSID), MATRIX PROTEIN, NUCLEIC ACID–BINDING PROTEIN, and PROLINE-RICH PROTEIN.

gamma globulin ■ A protein fraction from blood that is rich in antibodies. Gamma globulin pooled from many blood donors is sometimes used to prevent or reduce the symptoms of measles, chickenpox, and other diseases.

gastrointestinal (GI) tract ■ The stomach and intestines.

gene ■ A specific sequence of NUCLEOTIDES in DNA or RNA that specifies, or is encoded with, the structure of a PROTEIN. The array of genes that are active in a cell determines the cell's function. Genes in eggs and sperm pass parental characteristics to offspring. See also CHROMOSOME.

gene expression ■ The production of MESSENGER RNA (mRNA) or PROTEIN by a gene. If the mRNA or the protein encoded by a specific gene is detectable in a given cell, the gene is said to be expressed, or active. If no trace of a given mRNA or protein is detectable, the gene is said to be inactive.

gene product ■ General name for the mRNA or protein specified by a gene.

generic name ■ One of at least three names that can be used when referring to a drug. The generic name is the name used when referring to the drug during clinical trials, in medical-research papers, and usually in references by the media. The generic name of a drug is never capitalized; for example, the generic name of ddI is didanosine. Compare with BRAND NAME and CHEMICAL NAME.

genetic engineering ■ The process of removing one or more genes from one cell and splicing them into the chromosomes of another cell. The second cell can be of the same or a different species. See also RECOMBINANT PROTEIN.

genetic variability ■ The effect of chance mutations or the mixing of genes from two different organisms that results in genetic change from one generation to the next.

genital ■ Relating to the sexual organs.

genome ■ The complete set of one species' genes such as those that exist in the set of 23 chromosomes present in a human egg or sperm. Also, the complete set of genes for a virus or other microbe.

genomic RNA ■ RNA that carries genetic information in retroviruses and other RNA viruses.

genotype ■ The genetic makeup of an organism or group of related organisms. In HIV, the name for a genotypic subtype is CLADE.

germ cell ■ An egg or sperm cell.

gingiva ■ The gums of the mouth.

glycoprotein ■ A molecule that consists of protein and sugar. Abbreviated "gp."

glycosylation ■ The biochemical process in cells in which a sugar entity is added to a PROTEIN to make a GLYCOPROTEIN.

gonorrhea ■ A scxually transmitted disease that causes INFLAMMATION of the MUCOUS MEMBRANES of the sexual organs. It can also affect mucous membranes of the eye, mouth and throat, rectum, and joints.

gp41 ■ The GLYCOPROTEIN that anchors the GP120 glycoprotein in HIV's envelope.

gp120 ■ The GLYCOPROTEIN that forms the knobs that project from HIV's envelope.

gp160 ■ A POLYPROTEIN produced during HIV REPLICATION. The gp160 molecule is subsequently cleaved to form the gp120 and gp41 envelope proteins.

gram ■ A metric unit of weight equivalent to about 1/28th of an ounce.

granulocytes ■ WHITE BLOOD CELLS that when stained and examined under the microscope are shown to have granules in their cytoplasm. There are three types of granulocytes: NEUTROPHILS, EOSINOPHILS, and BASOPHILS.

granuloma ■ A capsule of immune-system cells, primarily MACROPHAGES, that forms around certain sites of infection to contain and control the infectious agent.

gray matter ■ Tissue of the brain and spinal cord that has a brownish-gray color and consists primarily of nerve-cell bodies.

helical virus ■ A virus with a CAPSID composed of repeating protein subunits (CAPSOMERS) that are stacked in a spiraling fashion to form a cylinder.

helper T lymphocyte ■ A type of lymphocyte that plays an important role in co-ordinating both ANTIBODY-MEDIATED and CELL-MEDIATED IMMUNE RESPONSES. Also known as CD4 lymphocyte. Helper T lymphocytes are rapidly killed by infection with HIV.

hemophilia ■ A disorder of the blood clotting system that is treated through the administration of CLOTTING FACTORS.

hemopoietic ■ An adjective that refers to blood-forming tissues and cells.

hepatitis ■ Inflammation of the liver usually caused by viral infection or some-times by exposure to a toxic substance. There are five types of viral hepatitis: A, B, C, D, and E, although hepatitis types D and E are uncommon in the United States.

hepato- ■ A prefix that refers to the liver.

herpes simplex virus (HSV) ■ A virus responsible for two common types of in-fections. HSV type 1 (HSV-1) is primarily responsible for cold sores or fever blis-ters that develop around the mouth and nose; HSV type 2 (HSV-2) is the most frequent cause of genital herpes.

herpesvirus ■ Any virus that belongs to the virus family Herpesviridae. They include HERPES SIMPLEX VIRUS type 1 (human herpesvirus 1), herpes simplex virus type 2 (human herpesvirus 2), VARICELLA-ZOSTER VIRUS (human her-pesvirus 3), EPSTEIN-BARR VIRUS (human herpesvirus 4), CYTOMEGALOVIRUS (human herpesvirus 5), and the virus associated with Kaposi's sarcoma (human herpesvirus 8).

high risk ■ An epidemiological concept that is useful for monitoring the spread of an epidemic. At each stage of the HIV epidemic, certain groups of people have been at higher risk for acquiring and transmitting the disease than others. These have included men who have sex with men, injection drug users and their sex partners, and, in the early years of the epidemic, hemophiliacs and transfusion recipients and their sex partners.

histoplasmosis ■ An OPPORTUNISTIC INFECTION caused by the fungus *Histo-plasma capsulatum* that primarily affects the lungs, although it can disseminate to other areas of the body.

HIV ■ The HUMAN IMMUNODEFICIENCY VIRUS.

HIV-1 ■ See HUMAN IMMUNODEFICIENCY VIRUS.

HIV-2 ■ See HUMAN IMMUNODEFICIENCY VIRUS.

HIV encephalopathy ■ See AIDS DEMENTIA COMPLEX.

HIV headache ■ A headache experienced during HIV disease, the cause of which is not understood. It sometimes indicates a systemic infection, or it may be due to blood-borne CYTOKINES that act on blood vessels in the brain.

HIV particle ■ A single HIV VIRION.

HIV positive ■ The immune status of a person who has been confirmed by two different tests to have ANTIBODIES or ANTIGENS to HIV in his or her blood. Such a person is infected with HIV and can transmit it to others.

HLA ■ See HUMAN LEUKOCYTE-ASSOCIATED ANTIGEN. Known today as MAJOR HISTOCOMPATIBILITY COMPLEX (MHC) MOLECULES.

home specimen-collection kits ■ Kits that are purchased over the counter from pharmacies for the self-collection, in the privacy of one's own home, of blood samples to be mailed in for HIV testing under conditions that protect the user's anonymity. Home specimen-collection kits are a form of ENZYME-LINKED IMMUNOSORBENT ASSAY (ELISA) known as a DOT BLOT.

horizontal transmission ■ Transmission of a PATHOGEN from one person to another in a population (as opposed to vertical transmission, which occurs from mother to child).

hospice ■ A program that provides pain control, symptom relief, and support services to dying persons and their families.

human immunodeficiency virus (HIV) ■ The VIRUS responsible for HIV disease and AIDS. There are two types of HIV, designated HIV-1 and HIV-2. HIV-1 is the virus that causes HIV disease and AIDS worldwide. HIV-2 is rare in the United States and is found primarily in West Africa. HIV-2 also causes an immune deficiency disease, but its rate of progression is slower.

human leukocyte-associated antigen (HLA) ■ Former name for MAJOR HISTOCOMPATIBILITY COMPLEX (MHC) MOLECULES.

humoral ■ Pertaining to blood or other bodily fluids, or to a substance found in a bodily fluid.

humoral immune response ■ Same as ANTIBODY-MEDIATED IMMUNE RESPONSE.

hypergammaglobulinemia ■ An increased production of GAMMA GLOBULIN proteins seen in HIV and other chronic infectious diseases.

hyperplasia ■ An increase in the number of cells in a tissue or organ.

hypoxia ■ An insufficient level of oxygen in the blood and tissues.

icosahedral virus ■ A virus with a CAPSID consisting of an icosahedron, a sphere-like structure composed of 20 identical triangular faces.

IL-2 ■ See INTERLEUKIN-2.

IL-12 ■ See INTERLEUKIN-12.

immune deficiency ■ An impairment of the immune system. In HIV disease, immune deficiency results from the loss of HELPER T CELLS and other immune-system cells, a loss of regulation of the immune system, and damage to the structure of LYMPH NODES, the THYMUS, and the SPLEEN.

immune response ■ The total reaction of the immune system to the presence of a foreign ANTIGEN in the body. It can include an ANTIBODY-MEDIATED IMMUNE RESPONSE, a CELL-MEDIATED IMMUNE RESPONSE, and other reactions.

immunogen ■ A substance capable of inducing an IMMUNE RESPONSE. Same as ANTIGEN.

immunoglobulins ■ General term for the antibody proteins. There are five families of immunoglobulins: IgA, IgD, IgE, IgG, and IgM.

immunosuppression ■ Prevention or interference with the development of an IMMUNE RESPONSE. It may be induced by drugs, radiation, or other agents, or by disease.

incidence ■ The number of new CASES of a disease occurring in a population during a specific period of time. For example, the worldwide incidence of HIV infection is 16,000 new cases per year.

indeterminate ■ The result of a CONFIRMATORY TEST for HIV that does not meet the criteria for either a positive test or a negative test result. For example, a WESTERN BLOT is positive for HIV if it detects antibodies to two of the following HIV proteins: P24, GP41, GP120, or GP160. If no bands are present, the result is negative. If only a single band is present or the wrong combination of bands is present, the result is indeterminate.

indirect immunofluorescence assay (IFA) ■ A type of test that like the WESTERN BLOT, is used to confirm the positive results of an ENZYME-LINKED IMMUNOSORBENT ASSAY (ELISA).

infection ■ The establishment and multiplication of a PATHOGEN in the body.

infectious disease ■ A disease caused by growth of a pathogenic organism in the body. An infectious disease may or may not be CONTAGIOUS.

inflammation ■ The body's reaction to tissue damage. Inflammation is characterized by swelling, redness, heat, and pain. WHITE BLOOD CELLS move into the damaged tissue to destroy infecting microbes and clean up biological debris. This sets the stage for tissue healing, but it can also lead to a pathological condition that requires treatment. The suffix "-itis" indicates inflammation (e.g., hepatitis is inflammation of the liver).

informed consent ■ The voluntary consent given by a person (or a parent or guardian) before participating in a CLINICAL TRIAL, or experimental immunization program after being informed of its purpose, procedures, risks, and benefits. Informed consent requires that the individual comprehend the explanation of the study or procedure, freely give his or her consent without duress or undue influence, and understand that he or she has the right to withdraw at any time.

injection drug user (IDU) ■ An individual who injects drugs because of addiction or other nonmedical purpose.

integrase ■ The HIV ENZYME that incorporates HIV's PROVIRUS into a CHROMOSOME of the host cell.

interferons ■ A group of diverse CYTOKINES produced by infected cells in response to viruses, foreign NUCLEIC ACIDS, or ANTIGENS. Interferons have mainly antiviral and cell-growth inhibitor activities.

interleukins ■ A family of diverse CYTOKINES released by LYMPHOCYTES and important to the regulation of IMMUNE RESPONSES.

interleukin-2 (IL-2) ■ A CYTOKINE that stimulates the proliferation of T LYMPHOCYTES, NATURAL KILLER CELLS, and B LYMPHOCYTES

interleukin-12 (IL-12) ■ A CYTOKINE that has a variety of effects on immune cells. IL-12 stimulates the activity of a subgroup of HELPER T CELLS known as helper T cells type 1, or TH1 cells. TH1 cells are important in activating CYTOTOXIC T CELLS and the CELL-MEDIATED IMMUNE RESPONSE, believed to be important in fighting HIV.

intracellular ■ Within the cell.

in vitro ■ Latin for "in glass." The study of biological systems, organs, cells, or parts of cells outside the body.

in vivo ■ Latin for "in the living body." The study of biological processes, organs, or cells in living organisms.

Kaposi's sarcoma (KS) ■ The most common form of CANCER in people with HIV disease, occurring predominately in homosexual males. KS is a MALIGNANCY of the cells of the walls of certain blood vessels. It produces one to many purple, pink, or red spots, patches, or nodules. The lesions usually occur on the face, neck, chest, or back, but they can arise in internal organs as well. KS has been linked to a HERPESVIRUS (human herpesvirus 8).

killer T cell ■ Same as CYTOTOXIC T LYMPHOCYTE.

kilobase ■ A unit of length along a molecule of SINGLE-STRANDED DNA or RNA that equals 1,000 BASES.

kilobase pairs ■ A unit of length along a molecule of DOUBLE-STRANDED DNA or RNA that equals 1,000 BASE PAIRS.

lactating ■ Breast-feeding.

lamivudine (3TC) ■ An ANTIRETROVIRAL drug and NUCLEOSIDE ANALOGUE REVERSE TRANSCRIPTASE INHIBITOR. Lamivudine is an analogue of the nucleoside cytidine.

Langerhans' cells ■ The historical name of DENDRITIC CELLS present in the skin.

late HIV disease ■ A term that is sometimes applied to HIV disease when the CD4 lymphocyte count drops below 50 to 100 cells per mm^3.

latent infection ■ A type of CHRONIC INFECTION in which a VIRUS or other microbe establishes a lifelong infection that remains ASYMPTOMATIC until certain circumstances reactivate it. Reactivation then produces an acute infection until the immune system again brings it under control. HERPES SIMPLEX VIRUS, for example, establishes a latent infection of nerve cells until conditions occur that activate the virus, which then produces cold sores or genital ulcers.

lean body mass ■ The nonfat tissue mass of the body, particularly the muscle. There are losses in lean body mass, along with fat tissue, during HIV-associated WASTING.

lentivirus ■ The subfamily of RETROVIRUSES to which HIV-1 and HIV-2 belong. Lentiviruses also include SIMIAN IMMUNODEFICIENCY VIRUS (SIV) and feline (cat) immunodeficiency virus (FIV).

lesion ■ An injury, wound, or change in a part of the body due to disease or injury. Examples of lesions include cuts, abrasions, vesicles, pustules, chancres, and tumors.

leukocytes ■ A generic name for WHITE BLOOD CELLS.

ligand ■ A substance or molecule that binds with a CELL-SURFACE RECEPTOR. For example, the cytokine interleukin-2 (IL-2) is the ligand for the IL-2 receptor; the chemokine SDF-1 is the ligand for the CXCR-4 receptor.

lipid bilayer ■ Fluid-like double layer of lipids that constitutes the CELL MEMBRANE and the envelope of HIV virions.

lipids ■ The category of organic molecules that includes the fats, oils, waxes, and steroids.

liposomes ■ Hollow, microscopic spheres of fat (i.e., LIPID) that are produced in the laboratory and are being tested as a means of encapsulating drugs and genes for use in the body.

living will ■ A document that directs a physician to use or withhold life-sustaining procedures if a person is permanently unconscious or in a terminal condition.

log ■ In mathematics, a log is a factor of ten. VIRAL-LOAD measurements are sometimes reported as a log of the number of copies of a viral genome (i.e., log copy number) per MILLILITER of blood. A 1-log change in viral load is the same as a tenfold change in the number of copies of the viral genome.

long terminal repeats (LTRs) ■ Extensions of genetic material at each end of the HIV PROVIRUS. The LTRs enable the provirus to be inserted into a host chromosome, and they play a major role in regulating the production of viral proteins.

long-term nonprogressors ■ HIV-infected individuals who show very low and steady levels of HIV in their blood, and normal or nearly normal CD4 cell counts for more than 10 to 15 years. Long-term nonprogressors make up 5% to 7% of all HIV-infected individuals.

lymph ■ Clear yellowish fluid that drains from the tissues and enters the vessels of the LYMPHOID SYSTEM.

lymphadenopathy ■ General term for disease that affects the LYMPH NODES.

lymphadenopathy-associated virus (LAV) ■ The original name given to the AIDS virus discovered by French researchers. Later renamed HIV.

lymph nodes ■ Organs of the lymphatic system consisting of rounded capsules that vary in size from that of a pinhead to that of an olive. Lymph nodes are the sites where the major events occur that lead to an immune response. Lymph nodes are located throughout the body, with clusters occurring in the neck, in the armpits, along the back wall of the abdomen, and in the groin. Together with the SPLEEN, lymph nodes contain about 95% of the adult body's lymphocytes.

lymphocyte count ■ The number of HELPER T LYMPHOCYTES in a cubic millimeter (mm^3) of blood. Helper T lymphocyte counts are used as a measure of the health of a patient's immune system. (Helper T lymphocytes are also known as CD4 lymphocytes or CD4 cells. Helper T lymphocyte count is also known as the CD4 cell count.)

lymphocytes ■ A class of WHITE BLOOD CELLS that have a major role in attacking pathogens in the body. See ANTIBODY-MEDIATED IMMUNE RESPONSE and CELL-MEDIATED IMMUNE RESPONSE.

lymphoid interstitial pneumonitis (LIP) ■ A disease that occurs primarily in children with HIV disease. It is characterized by the gradual accumulation of lymphoid cells and other white blood cells in the tissues of the lung. It produces a chronic, diffuse pneumonia.

lymphoid system ■ The lymphoid system consists of the primary lymphoid organs, the secondary lymphoid organs, and the lymphatic fluid and vessels. Primary lymphoid organs are the LYMPH NODES and SPLEEN. Secondary lymphoid organs include the tonsils and adenoids and the diffuse lymphoid tissue (collections of lymphocytes in the skin and beneath the membranes that line the digestive and respiratory systems; Peyer's patches are examples of diffuse lymphoid tissues in the intestines).

lymphokine ■ A CYTOKINE secreted by a LYMPHOCYTE.

lymphoma ■ A form of cancer that arises in T LYMPHOCYTES and B LYMPHOCYTES. Lymphomas that occur in B lymphocytes are known as B-cell lymphomas; lymphomas that occur in T lymphocytes are known as T-cell lymphomas.

lyse ■ To break apart or open. Certain viruses lyse cells when they escape from them.

lysosome ■ Vesicles in the CYTOPLASM of cells that contain ENZYMES for the digestion of substances taken up by the cell.

lytic viruses ■ Viruses that rupture, or lyse, the host cell during their release from the cell.

MAC ■ See *MYCOBACTERIUM AVIUM* COMPLEX.

macrophage ■ An immune-system cell derived from MONOCYTES that travels through the tissues of the body and plays important roles in the CELL-MEDIATED IMMUNE RESPONSE. Macrophages are both ANTIGEN-PRESENTING CELLS and PHAGOCYTES. As a phagocyte, macrophages engulf microbes and other antigens. As antigen-presenting cells, macrophages display antigens on their surface where the antigen can be detected by helper T cells and thereby stimulate an immune response.

maintenance therapy ■ Therapy given to prevent the recurrence of any disease, including OPPORTUNISTIC INFECTION. Same as SECONDARY PROPHYLAXIS or SUPPRESSIVE THERAPY.

major histocompatibility complex (MHC) ■ The group of genes that produce MAJOR HISTOCOMPATIBILITY COMPLEX (MHC) MOLECULES.

major histocompatibility complex (MHC) molecules ■ Molecules that display ANTIGENS on the surface of cells. There are two classes of MHC molecules, class

I MHC and class II MHC. Class I MHC molecules are produced by all cells; they display bits of proteins that are produced within the cell. Class II MHC molecules are found only on ANTIGEN-PRESENTING CELLS; they display proteins that have come from outside the cell.

malabsorption ■ Inadequate absorption of nutrients by the GASTROINTESTINAL TRACT.

malignancy ■ A MALIGNANT TUMOR. Same as CANCER.

malignant tumor ■ A tumor that can invade other tissues and spread to other areas of the body, and lead to death. CANCER is a general name for a malignant tumor.

malnutrition ■ Condition resulting from inadequate nutrition, or malabsorption of foods.

matrix protein ■ The layer of viral protein that lies between the VIRAL ENVELOPE and the CAPSID and that maintains the structure of the VIRION. In HIV, the matrix protein (MA) is p17.

mediate ■ To bring about or influence. Used in a variety of biological situations. Cells, hormones, and CYTOKINES can mediate biological events. For example, helper T cells mediate immune responses.

memory lymphocytes/memory cells ■ Lymphocytes produced during an ANTIBODY-MEDIATED IMMUNE RESPONSE that do not produce large amounts of ANTIBODY, but instead serve to maintain a molecular record of an ANTIGEN. They remain in the body, ready to promote a prompt immune response should the antigen enter the body again.

meninges ■ The membranes that surround the brain and spinal cord.

messenger RNA (mRNA) ■ A copy of a gene. It is assembled in the nucleus during TRANSCRIPTION, the first phase of PROTEIN SYNTHESIS. The molecule of mRNA then travels to the cell CYTOPLASM where the genetic information it carries is used to assemble a PROTEIN during the phase of protein synthesis known as TRANSLATION.

metabolism ■ The sum of all chemical processes through which cells obtain energy and building materials from food and respiration to grow, divide, and maintain life. Metabolism occurs through thousands of precisely regulated chemical reactions that take place simultaneously throughout life.

metastatic tumor ■ A tumor that has spread from its original site to LYMPH NODES or other sites in the body. Metastatic tumors arise when cancer cells are carried by the LYMPHOID SYSTEM or blood system from the original, or primary, tumor to other organs.

MHC molecules ■ See MAJOR HISTOCOMPATIBILITY COMPLEX (MHC) MOLECULES.

microbe ■ Any single-celled organisms such as bacteria and protozoa. Although they are not cells, viruses can be called microbes.

microglial cells ■ MACROPHAGES that are found in the brain.

micron ■ A metric unit of length that equals one-millionth of a meter (10^{-6} meter). Represented by the Greek letter μ.

microsporidiosis ■ A protozoal infection that is thought to be a cause of diarrhea in many HIV-positive patients.

milligram (mg) ■ A metric unit of weight that equals one-thousandth of a gram. A gram is about 1/28th of an ounce.

milliliter (ml) ■ A metric measure of volume equal to one-thousandth of a liter (i.e., there are 1,000 ml in a liter). One milliliter is about one-fifth of a teaspoon.

molecule ■ The smallest unit of a substance that carries the properties of that substance. Molecules are made up of atoms; for example, two atoms of hydrogen combine with one atom of oxygen to form H_2O, or one molecule of water. At the level of the cell, many substances exist as individual molecules.

monocyte ■ A WHITE BLOOD CELL that can leave blood vessels and undergo changes in function and appearance to become a MACROPHAGE.

mononuclear cells ■ A generic name for LYMPHOCYTES and MONOCYTES; all WHITE BLOOD CELLS that have a single, nearly round NUCLEUS.

monotherapy ■ The use of a single drug to treat a disease. An example of monotherapy is the previous use of AZT alone to treat HIV infection.

mucous membrane ■ A tissue that lines the various cavities and tubular organs of the body (like the mouth, rectum, digestive tract, and the internal passages of genital tract). It consists of several layers, the topmost thin layer consists of an EPITHELIUM that secretes MUCUS.

mucus ■ A clear, viscous fluid produced by MUCOUS MEMBRANES. When used as an adjective, the word is spelled "mucous."

multidrug therapy ■ The use of two or more drugs to treat a disease. Same as COMBINATION THERAPY.

mutation ■ Spontaneous or induced change in the genetic material of cells; specifically, a mutation is a change in the sequence of DNA BASE PAIRS in a GENE.

mycobacteria ■ Bacteria belonging to the genus *Mycobacterium*, which are responsible for TUBERCULOSIS and MYCOBACTERIUM AVIUM COMPLEX.

Mycobacterium avium complex (MAC) ■ The most common bacterial OPPORTUNISTIC INFECTION in people with advanced HIV disease. It is also one of the last opportunistic infections to develop. MAC is caused by two species of bacteria, *Mycobacterium avium* and *Mycobacterium intracellulare*, which are collectively referred to as *Mycobacterium avium* complex.

myelosuppression ■ A drop in the production of WHITE BLOOD CELLS.

myristate ■ A fatty acid-containing molecule that is added to HIV's Gag POLYPROTEIN during its production in HIV-infected cells. The process of adding the fatty acid to the protein is known as myristylation. If myristylation is blocked, mature HIV particles are not formed.

myristylation ■ See MYRISTATE.

nanometer (nm) ■ A metric unit of length equal to one-billionth of a meter (1 $\times 10^{-9}$ meter). A red blood cell is about 7,000 nm in diameter.

natural immunity ■ Components of the immune system that do not require activation by ANTIGENS. They include complement proteins, NEUTROPHILS, MACROPHAGES, and NATURAL KILLER CELLS. Also known as innate or native immunity. Compare with SPECIFIC IMMUNITY.

natural killer (NK) cells ■ WHITE BLOOD CELLS that resemble LYMPHOCYTES. NK cells play an important role in destroying tumor cells and virus-infected cells.

Nef protein ■ An HIV regulatory protein produced by HIV's *nef* gene. Its role in HIV is not clearly defined.

neoplasm ■ Literally means new (neo-) growth (-plasm). An abnormal growth of cells that may or may not be precancerous. A malignant neoplasm is a cancerous tumor.

neuralgia ■ Pain that radiates from a nerve.

neurons ■ Cells of the nervous system that conduct nerve impulses.

neutralizing antibody ■ An antibody that renders a PATHOGEN noninfectious. For example, neutralizing antibodies can inhibit the ability of a virus to infect cells (note: not all antibodies that can bind to a virus can also neutralize it).

neutropenia ■ An abnormally low number of NEUTROPHILS in the blood.

neutrophil ■ A WHITE BLOOD CELL that is a PHAGOCYTE. Also known as a POLY-MORPHONUCLEAR LEUKOCYTE (i.e., a white blood cell with a nucleus that can have many shapes). Neutrophils are a type of GRANULOCYTE.

NF-κB ■ See NUCLEAR FACTOR KAPPA B.

NK cells ■ See NATURAL KILLER CELLS.

nonenveloped viruses ■ Viruses that have a naked CAPSID; that is, they do not have an outer ENVELOPE. Also known as naked viruses.

non-Hodgkin's lymphoma (NHL) ■ A form of LYMPHOMA that is the second most common cancer (after KAPOSI'S SARCOMA) in people with HIV disease.

nonnucleoside reverse transcriptase inhibitors (NNRTIs) ■ A class of ANTI-RETROVIRAL drugs that work by binding to the viral enzyme REVERSE TRANSCRIP-TASE, thereby blocking the enzyme's action.

nonproductive infection ■ An infection that is stopped by the immune system before it causes disease. Same as an ABORTIVE INFECTION.

nuclear factor kappa B (NF-κB) ■ A DNA-BINDING PROTEIN that helps regulate PROTEIN SYNTHESIS in cells. Nuclear factor kappa B also helps activate PROTEIN SYN-THESIS in the HIV PROVIRUS.

nuclear RNA ■ See RIBOZYMES.

nucleic acid ■ The family of organic molecules to which DNA and RNA belong. A general name for DNA and RNA.

nucleic acid–binding protein ■ A protein in HIV that is important for packing the RNA GENOME during assembly of new VIRIONS. The p9 protein, also known as nucleocapsid protein.

nucleoid ■ The core of a virus. Another name for CAPSID.

nucleoside ■ A nucleoside is a DNA BASE plus a molecule of ribose or deoxyri-bose sugar. See also NUCLEOTIDE.

nucleoside analogue reverse transcriptase inhibitors ■ Class of ANTIRETROVIRAL drugs that includes AZT, ddI, ddC, d4T, and 3TC. These drugs work by mimic-king nucleosides, which are needed by the HIV enzyme REVERSE TRANSCRIPTASE to build a viral DNA strand. The incorporation of a nucleoside analogue in viral DNA halts its further assembly, thereby blocking viral REPLICATION.

nucleotide ■ A nucleotide is a DNA BASE plus a molecule of ribose or deoxyri-bose sugar plus a phosphate group (an atom of phosphorus and four atoms of oxygen). Nucleotides are building blocks of DNA and RNA. See also NUCLEOSIDE.

nucleus ■ The region of the cell that contains the CHROMOSOMES. The nucleus is bound by a porous membrane, the nuclear membrane, that separates it from the other main region of the cell, the CYTOPLASM.

occupational exposure ■ Exposure to HIV or other PATHOGENS that occurs in the course of one's job.

oligonucleotide ■ A short fragment of DNA or RNA.

oncoviruses ■ The subfamily of RETROVIRUSES that contains the RNA tumor viruses. Examples include HTLV-I, HTLV-II, Rous sarcoma virus, and the feline leukemia virus.

oocyst ■ Spore-like stage in the life cycle of *Cryptosporidium,* which causes the opportunistic infection CRYPTOSPORIDIOSIS. *Cryptosporidium* infection begins with ingestion of oocysts. The parasite then passes through a multistage life cycle that ends with the production of more oocysts. These are released into the intestine to reinfect the same individual or pass out in the feces to infect new hosts.

opportunistic infections ■ Infections that arise when the immune system is suppressed. Opportunistic infections are responsible for up to 90% of all AIDS-related deaths.

oral candidiasis ■ A CANDIDIASIS infection of the mouth. Also called thrush.

oral hairy leukoplakia ■ A benign condition that produces white patches on the sides and surface of the tongue and other areas of the mouth of many individuals with HIV disease.

organelles ■ Components of cells that generate energy, process food and waste, produce proteins, and carry out specific cell functions. Cellular organelles include mitochondria, lysosomes, Golgi apparatus, and endoplasmic reticulum.

p17 (MA) ■ The HIV MATRIX PROTEIN.

p24 ■ The HIV CAPSID protein.

P450 enzyme system ■ A group of enzymes in liver and other cells that metabolizes many drugs and toxins (see METABOLISM).

pandemic ■ An epidemic that occurs worldwide.

Pap test ■ An important test for detecting cervical cancer. It involves the microscopic examination of cells scraped from the CERVIX.

parenteral ■ Occurring outside the intestine. Refers to the introduction of drugs into the body in ways other than through the mouth and the intestines, such as by injection.

pathogen ■ A virus, bacterium, protozoan, fungus, or other organism or substance that causes disease.

PBMC ■ See PERIPHERAL BLOOD MONONUCLEAR CELLS.

PCP ■ See *PNEUMOCYSTIS CARINII* PNEUMONIA.

-penia ■ A suffix that refers to a deficiency in the entity mentioned in the main body of the word. For example, leukopenia is a below-normal number of white blood cells (which is signified by the prefix "leuko-"). Neutropenia is an insufficient number of neutrophils.

peptide ■ A short chain of amino acids. See PROTEIN.

percutaneous ■ Applied or removed through the skin, such as given through injection or inoculation, or removed using a needle and syringe.

percutaneous exposure ■ Exposure to an infectious agent through a cut, abrasion, or bite that breaks the skin.

perforin ■ A PROTEIN used by CYTOTOXIC T LYMPHOCYTES and NATURAL KILLER CELLS to produce holes in the cell wall of bacteria, thereby killing them.

perianal ■ The area of anus and the surrounding skin.

perinatal ■ Occurring during birth or within a few weeks before or after birth.

perinatal HIV transmission ■ Transmission of HIV from mother to infant.

peripheral blood ■ The blood in circulation outside of the chest cavity. Also known as peripheral circulation. (The circulation of blood through the heart and lungs is known as the central circulation.)

peripheral blood mononuclear cells (PBMCs) ■ The LYMPHOCYTES, MONOCYTES, and NATURAL KILLER CELLS (all cells that have a round nucleus) found in circulating blood, as opposed to those in lymphatic organs.

peripheral nerves ■ The sensory and motor nerves outside of the CENTRAL NERVOUS SYSTEM (i.e., the brain and spinal cord).

peripheral neuropathy ■ Pain resulting from damage to PERIPHERAL NERVES, especially those of the feet and legs.

persistent generalized lymphadenopathy (PGL) ■ Chronic, generalized swelling of the LYMPH NODES. This condition occurs in many persons infected with HIV.

persistent infection ■ A chronic infection in which a VIRUS or some other PATHOGEN escapes immune system defenses and causes long-term illness.

phagocytes ■ Immune cells that engulf viruses, bacteria, and cellular debris in the blood and tissues by PHAGOCYTOSIS. Phagocytes play an important role in INFLAMMATION, wound healing, and immune defenses. NEUTROPHILS and MACROPHAGES are phagocytes.

phagocytosis ■ The cellular process through which PHAGOCYTES engulf material.

phase I clinical trial/phase I testing ■ The first stage in the clinical evaluation process. A phase I trial is the first test of an experimental drug or vaccine in humans. Its objective is to determine a safe dose of the agent in a small group of usually healthy volunteers.

phase II clinical trial/phase II testing ■ The second stage in the clinical evaluation of an experimental drug or vaccine in humans. In addition to the safety of the agent, phase II trials study its effectiveness using a small group of patient volunteers.

phase III clinical trial/phase III testing ■ The third stage in the clinical evaluation of an experimental drug or vaccine in humans. Phase III clinical trials are designed to determine the safety and efficacy of an experimental agent in a much larger number and a broader cross section of patients from those used during PHASE I and PHASE II CLINICAL TRIALS.

plasma ■ The liquid portion of blood (blood minus the cells) before the blood has time to clot.

plasma cell ■ A B LYMPHOCYTE that is producing a large quantity of antibody.

***Pneumocystis carinii* pneumonia (PCP)** ■ The most common AIDS-associated type of pneumonia. PCP is an OPPORTUNISTIC INFECTION caused by a fungus. Left untreated, PCP is life-threatening.

pneumonia ■ An inflammation of the lungs that involves the accumulation of fluid, inflammatory cells, or fibrous material in the lung's air spaces. There are more than 50 different causes of pneumonia, the most common of which are bacterial and viral infections. Some diseases (e.g., LYMPHOID INTERSTITIAL PNEUMONITIS [LIP], syphilis, rheumatic fever) are also accompanied by pneumonia.

***pol* gene** ■ HIV gene that carries information for the three viral enzymes: REVERSE TRANSCRIPTASE, INTEGRASE, and PROTEASE.

polymerase ■ An ENZYME that combines individual molecular building blocks into a long chain, or polymer. The cell uses the enzyme DNA polymerase to construct new molecules of DNA during DNA REPLICATION, and RNA polymerase to construct molecules of MESSENGER RNA during PROTEIN SYNTHESIS. HIV uses the same cellular polymerases for its own replication.

polymerase chain reaction (PCR) ■ A technique that reveals the presence of minute amounts of DNA in cells and other kinds of samples. PCR has been adapted for use as a VIRAL GENOME TEST for detecting the presence of HIV in blood and serum samples. It is so sensitive that it can detect the presence of a single HIV PROVIRUS in 100,000 cells.

polymorphonuclear leukocytes ■ Another name for NEUTROPHILS, BASOPHILS, and EOSINOPHILS because the nucleus of these cells takes many shapes.

polypeptide ■ See PROTEIN.

polyprotein ■ A short string of protein molecules that is produced from a single long mRNA. Polyproteins are sometimes referred to as pre-proteins.

positive predictive value ■ The probability that a positive result of a medical test is truly positive.

post-test counseling ■ Counseling given when someone is being told the result—whether positive or negative—of a blood test for HIV infection.

power of attorney ■ A legal document that authorizes a person to make health-care decisions for someone who is unable to make such decisions for himself or herself.

PPD test ■ The tuberculin skin test. PPD stands for purified protein derivative, which refers to proteins derived from dead tuberculosis bacteria that are used in the test.

precancerous ■ Cells that show an abnormal growth pattern or changes in appearance that indicate that they could become cancerous with time.

preclinical testing/preclinical research ■ The testing of a drug, vaccine, or other agent in cultured cells and animals. Preclinical testing helps determine the safety, toxicity, tolerated dose, side effects, and mechanism of action of experimental agents prior to trials in humans.

pre-protein ■ Same as a POLYPROTEIN.

pretest counseling ■ Counseling given to someone prior to a blood test for HIV infection.

prevalence ■ The proportion or percent of a population that has a disease (or some other characteristic) at a specific point in time. See INCIDENCE.

primary infection ■ Another name for the ACUTE STAGE of HIV infection.

primary prophylaxis ■ Treatment or any public health measure used to prevent an initial infection.

primary tumor ■ A malignant tumor found in the tissue in which it originated. Compare with METASTATIC TUMOR.

prognosis ■ Prediction of the course of a disease and the prospect for recovery.

progressive multifocal leukoencephalopathy (PML) ■ An OPPORTUNISTIC INFECTION of the white matter of the brain caused by the JC virus (the initials are those of the patient from whom the virus was first isolated).

proline-rich protein ■ An HIV protein that is important for assembly and release of VIRIONS.

promoter ■ A region within the REGULATORY SEGMENT of a gene that is the primary on-off switch for the gene. A gene is activated when DNA-BINDING PROTEINS bind to the promoter. The promoter region is also where gene TRANSCRIPTION begins.

prophylactic therapy ■ The use of a treatment to prevent a disease from occurring (prophylactic means "preventative"). Also known as chemoprophylaxis when drugs are used. See also PRIMARY PROPHYLAXIS and SECONDARY PROPHYLAXIS (the latter is also known as suppressive therapy).

prophylaxis ■ The use of PROPHYLACTIC THERAPY.

protease ■ Any ENZYME that cleaves a larger protein into smaller pieces. HIV has a protease enzyme that is necessary for the production of new viable VIRIONS. Cells also have their own protease enzymes.

protease inhibitors ■ A class of ANTIRETROVIRAL drugs that block the production of infectious HIV virions by inhibiting the action of HIV's PROTEASE enzyme.

protein ■ A molecule made up of one or more chains of amino acids. Proteins may have from approximately 50 to several thousand amino acids. Molecules consisting of only a few amino acids are called PEPTIDES; extra long and complex proteins are POLYPEPTIDES.

protein synthesis ■ The production of proteins in cells.

protocol ■ A document outlining precisely how a clinical trial has to be conducted. It describes such things as which patients are eligible for the trial, how and when patients are scheduled to receive treatment, what laboratory tests are required, and how the trial's outcome is to be evaluated.

protozoa ■ One-celled animals, some species of which cause disease. A number of OPPORTUNISTIC INFECTIONS are caused by certain protozoa that live in cells as parasites.

provirus ■ HIV DNA that has fused with and become a permanent part of a CHROMOSOME in a host cell.

pseudovirions ■ HIV-like particles that are being tested for use as protective vaccines. Pseudovirions have much of the outer structure of a normal HIV particle but do not contain viral genes.

purine ■ Chemical group to which the BASES adenine and guanine belong.

pyrimidine ■ Chemical group to which the BASES cytosine, thymine (found in DNA), and uracil (found in RNA) belong.

quantitative competitive PCR (QC-PCR) ■ A VIRAL GENOME TEST that is a modified form of the POLYMERASE CHAIN REACTION (PCR). It differs from the PCR test in that it also reveals the amount of virus present.

receptor molecule ■ A molecule on or inside the cell that binds with another molecule to cause a change to occur inside the cell. There are two categories of receptor molecules: CELL-SURFACE RECEPTORS are found on the outside surface of cells; steroid receptors are located in the cell NUCLEUS and are triggered by steroid hormones. A molecule that binds with a receptor is a LIGAND.

recognition proteins ■ Proteins on the surface of a cell that identify it to other cells. Recognition proteins are used by immune cells to recognize the cells with which they come in contact.

recombinant DNA technology ■ The body of techniques that enable the production of RECOMBINANT PROTEINS.

recombinant protein ■ A protein obtained by removing the gene responsible for that protein from the animal in which it is normally found and transplanting it into the chromosome of a bacterium or other cell. The bacterium, which can easily be grown in large quantities, then produces the protein in large amounts for use in research as a vaccine or as a drug. This technology is also known as recombinant DNA technology, or, more loosely, as GENETIC ENGINEERING.

regimen ■ A program of treatment.

regulatory cells ■ General term for HELPER T LYMPHOCYTES because they regulate IMMUNE RESPONSES.

regulatory proteins ■ Proteins that play a role in activating and deactivating genes.

regulatory segment (of a gene) ■ The region of a gene that controls the activity of the gene and contains the PROMOTER and ENHANCER regions. Compare with STRUCTURAL SEGMENT.

replication ■ In DNA replication, the process by which cellular DNA is duplicated prior to cell division. In viral replication, the process by which a virus produces new virus particles, or VIRIONS.

respite care ■ A community or HOSPICE program that provides relief to someone caring for a seriously ill person in the home. Respite care provides time for the caregiver to attend to other responsibilities or to get much-needed rest.

retina ■ The light-sensitive tissues that line the back of the eye.

retinitis ■ Inflammation or infection of the eye. CMV RETINITIS is an infection of the eye by CYTOMEGALOVIRUS. Left untreated, it results in blindness.

retrovirus ■ A virus with an RNA genome retro-transcribed into DNA during its REPLICATION cycle. The strand of DNA then becomes integrated into a CHROMOSOME of the infected cell, where it remains for the life of the cell.

reverse transcriptase ■ An enzyme found in RETROVIRUSES and a few other viruses that enables them to make a DNA copy of their RNA genome.

reverse transcriptase inhibitor ■ An ANTIRETROVIRAL drug that works by inhibiting the enzyme REVERSE TRANSCRIPTASE. Includes NUCLEOSIDE ANALOGUE REVERSE TRANSCRIPTASE INHIBITORS (e.g., AZT) and NONNUCLEOSIDE REVERSE TRANSCRIPTASE INHIBITORS (e.g., delavirdine).

ribonucleic acids (RNAs) ■ Ribonucleic acids are molecules built of the BASES adenine, cytosine, guanine, and uracil and a backbone of ribose sugar molecules linked by phosphate groups. Human cells contain four main forms of RNA: MESSENGER RNA, ribosomal RNA, TRANSFER RNA, and RIBOZYMES, all of which are involved in PROTEIN SYNTHESIS. The GENOME of certain viruses is also composed of RNA.

ribosomes ■ Submicroscopic structures found in the cell's CYTOPLASM that play a major role in PROTEIN SYNTHESIS. Ribosomes travel along a strand of MESSENGER RNA (mRNA), read its message, and help link amino acids in the proper order to build a protein molecule.

ribozymes ■ Enzyme-like molecules found in the cell nucleus that contain RNA. Ribozymes process and "edit" MESSENGER RNA (mRNA) before it leaves the nucleus during PROTEIN SYNTHESIS.

RNA ■ See RIBONUCLEIC ACIDS.

RNase H ■ An enzyme that is part of HIV's REVERSE TRANSCRIPTASE enzyme. RNase H degrades the virus's original RNA genome after it is copied as DNA during replication.

RT inhibitor ■ See REVERSE TRANSCRIPTASE INHIBITOR.

safer sex ■ Sexual practices, such as the use of condoms during every act of sexual intercourse and barriers during oral sex, that greatly reduce the risk of HIV transmission.

sarcoma ■ A malignancy that arises in muscle, connective tissue, bone, and organs that include the liver, lungs, spleen, and kidneys. KAPOSI'S SARCOMA is a malignancy of the lining of certain blood vessels.

scabies ■ A skin eruption caused by the mite *Sarcoptes scabiei.*

screening test ■ A test that is relatively fast and easy to perform and that can detect the presence or possibility of disease in a population.

secondary prophylaxis ■ Treatment that is used to prevent an infection from recurring. Same as suppressive therapy.

secondary tumor ■ Same as a METASTATIC TUMOR.

sense ■ A property of viruses with a GENOME made of a single strand of RNA (ssRNA). Sense refers to whether the single strand of RNA can by itself direct viral protein synthesis in host cells. The sense of a SINGLE-STRANDED RNA (ssRNA) virus can be positive (+) or negative (−). When a ssRNA genome with positive sense is injected into a cell, it will produce new virions as if the entire virus had entered the cell; that is, the viral genome behaves as if it were a MESSENGER RNA (mRNA), and it is translated into viral proteins. When a ssRNA genome with negative sense is injected into a cell, no viral proteins are produced.

sensitivity (of a test) ■ A measure of the number of false negatives a diagnostic test is estimated to produce. A test with high sensitivity produces a low number of false-negative results. Compare with SPECIFICITY.

septicemia ■ The presence of bacteria, other infectious organisms, or their toxins in the blood. Sometimes also known as blood poisoning.

sero- ■ A prefix referring to blood serum.

seroconversion ■ The development of detectable antibody in blood serum. Following infection with HIV, a person will test positive by the standard antibody ENZYME-LINKED IMMUNOSORBENT ASSAY for HIV.

seronegative ■ The absence of a specific ANTIBODY in the blood. Being seronegative for an antibody is taken to mean that the person has never been infected by a specific agent. A person who is serogenative for VARICELLA-ZOSTER VIRUS (VZV) lacks antibodies to the virus and is therefore at risk for developing either chickenpox or SHINGLES from someone who has either of those diseases, both of which are caused by VZV.

seropositive ■ The presence in the blood of antibodies against a specific pathogen; indicative of infection with this pathogen.

serum ■ The watery portion of the blood that remains after blood has clotted. See PLASMA.

set point ■ A persistent and fairly stable level of HIV in the blood (VIRAL LOAD) that is established usually six months to a year after HIV infection. The set point varies with the individual. High set points are correlated with faster loss of CD4 cells, more rapid disease progression, and shorter survival.

shedding, virus ■ The release of viruses into an area of the body that enables them to spread from one person, or host, to another. The site of virus shedding depends on the virus. Respiratory viruses are usually shed into the respiratory tract, whereas sexually transmitted viruses are shed primarily into semen and vaginal secretions.

shingles ■ Eruption of skin vesicles on an area of the body served by a nerve. Shingles is caused by the VARICELLA-ZOSTER VIRUS (VZV), which is also responsible for chickenpox. The eruptions result from the activation of a latent VZV infection acquired during a childhood case of chickenpox.

side effect ■ An action or effect of a drug or treatment that occurs in addition to the desired effect. It is usually, but not always, an undesirable effect such as nausea, headache, or a drop in the number of WHITE BLOOD CELLS.

simian immunodeficiency virus (SIV) ■ A RETROVIRUS that occurs harmlessly in many African monkeys and in chimpanzees but that causes an AIDS-like illness in Asian monkeys.

single-stranded DNA (ssDNA) ■ A form of DNA that consists of a single strand. The GENOME of some DNA viruses consists of ssDNA (compare with DOUBLE-STRANDED DNA).

single-stranded RNA (ssRNA) ■ An RNA molecule that consists of a single strand. The GENOME of many RNA viruses consists of ssRNA.

sinusitis ■ Inflammation of the sinuses.

SIV ■ See SIMIAN IMMUNODEFICIENCY VIRUS.

slow progressors ■ HIV-infected individuals who for more than ten years after infection have developed few or no symptoms of HIV disease and only a small, slow drop in CD4 lymphocyte numbers. Fewer than 5% of people who are HIV positive are slow progressors.

somatic cells ■ All cells in the body that contain two sets of CHROMOSOMES (red blood cells, which have no nucleus, and therefore no chromosomes, are also somatic cells). All cells in the body except eggs and sperm (which are known as germ cells and have only one set of chromosomes) are somatic cells.

specific immunity ■ Immune responses that are induced or stimulated by exposure to an ANTIGEN, and are specifically mounted against it. Includes both antibody-mediated immunity and cell-mediated immunity. Also known as acquired immunity. Compare with NATURAL IMMUNITY.

specificity (of a test) ■ A measure of the number of false positives a diagnostic test produces. A test with high specificity produces a low number of false-positive results. Compare with SENSITIVITY.

spinal cord ■ A column of nervous tissue that runs from the brain down most of the length of the spinal column (i.e., backbone). All the nerves that serve the chest, abdomen, arms, and legs issue from the spinal cord.

spleen ■ A soft, spongy organ of the immune system that lies on the left side of the body somewhat behind the stomach. The spleen has a rich blood circulation and is the primary site of IMMUNE RESPONSES to ANTIGENS that occur in the bloodstream.

splenomegaly ■ Enlarged spleen.

spore ■ A reproductive cell produced by fungi and some protozoans. Spores usually possess a thick wall that enables them to tolerate harsh environmental conditions.

stavudine (d4T) ■ An ANTIRETROVIRAL drug and NUCLEOSIDE ANALOGUE REVERSE TRANSCRIPTASE INHIBITOR. An analogue of the nucleoside thymidine.

stem cell ■ A cell that gives rise to other cells. Blood cells, for example, are derived from HEMOPOIETIC stem cells present in the BONE MARROW.

stomatitis ■ Inflammation of the MUCOUS MEMBRANES of the mouth.

structural segment (of a gene) ■ The region of a gene that codes for (contains the information for) the amino acid sequence of a protein (compare with REGULATORY SEGMENT).

suppressive therapy ■ Same as SECONDARY PROPHYLAXIS.

surrogate markers/end points ■ A change in a laboratory measurement or in a disease sign, other than a clinical response such as longer survival or fewer OPPORTUNISTIC INFECTIONS, that signals a response to treatment. Examples of surrogate markers in HIV disease are CD4 lymphocyte count and VIRAL LOAD. If a patient's average CD4 count remains stable or increases following treatment, it is regarded as a sign that the treatment is effective. An increase in viral load (the amount of free virus in the blood) is regarded as an indication of disease progression. Surrogate markers are often used to measure responses to experimental treatments during a clinical trial because changes in a surrogate marker occur more quickly than do changes in a clinical outcome such as survival, which is the most accurate indicator of treatment effectiveness. Whether a surrogate marker also indicates better survival requires testing through long-term clinical trials that measure patient survival.

surveillance system ■ The ongoing systematic collection, analysis, interpretation, and dissemination of data to follow the demographic and geographic spread of a disease in a population. The information is used to help understand disease transmission prevention methods and allocate public resources to its control. Surveillance is carried out by the Centers for Disease Control and Prevention.

syncytia-forming viruses ■ Strains of HIV that promote the formation of syncytia.

syncytium (plural: syncytia) ■ The fusion of two or more cells into one giant cell with multiple nuclei. Some strains of HIV promote the formation of syncytia among lymphocytes. Most human cells, including lymphocytes, cannot survive as a syncytium. Some researchers believe that the formation of syncytia from the merging of infected cells with uninfected cells is partially responsible for the increasing loss of helper T cells as HIV disease progresses.

syndrome ■ A group of signs and symptoms that together characterize a particular disease or abnormal condition.

syphilis ■ An infectious chronic disease usually transmitted through sexual intercourse, but also by contact with infected blood and from mother to infant during pregnancy. Syphilis is caused by the bacterium *Treponema pallidum*.

systemic ■ Occurring throughout the body.

systemic treatment ■ A drug or medication given by mouth or by injection that is carried throughout the body by the circulating blood.

Tat protein ■ A regulatory protein produced by HIV's *tat* gene. The Tat protein binds to the Tat-responsive element (TAR), which is present on all MESSENGER RNAs (mRNAs) produced by an HIV PROVIRUS. High levels of Tat can increase the TRANSCRIPTION of all HIV genes by 1,000 times.

testosterone ■ The most potent naturally occurring male sex hormone. A synthetic version of the hormone is being tested for the treatment of HIV-related WASTING syndrome.

therapeutic index ■ A measure of the relative desirability of a drug for attaining a particular medical end. It is the largest dose that produces no toxic symptoms divided by the smallest dose that regularly produces a cure.

therapy ■ The treatment of disease for curative purposes by various methods.

thrush ■ Same as ORAL CANDIDIASIS.

thymus ■ A lymphoid organ in which T LYMPHOCYTES mature. It rests above the heart.

T lymphocytes ■ Lymphocytes that mature in the thymus. They include HELPER T LYMPHOCYTES (CD4 lymphocytes) and CYTOTOXIC T LYMPHOCYTES (CD8 lymphocytes).

toxoplasmosis ■ An OPPORTUNISTIC INFECTION caused by the protozoan *Toxoplasma gondii*. Toxoplasmosis most often occurs in the brain, where it causes cerebral toxoplasmosis, or toxoplasmic encephalitis.

transfer RNA (tRNA) ■ A cloverleaf-shaped form of RNA that transports AMINO ACIDS to RIBOSOMES during PROTEIN SYNTHESIS.

transcription ■ The first phase of PROTEIN SYNTHESIS. During transcription, a copy of a gene is made in the form of MESSENGER RNA (mRNA).

treatment ■ Medical or surgical management of a patient. Often used interchangeably with therapy.

treatment IND program ■ An FDA EXPANDED-ACCESS PROGRAM that allows certain patients with serious illness to obtain an experimental drug at cost and prior to FDA approval because extensive clinical testing has shown it likely to provide clinical benefit. ("IND" stands for "investigational new drug.")

trichomoniasis ■ A protozoal infection of the vagina that causes inflammation.

tropism ■ As used in reference to viruses, relates to the ability of a virus to infect one type of cell more efficiently than another. For example, some isolates of HIV are 10 to 100 times more efficient at infecting MACROPHAGES than are other isolates.

tuberculin skin test ■ See PPD TEST.

tuberculosis (TB) ■ An infection caused by the bacterium *Mycobacterium tuberculosis*. TB can affect any organ, though the primary site of infection is usually the lungs. TB also occurs as an OPPORTUNISTIC INFECTION in people with AIDS.

U.S. Public Health Service ■ The arm of the federal government primarily charged with leading and supporting national efforts to prevent disease and promote health through policy development and programs. It is made up of eight agencies, including the CENTERS FOR DISEASE CONTROL AND PREVENTION (CDC), the FOOD AND DRUG ADMINISTRATION (FDA), the National Institutes of Health (NIH), the Health Resources and Services Administration (HRSA), and the Substance Abuse and Mental Health Services Administration (SAMHSA).

V3 loop ■ A loop-like region of HIV's GP120 molecule that plays an important role in the fusion of HIV's envelope with the cell membrane when the virus infects a cell. The name stands for the third variable region of the gp120 molecule. "Variable" refers to the fact that the amino-acid sequence in this area of the molecule is frequently different from one HIV particle to the next. There are several variable regions in the HIV gp120 protein, with this region being the third.

vaccine ■ A preparation that is designed to stimulate an IMMUNE RESPONSE against a disease-causing microbe so as to prevent future infection and illness caused by that microbe.

vaginal candidiasis ■ A yeast infection of the vagina caused by the yeast-like fungus *Candida albicans*, which is also responsible for ORAL CANDIDIASIS (i.e., thrush).

varicella-zoster virus (VZV) ■ The HERPESVIRUS that causes chickenpox and SHINGLES. Also known as human herpesvirus 3.

vector (for vaccines) ■ An AVIRULENT VIRUS that serves as a vehicle to carry selected genes of a virulent virus (like HIV) into body cells. There, the avirulent virus produces both its own proteins and those of the virulent virus. In theory, all the viral proteins should elicit an IMMUNE RESPONSE, including a response against the virulent virus. This is the concept behind live recombinant vector vaccines.

veneral disease ■ A disease contracted through sexual intercourse.

vertical transmission ■ Transmission of a VIRUS or other PATHOGEN from mother to infant.

viral coculture ■ A method of determining whether a person is infected with HIV. The method involves growing LYMPHOCYTES from a person to be tested along with lymphocytes from an uninfected donor. The cells are grown under conditions that encourage the growth of both lymphocytes and HIV.

viral envelope ■ A lipid membrane, similar to the CELL MEMBRANE, that surrounds the CAPSID of enveloped viruses. HIV's envelope also contains the viral GP120 and GP41 envelope proteins.

viral genome tests ■ Tests that measure VIRAL LOAD by detecting copies of the viral GENOME in blood or in infected lymphocytes. Viral genome tests include the POLYMERASE CHAIN REACTION (PCR), QUANTITATIVE COMPETITIVE PCR (QC-PCR), and BRANCHED-CHAIN DNA AMPLIFICATION.

viral load ■ The relative amount of free virus in blood plasma.

viremia ■ The presence of virus in the blood.

virion ■ An individual virus particle.

virucidal ■ A substance or chemical compound that kills viruses.

virulence ■ The relative disease-causing power of a PATHOGEN.

virus ■ An infectious agent that usually cannot be seen under a light microscope, passes through fine filters that retain most bacteria, and cannot grow or reproduce outside of living cells.

virus particle ■ Complete, free-floating viral units as found in body fluids. Same as a VIRION.

virustatic ■ A drug that stops a virus from replicating but does not kill it.

wasting ■ The involuntary loss of 10% of baseline body weight associated with diarrhea (more than two stools a day) for more than 30 days. Wasting involves loss of lean muscle mass as well as fat. Also known as cachexia. Rapid weight loss—wasting—is usually due to an OPPORTUNISTIC INFECTION of the intestines.

Western blot ■ A test that is frequently used to confirm a positive result obtained on an HIV screening test.

white blood cell (WBC) ■ Cell found in the bloodstream that, unlike red blood cells, has a NUCLEUS and lacks hemoglobin. White blood cells are all members of the immune system. They include T and B LYMPHOCYTES, MONOCYTES/MACROPHAGES, NATURAL KILLER CELLS, NEUTROPHILS, BASOPHILS, and EOSINOPHILS.

white matter ■ Tissue of the brain and spinal cord that has a whitish color and consists of nerve fibers that are sheathed in myelin (a fatty substance that insulates the fiber, speeds the conduction of nerve impulses, and gives white matter its color).

wild type ■ Designation given to strains of viruses and other microbes found in nature as opposed to strains that have undergone mutations in the laboratory or, after a period of time, in the human body.

window period ■ The time between initial infection and the appearance of detectable antibody. In HIV, the window period is four to six weeks on average but can be up to 18 months. An HIV-infected individual can infect others during the window period.

works ■ Street term for the equipment used by injection drug users to prepare and inject drugs.

zalcitabine (ddC) ■ An ANTIRETROVIRAL drug and NUCLEOSIDE ANALOGUE REVERSE TRANSCRIPTASE INHIBITOR. It is an analogue of the nucleoside cytidine.

zidovudine (ZDV) ■ ANTIRETROVIRAL drug and NUCLEOSIDE ANALOGUE REVERSE TRANSCRIPTASE INHIBITOR that is an analogue of thymidine. Also known as AZIDOTHYMIDINE (AZT).

APPENDIX 1:
MORE INFORMATION ABOUT HIV/AIDS

There is an abundance of information on HIV/AIDS. The task facing an individual in need of it is not so much where to find it as it is how to select what will be most helpful and reliable. Sources of information about HIV/AIDS include books, hotlines, newsletters, and Internet sites on the World Wide Web. Some readers may also wish to read original scientific research papers and journal articles to examine research results that relate to treatment or other developments. For those who are unfamiliar with the medical literature, an explanation of how the two most common types of research papers are organized is included at the end of this appendix.

Books
AIDS: Etiology, Diagnosis, Treatment and Prevention. Vincent T. DeVita, Jr., Samuel Hellman, Steven A. Rosenberg, eds.; James Curran, Max Essex, and Anthony S. Fauci, associate eds. 4th edition, 1997. Philadelphia: Lippincott-Raven.

AIDS in the World II: Global Dimensions, Social Roots, and Responses/The Global AIDS Policy Coalition. Jonathan M. Mann and Daniel J. M. Tarantola, eds. 1996. New York: Oxford University Press.

AIDS/HIV Treatment Directory. Published by AmFAR, the *AIDS/HIV Treatment Directory* describes AIDS-related clinical trials, including vaccine trials, and gives comprehensive information on experimental treatments for HIV and HIV-related disorders. It is updated twice a year. Available through the National AIDS Clearinghouse, or from AmFAR (to order, call 1-800-764-9346; to order by e-mail, write to txdir@amfar.org). *The AIDS/HIV Treatment Directory* is also available on AmFAR's Web site, listed below.

HIV and the Pathogenesis of AIDS. Jay A. Levy. 2nd edition, 1998. Washington, DC: ASM Press.

The Hospice Handbook: A Complete Guide. Larry Beresford. 1993. Boston: Little, Brown. A good overview of hospice care and hospice programs.

Living Well with HIV and AIDS. A. L. Gifford, K. Lorig, D. Laurent, and V. Gonzalez. 1997. Palo Alto: Bull Publishing Company. A guide to help people with HIV/AIDS manage their illness. Topics include evaluating and controlling symptoms; exercise, diet, and food safety; and managing the tasks of daily life with a chronic illness.

The OI Report: A Critical Review of the Treatment and Prophylaxis of HIV-Related Opportunistic Infections. Michael Marco et al. 1998. The Treatment Action Group (TAG), 200 E. Tenth Street #601, New York, NY 10003. 1-212-260-0300.

Taber's Cyclopedic Medical Dictionary. 18th edition, 1997. Philadelphia: F.A. Davis Company. A good, affordable medical dictionary.

World Wide Web (WWW) Sites, Hotlines, Newsletters

A bewildering amount of information on almost any subject—including HIV/AIDS—is available on the World Wide Web. And one need not own a computer to take advantage of it: Most public libraries now provide Web access to their patrons.

Many of the organizations that provide the Web sites listed here also have hotlines and newsletters. Most of the publications are available free or at little cost to persons with AIDS/HIV.

Also note that many documents disseminated through U.S. Public Health Service Web sites (e.g., HIV/AIDS Treatment Information Service,

National AIDS Clearinghouse) are posted as PDF (Portable Document Format) files. PDF reproduces documents in a format identical to their published version. PDF files are opened and printed using Adobe Acrobat, which can be downloaded for free from the ATIS site as well as other sites. If you have trouble with downloading this program, click on the hyperlink to the Adobe Acrobat Web page, and then click on "Getting Help." This section answers commonly asked questions about how to download this program. The Adobe company also provides on-line help and a toll-free telephone number to aid people installing Acrobat on home computers. Information about one-to-one technical assistance is also accessed through the "Getting Help" section of the Adobe Acrobat Web site.

Last, while much of the information on the Web is accurate and reliable, some of it can be questionable. Web sites can be set up by anyone with the appropriate hardware and software, and a flashy looking Web page is by itself no guarantee of the quality of information presented there. When investigating an unfamiliar Web site, click to its home page and look for the following information:

- Who is sponsoring and maintaining it (this is usually made clear, but not always)

- Its editorial policy, if it has one

- A listing of its board of directors or advisory board

If these elements are missing, be sure to verify the information you take from the site with a health-care professional or other reliable source. The sites listed below all provide a range of accurate, reliable information. They also include links to additional sites.

ACLU Lesbian and Gay Rights Project
http://www.aclu.org

The American Civil Liberty Union's (ACLU) national Lesbian and Gay Rights Project undertakes precedent-setting litigation, public policy advocacy, and public education on issues of national importance related to lesbian and gay rights.

For information by telephone, call 1-212-549-2627.

AIDS Clinical Trials Information Service (ACTIS)
http://www.actis.org/

Sponsored by the U.S. Public Health Service (PHS), ACTIS provides current information on federally and most industry-sponsored clinical trials for adults and children in any stage of HIV infection. This includes vaccine trials. Information is available in English and Spanish. This site is run by the same staff as, and in parallel with, the HIV/AIDS Treatment Information Service, described below.

For information by telephone, call toll-free: 1-800-TRIALS-A (1-800-874-2572); hearing-impaired callers: 1-800-243-7012 (TTY/TTD); Fax: 1-301-519-6616; e-mail: actis@cdcnac.org

AIDS Data Treatment Network
http://www.aidsnyc.org/network

The AIDS Treatment Data Network is a national, nonprofit, community-based organization. The site includes information on clinical trials for HIV and opportunistic infections, fact sheets, and information about access to government- and pharmaceutical company–sponsored treatments nationwide. The organization also publishes the newsletter, *Treatment Review.*

For information by telephone, call toll-free: 1-800-734-7104.

AIDS Project Los Angeles (APLA)
http://www.apla.org/

The AIDS Project Los Angeles is a nonprofit, community-based organization that provides HIV/AIDS services and information.

American Foundation for AIDS Research (AmFAR)
http://www.amfar.org

AmFAR's Web site includes a description of the foundation and its programs, information on upcoming conferences and special events, and a listing of AmFAR publications. Includes a link to the *AIDS/HIV Treatment Directory.*

The Body: An AIDS and HIV Information Resource
http://www.thebody.com

The Body is presented by Body Health Resources Corporation, which is gay owned and operated. The Body's content is provided by more than 40 AIDS-related organizations. It includes interactive question-and-answer forums in which visitors can submit questions about treatment and a range of other issues to HIV experts.

CancerNet
http://cancernet.nci.nih.gov/

Presented by the National Cancer Institute (a component of the National Institutes of Health), CancerNet provides a wide range of accurate cancer information for the public, clinicians, and researchers, including information on cancer in people with HIV disesase.

Critical Path
http://www.critpath.org/critpath.htm

The Critical Path AIDS Project is a Philadelphia-based organization founded by people with AIDS (PWAs). The site includes treatment, resources, and prevention information in levels of detail useful to PWAs, and names of researchers and service providers.

Centers for Disease Control and Prevention (CDC), National Center for HIV, STD, and TB Prevention, Division of HIV/AIDS Prevention
http://www.cdc.gov/nchstp/hiv__aids/dhap.htm

The CDC's Division of HIV/AIDS Prevention (DHAP) Web site provides statistics relating to HIV transmission, a description of the CDC's HIV/AIDS Fax Information Service (which enables one to receive CDC information via a fax machine), links to other sites, and access to government fact sheets and other information.

Gay Men's Health Crisis (GMHC)
http://www.gmhc.org/index.html

GMHC was founded in 1981, and it is the oldest and largest nonprofit AIDS service organization in the United States. The site also posts GMHC's monthly newsletter, *Treatment Issues.*

HIV/AIDS Treatment Information Service (ATIS)

http://www.hivatis.org

ATIS is operated by the PHS, and it is an important dissemination point for PHS information on the treatment of HIV in adults, children, and pregnant women. All PHS treatment guidelines can be found here, along with updates and revisions.

For information by telephone, call toll-free: 1-800-448-0440 (English and Spanish); hearing-impaired callers: 1-800-243-7012 (TTY/TDD); Fax: 1-301-519-6616; e-mail: atis@cdcnac.org/

HIV InSite

http://hivinsite.ucsf.edu

This site is maintained by the University of California, San Francisco (UCSF) AIDS Program in conjunction with San Francisco General Hospital, and the UCSF Center for AIDS Prevention Studies. HIV InSite is designed to be a gateway to in-depth information about HIV/AIDS. It includes balanced viewpoints on many controversial aspects of AIDS.

JAMA HIV/AIDS Information Center

http://www.ama-assn.org/special/hiv/hivhome.htm

Presented by the American Medical Association, the JAMA HIV/AIDS Information Center is an easy-to-use site for both health-care professionals and the public. It provides clinical updates, news, and information on a broad range of social and policy issues.

National AIDS Clearinghouse

http://www.cdcnac.org

The National AIDS Clearinghouse, operated by the CDC, provides a wide range of information on HIV, sexually transmitted diseases, and tuberculosis. The site includes links to ACTIS, ATIS, and the CDC's Business and Labor Resource Service, which offers information on setting up programs to deal with HIV/AIDS issues in the workplace.

For information by telephone, call toll-free: 1-800-458-5231; hearing-impaired callers: 1-800-243-7012; international callers: 1-301-519-0459; e-mail: aidsinfo@cdcnac.org

National AIDS Hotline

This toll-free hotline provides answers to questions and clear and accurate information about HIV/AIDS. The service sends free written material upon request. It provides treatment information, referrals to testing, and support services.

English: 1-800-342-AIDS (1-800-342-2437), seven days a week, 24 hours a day; Spanish: 1-800-344-7432, seven days a week, 8 AM–2 AM Eastern time; Deaf Community and other TTY users: 1-800-243-7889, Monday–Friday, 10 AM–10 PM Eastern Standard Time; e-mail: hivnet@ashastd.org

National Hemophilia Foundation
http://www.infonhf.org

This site includes information on hemophilia and other bleeding disorders in which the blood does not clot normally. It also includes information on the symptoms and treatment of clotting disorders, medical news, congressional updates, and HIV compensation updates.

For information by telephone, call toll-free: 1-800-424-2634 (1-800-42-HANDI), Monday–Friday, 9 AM–6 PM Eastern Standard Time.

National Hospice Organization (NHO)
http://www.nho.org/general2.htm

NHO is the oldest and largest nonprofit public benefit organization devoted exclusively to hospice care. The site includes basic information about hospices, as well as information on how to find a hospice, reimbursement, and frequently asked questions.

For information by telephone, call toll-free: 1-800-658-8898.

National Institute of Allergy and Infectious Diseases (NIAID), Division of Acquired Immune Deficiency Syndrome
http://www.niaid.nih.gov/research/Daids.htm

This site contains an overview of the division's mission, summaries of conferences and meetings, NIAID resources available to researchers, and information on NIAID research activities in HIV/AIDS.

Oncolink

http://oncolink.upenn.edu/

Oncolink, offered by the University of Pennsylvania Cancer Center, was the first multimedia oncology information resource placed on the Internet. The site includes information on specific types of cancer, cancer treatments, psychosocial support, frequently asked questions about cancer, and support services for those with cancer.

Project Inform

http://www.projinf.org/

Project Inform is a national, nonprofit, community-based organization founded in 1985. The organization's Web site provides up-to-date information on the diagnosis and treatment of HIV disease for HIV-infected individuals, caregivers, and health-care and service providers.

Project Inform National HIV/AIDS Treatment Hotline. For confidential treatment information, to request publications, and for other HIV-related questions, call toll-free: 1-800-822-7422 or 415-558-9051 (San Francisco Bay Area or international calls), Monday–Friday, 9 AM–5 PM and Saturday, 10 AM–4 PM Pacific Time.

Resources of Interest to Women

Women's Treatment Information Resources

International Community of Women Living with HIV/AIDS (ICW). Livingstone House, 11 Carteret Street, London SW1H 9DL. Telephone: 011 44 171 222-1333. An international network run by women who are HIV positive.

LAPNOTES. A quarterly newsletter of the Lesbian AIDS Project, GMHC, 129 West 20th Street, New York, NY 10011. Free. Telephone: 1-212-367-1000.

Lovenotes. A quarterly newsletter published by Sisterlove featuring treatment information and calendar of upcoming events. Free. 1432 Donnelly Avenue, Atlanta, GA 30310. Telephone: 1-404-753-7733.

Women Alive—Knowledge, Action, Health—A Woman's Guide to HIV Treatments. A pocket-sized treatment guide for women, with "action steps and scorecards" to help readers evaluate information. Color illustrations, charts, and worksheets to enable readers to better understand treatment options, and to monitor and analyze their CD4 counts, viral-load tests, and drug side effects. To obtain a copy, contact Women Alive, 1566 Burnside Avenue, Los Angeles, CA 90019. Telephone: 1-213-965-1564.

Women's Hotlines

Lesbian AIDS Project (LAPS), GMHC, New York, NY. Telephone: 1-212-807-6655.

Women and HIV/AIDS, Sister Connect, NJ. Telephone: 1-800-747-1108.

Other Useful Phone Numbers

To learn about HIV/AIDS resources in your area, call the 24-hour National AIDS Hotline at 1-800-342-2437; for Spanish-speaking callers, call 1-800-344-7432.

Consumer Nutrition Hotline: 1-800-366-1655. American Dietetic Association hotline. Callers can speak with a registered dietitian about HIV/AIDS and nutrition, or ask for a referral to a registered dietitian.

Lamda Legal Defense and Education Fund: 1-212-809-8585. A national organization dedicated to improving life and liberty for lesbians, gay men, and people with HIV and AIDS through impact litigation, education, and public policy work.

National Patient Air Transport Hotline: 1-800-296-1217. Provides information on compassionate travel programs of the airline industry and volunteer organizations for individuals traveling for medical treatment.

National Pediatric and Family HIV Resource Center: 1-800-362-0071.

Native American AIDS Information Hotline: 1-800-283-2437. Monday–Friday, 8:30 AM–12:00 NOON Pacific Time. Provides education and information.

Pediatric AIDS Coalition: 1-800-336-5475.

Social Security Administration, Benefits: 1-800-772-1213.

State Drug Assistance Programs

The following is a list of phone numbers for state departments of health and their pharmacy-assisted services to people with HIV/AIDS. Eligibility requirements and drugs/services covered vary from state to state. Questions regarding the reimbursement programs should be directed to your state department of health.

Alabama: 1-334-613-5364

Alaska: 1-907-269-8058

Arizona: 1-602-230-5819

Arkansas: 1-501-661-2292

California: 1-916-324-8429

Colorado: 1-303-866-2445

Connecticut: 1-800-238-2503

Delaware: 1-302-739-3032

District of Columbia:
1-202-347-8888

Florida: 1-904-413-0674

Georgia: 1-404-657-3129

Hawaii: 1-808-732-0315

Idaho: 1-208-334-6657

Illinois: 1-800-825-3518

Indiana: 1-800-659-7580

Iowa: 1-515-242-5838

Kansas: 1-913-296-8891

Kentucky: 1-502-564-6539

Louisiana: 1-504-568-7474

Maine: 1-207-287-5060

Massachusetts: 1-617-566-8358

Michigan: 1-517-335-9333

Minnesota: 1-612-297-3344

Mississippi: 1-601-960-7723

Missouri: 1-314-751-6439

Montana: 1-406-444-4744

Nebraska: 1-402-559-4673

Nevada: 1-702-687-4800

New Hampshire:
1-603-271-4576

New Jersey: 1-609-588-7038

New Mexico: 1-505-827-8426

New York: 1-800-542-2437

North Carolina: 1-919-773-3091

North Dakota: 1-800-472-2180

Ohio: 1-614-466-4669

Oklahoma: 1-405-271-4636

Oregon: 1-503-731-4029

Pennsylvania: 1-800-922-9384

Puerto Rico: Available only through enrollment in a public-health clinic

Rhode Island: 1-401-464-2183

South Carolina: 1-803-734-6033

South Dakota: 1-605-773-3737

Tennessee: 1-615-741-8530

Texas: 1-800-255-1090

Utah: 1-801-538-6096

Vermont: 1-802-241-2880

Virginia: 1-804-225-4844

Virgin Islands: 1-809-776-8311

Washington: 1-360-753-3493

West Virginia: 1-304-242-9443

Wisconsin: 1-608-267-6875

Wyoming: 1-307-777-5800

Tips on Reading Medical-Research Papers

New medical findings are first published in scientific journals. Many people with HIV often wish to read a study firsthand. In addition, one or more of the major medical journals—such as the *Journal of the American Medical Association (JAMA)*, the *New England Journal of Medicine*, and *The Lancet*—are available at many public libraries. Other journals, including those devoted exclusively to HIV and AIDS research, are available at university and medical school libraries (community hospitals also often have small libraries that are sometimes available for use with permission). The following information is provided in the belief that having some familiarity with how scientific papers are organized can make it easier to use them.

Most journal articles fall into one of two main categories: review papers, which provide an overview of an area of research or treatment, and research papers, which describe the results of a study or clinical trial.

Research Papers

Research papers concisely describe why a study was done, how it was done, what it found, and what the implications of the results are. Research papers are usually divided into sections that present each of these areas of information:

- Title. The title identifies the topic of the paper. It is followed by a byline that lists the authors of the paper and the universities or companies with which the authors are affiliated.

- Abstract. The abstract summarizes the content, findings, and conclusions described by the paper.

- Introduction. It explains why the study was done, and states the question the study sought to answer or the problem the study sought to solve.

- "Materials and Methods" section. This section describes the types and sources of materials used in the study, how the study was done, and the statistical tests employed.

- "Results" section. This section presents the study's findings. It does not include an interpretation of the results or their significance. The Results section usually often includes tables, graphs, or charts that summarize the data collected and their statistical significance.

- "Discussion" section. The section interprets the study's results and compares them to the findings of similar studies. It often closes with the more far-reaching implications of the study and its conclusions.

- "Literature-Cited" section. This section lists the scientific literature referred to in the paper, along with the bibliographic information needed to track down the scientific papers used by the authors of the study.

It is usually not necessary to read a research paper cover to cover. It is often helpful to first read the abstract to get an overview of the study, then read the section of greatest interest, usually the "Results" and, for lay readers in particular, the "Discussion" sections.

Review Papers

Review papers summarize the state of the art of an area of research or treatment. They are useful for gaining a quick overview of a subject. The area covered might be as broad as "Cancer and HIV Disease" or as narrow as "A Review of the Treatment of Lymphoma in HIV Patients."

Review papers are not usually broken down into titled sections as are research papers. Many of them do follow a pattern, however, in which they begin with an introduction, followed by the body of the article. They often close with a summary of the author's (or authors') conclusions about the subject reviewed, including what important questions remain unresolved. Review papers also end with a long literature-cited section. There is a lag time involved in publishing review papers so that a paper published in 1997 will primarily cover research published through 1996.

APPENDIX 2: THE 1993 CLASSIFICATION SYSTEM FOR HIV/AIDS

The surveillance case definition currently in use for HIV disease and AIDS was introduced by the U.S. Public Health Service in 1993. It expanded the number of AIDS-defining conditions to include pulmonary tuberculosis, recurrent pneumonia, and invasive cervical cancer. It also combined CD4 T-cell counts and the presence of AIDS-defining illnesses as a way of identifying the various stages of disease in HIV-infected individuals. The system works as follows:

CD4 T-Cell Categories	Clinical Categories		
	A *Asymptomatic Acute (Primary) HIV or PGL*	B *Symptomatic (not 'A' or 'C' Conditions)*	C *AIDS-Indicator Conditions*
1. ≥ 500/μl	A1	B1	C1
2. 200–499/μl	A2	B2	C2
3. < 200/μl (AIDS-indicator T-cell count)	A3	B3	C3

The shaded cells indicate cases that are officially defined as AIDS. The clinical categories are defined as follows:

Category A includes individuals 13 years or older who have documented HIV infection, and who have one or more of the following conditions:

- Asymptomatic HIV infection

- Persistent generalized lymphadenopathy (PGL)

- Acute (i.e., primary) HIV infection with accompanying illness or history of acute HIV infection

Category B consists of infections and conditions that produce HIV-related symptoms but are not included among those listed in Category C. Formerly, individuals with Category B symptoms were said to have AIDS-related complex, or ARC. Conditions in clinical Category B include the following:

- Bacillary angiomatosis

- Oral candidiasis (thrush)

- Constitutional symptoms such as fever or diarrhea lasting more than one month

- Oral hairy leukoplakia

- Shingles (herpes zoster infection) that is widespread or involves at least two distinct episodes

- Peripheral neuropathy

Additional conditions that can occur in women (see also Chapter 11):

- Vulvovaginal candidiasis that is persistent, is frequent, and does not respond well to treatment

- Pelvic inflammatory disease, particularly if complicated by tubal or ovarian abscess

- Cervical dysplasia that is moderate or severe, or cervical carcinoma in situ

An HIV-infected individual who develops a Category B condition is thereafter regarded as having Category B disease, even if that condition clears up. Similarly, once an HIV-infected person develops a Category C disease, described below, the person is then classified as having Category C disease. Category C conditions include the following:

- Candidiasis of the bronchi, trachea, or lungs.

- Candidiasis of the esophagus.

- Cervical cancer that is invasive.

- Coccidioidomycosis that is disseminated through the body or that is extrapulmonary (i.e., it occurs outside the lungs).

- Cryptococcosis that is extrapulmonary.

- Cryptosporidiosis that causes an intestinal infection for more than one month.

- Cytomegalovirus (CMV) disease that occurs outside the liver, spleen, and lymph nodes.

- Cytomegalovirus retinitis, with loss of vision.

- Encephalopathy—dysfunction of the brain—that is HIV-related.

- Herpes simplex virus infection that produces ulcerous sores that last more than one month, or that causes bronchitis, pneumonitis, or esophagitis.

- Histoplasmosis that is disseminated or extrapulmonary.

- Isosporiasis, intestinal, for more than one month. Isosporiasis is an infection caused by the protozoan *Isospora belli* that can cause severe, chronic diarrhea in people with HIV infection.

- Kaposi's sarcoma.

- Lymphoma, Burkitt's. Lymphomas are cancers of the cells and tissues of the lymphatic system.

- Lymphoma, immunoblastic. This is a cancer of lymphocytes associated with lymph nodes.

- Lymphoma, primary, of the brain. This is a lymphoma that originates in the brain.

- *Mycobacterium avium* complex (MAC) or *Mycobacterium kansasii,* disseminated or extrapulmonary. These are bacterial infections that cause a variety of problems in people with HIV disease.

- *Mycobacterium tuberculosis* (the bacterium responsible for tuberculosis) infection, regardless of where it occurs anywhere in the body.

- Infection with *Mycobacterium* species other than those listed above, including unidentified species that cause disseminated or extrapulmonary infection.

- *Pneumocystis carinii* pneumonia (PCP).

- Pneumonia, recurrent, and other than PCP.

- Progressive multifocal leukoencephalopathy (PML), an opportunistic infection of the brain caused by the human JC virus. It occurs in about 4% of AIDS patient and results in the destruction of white matter in the brain.

- *Salmonella* septicemia, recurrent. This is an infection of the blood by *Salmonella* bacteria. It is not often seen in HIV patients today.

- Toxoplasmosis of the brain.

- Wasting syndrome due to HIV. Wasting is the involuntary loss of more than 10% of body weight over a period of six to eight weeks.

In the 1993 CDC definition, the CD4 T-cell counts and the three clinical categories are combined to describe the stage of HIV infection in a patient. For example, an HIV-infected person with CD4 cell counts of 300 who is asymptomatic will be classified as having A2 disease. Similarly, an HIV-infected person with average CD4 lymphocyte counts of 600 and who develops thrush is classified as having B1 HIV disease. Or, a person with CD4 counts of 150 and who has toxoplasmosis of the brain will be classified with C3 disease, which is AIDS. Note that any HIV-infected person with CD4 counts below 200 is considered to have AIDS, as does anyone, regardless of CD4 counts, who develops a Category C condition. For this reason, the infections, cancers, and other conditions included in Category C are known as AIDS-defining conditions. Most commonly, these conditions develop in patients with severely depressed immune systems and with CD4 counts that are well below 200 or rapidly declining.

Percentages of CD4 lymphocytes (i.e., CD4 lymphocytes as a percentage of total lymphocytes) are used by some physicians to classify patients with HIV infection. The percentages of CD4 T cells that are equivalent to total numbers of CD4 cells are as follows:

CD4 T-Cell Category	CD4 T Cells/µl	CD4 Percentage (%)
1	≥ 500	≥ 29
2	200–499	14–28
3	< 200	< 14

INDEX

Hispanic, 215–16, 384
as IDUs, 215, 217
medical care for, 12, 223–27
mortality of men vs., 220
as primary caregivers, 220, 230
see also pregnant women, HIV-infected
World Wide Web, 255

yeast infection, 10, 12, 38, 54, 57, 124, 130–35

zalcitabine (ddC), 64, 71, 116, 119, 293, 294, 351
zidovudine (ZDV), *see* azidothymidine
zinc finger inhibitor (CI-1012), 95
zintevir (AR-177), 95
zoster immune globulin, 153

The American Foundation for AIDS Research (AmFAR) is a national not-for-profit organization exempt from federal income tax under section 501(c)3 of the United States Internal Revenue Code and is therefore eligible to receive tax-deductible contributions. It is the legal successor to the AIDS Medical Foundation incorporated in New York State in 1983.

In the fight against HIV/AIDS, AmFAR identifies unmet needs in biomedical research (both laboratory and clinical research), prevention, public policy, and public information. AmFAR strives to meet these needs by awarding grants to researchers and by undertaking independent advocacy and educational activities. These activities foster rational, compassionate, and effective responses to the epidemic and enhance standards of medical care and other services for people with HIV/AIDS.

Funded by private contributions from caring individuals and corporations, AmFAR has invested nearly $150 million in its programs since 1985, primarily through grants to fund some 1,700 research projects which, through a process of stringent peer review, were carefully selected for promise, technical excellence, and relevance.

AmFAR's work has made significant contributions to progress in the medical treatment of HIV disease and its complications, the prevention of HIV transmission, the enactment of sound HIV/AIDS-related federal and state legislation, and the education of health care professionals and the public about the nature of the disease and its epidemic spread.

AmFAR believes that continuing—and expanding—cooperative efforts by the public and private sectors in biomedical research and development, particularly in the fields of antiretroviral therapy, immune reconstitution, and the correlates of anti-HIV immunity, will provide the means needed to end the global epidemic of HIV/AIDS. AmFAR is committed to helping humankind reach this goal at the earliest possible time.

AmFAR's national office is in the Association Center at 120 Wall Street, 13th Floor, New York, New York 10005-3902. Information about AmFAR and its work may be obtained from that office, (212) 806-1600, or from its Web site at www.amfar.org.